Introduction to the principles of drug design

Preface

Paul Ehrlich's concept that protozoal diseases could be cured by the administration of synthetic chemicals which selectively reacted with the target tissue of the protozoa rather than that of the host, and Domagk's later expansion of this view to the treatment of bacterial diseases with the introduction of prontosil, set the scene for a major breakthrough in the treatment by drugs of other types of disease, ailments and conditions where the target tissue may be an enzyme, a macromolecular structure such as DNA, RNA, or even a structure of unknown constitution. This approach has been so well developed that, with the expanding knowledge of the biochemical and physiological processes occurring in both the healthy and diseased state, it has become possible to select a target tissue and, from a knowledge of its characteristics, to design drugs with the correct size, shape, hydrophilic–lipophilic ratio, disposition of functional groups to selectively react with it to elicit the required clinical response. This procedure, however, involves considerable ingenuity on the part of the designer. This is despite the fact that he has currently at his command an array of established manipulative procedures enabling him to develop a clinically effective drug by modification of a parent drug lacking the essential requirements (such as selectivity for the target site, chemical stability, resistance to premature metabolism) necessary for evoking an optimal therapeutic response.

This introduction to the principles of drug design is intended for use in undergraduate pharmacy courses in medicinal chemistry and as an aid in similar courses in pharmacology and biochemistry where there is a need to appreciate the rationales behind the design of drugs. Graduates in chemistry just entering the pharmaceutical industry would find that it provides a suitable background for their future work.

The emphasis in this book is on principles, which are appropriately illustrated by groups of drugs in current (or even future) use. It is not our intention to deal comprehensively with all conceivable groups of drugs, or to consider drugs grouped on the basis of particular pharmacological actions. This would require repeated descriptions of a range of design aspects relevant to each group so that design considerations would become subservient to the biologically observable actions. We aim to provide a framework of basic drug design/principles into which current drugs, and more importantly future drugs following on new developments, may be fitted. This approach should provide the newly qualified graduate with an understanding of new developments as they become elaborated in future years.

We wish to thank Dr J. Dearden and Dr W. Hugo for reading the manuscripts for Chapters 8 and 9 respectively and providing helpful comments.

HJS. HW

List of contributors

K. C. James M Pharm, Ph D (Wales), C Chem, FRSC, FPS
Senior Lecturer in Pharmaceutics

I. W. Kellaway B Pharm, Ph D (London), MPS
Professor of Pharmaceutics

D. K. Luscombe B Pharm, Ph D (London), MPS, M I Biol
Senior Lecturer in Applied Pharmacology

P. J. Nicholls B Sc (Birmingham), Ph D (Wales), C Chem, FRSC, F I Biol
Reader in Pharmacology

A. D. Russell B Pharm (Wales), Ph D (Nottingham), D Sc (Wales), FPS, FRC Path
Reader in Pharmaceutical Microbiology

H. J. Smith B Pharm, Ph D (London), C Chem, FRSC, FPS
Senior Lecturer in Medicinal and Pharmaceutical Chemistry

H. Williams M Sc (Wales), C Chem, FRSC
Senior Lecturer in Medicinal and Pharmaceutical Chemistry

All are teachers in the Welsh School of Pharmacy, University of Wales Institute of Science and Technology, Cardiff.

Contents

Chapter 1

Processes of drug handling by the body

Processes of drug handling by the body

1.1 INTRODUCTION

To produce a pharmacological or therapeutic effect, a drug must reach its site or sites of action in a concentration sufficient to initiate a response. The concentration achieved, whilst being related to the amount of drug administered, will also depend on the extent and rate at which the drug is absorbed from its site of administration and its distribution by the bloodstream to other parts of the body. The characteristic effect of a drug will disappear when the drug is removed from the body and consequently from its site of action, either in an unchanged form or after metabolism of the drug has taken place giving metabolites which are removed by the process of excretion. Information on how the body handles a drug in terms of absorption, distribution, metabolism and excretion is therefore essential when selecting the dose, route and form of drug administration if a desired therapeutic effect is to be produced with minimal unwanted or toxic effects.

1.2 ABSORPTION

A drug may enter the body either by enteral or by parenteral administration. The enteral route refers to oral, sublingual and rectal administration whilst parenteral includes routes such as intravenous, intramuscular and subcutaneous injections; inhalation; and topical application to the skin and eye. Apart from drugs introduced directly into the systemic circulation by intravenous injection, absorption from the site of administration is essential if a drug is to gain entry to the bloodstream and thus reach its site of action. The process of absorption is consequently of fundamental importance in determining the pharmacological and therapeutic activity of a drug. Delays or losses of drug during absorption may contribute to variability in drug response or may result in a failure of drug therapy.

For the process of absorption to take place, a drug must cross at least one cell membrane and the ease with which it does so will reflect the concentration of drug achieved in the tissues and body fluids. It is therefore necessary to consider briefly the structure of cell membranes and the physico-chemical mechanisms involved in the passage of drugs across these membranes, together with the variety of factors which influence this process. It should be emphasized that as well as drug absorption, the processes of distribution, metabolism and excretion likewise involve the passage of drugs or their breakdown products across cell membranes.

1.2.1 Structure of cell membranes

Living cells are surrounded by membranes whose function is to maintain the integrity of the cell and to regulate the transfer of nutrients, waste products and

2

regulatory substances to and from the cytoplasm. The membrane is thus semiper-meable, measuring approximately 8 nm in total thickness.

Overton suggested that the rate at which various substances enter cells is proportional to the distribution of the substance between lipid and water, the lipid-soluble substance entering the cell more readily. This suggestion was supported by other workers and led to the theory that the cell is surrounded by a thin layer of lipid-like material interdispersed with minute water-filled channels. Membranes are now considered to be composed of bimolecular layers of phospholipid molecules enclosing a central fluid matrix. The cationic heads of the phospholipid molecules are orientated to form an almost continuous polar layer on both the inside and outside of the cell membrane. In contrast, the long hydrophobic chains of the phospholipid molecules extend into the central core of the membrane. Since these chains are in a state of flux in the living cell, the matrix can be considered to consist of a sea of liquid lipid. Globular proteins are embedded in the membrane matrix often extending through all three layers of the membrane. Pores or channels through which water-soluble molecules (such as alcohol and water itself) can pass may be associated with these proteins.

1.2.2   Modes of transfer across cell membranes

The transfer of substances across cell membranes can occur by a number of possible mechanisms. The most important are: (*a*) direct passage through its lipid or aqueous channels down a concentration gradient, often called passive diffusion; and (*b*) carrier-mediated transfer of polar molecules called facilitated diffusion or, in some instances, active transport. Other modes of transfer include pinocytosis, in which invaginations of the cell membrane engulf drops of extracellular fluid enabling solute to be carried through in the resulting vacuoles of water; per-sorption; filtration or aqueous diffusion; and finally diffusion of ions.

1.2.2.1   *Passive diffusion*

Most drugs are transferred across cell membranes by passive diffusion from a region of higher concentration to one of lower concentration. Passive transfer is described by Fick's first law which states that the rate of diffusion across a membrane (dC/dt) is proportional to the difference in drug concentration either side of the membrane (ΔC), i.e.

$$\frac{dC}{dt} = -k\Delta C = -k(C_1 - C_2), \qquad (1.1)$$

where C_1 and C_2 denote the concentrations of drug on each side of the membrane, C_1 being greater than C_2 and k representing the rate constant for diffusion. This is a proportionality constant incorporating the diffusion coefficient of the drug, the surface area of the membrane and the permeability of the membrane to the specific drug. If a large concentration gradient is maintained throughout the absorption phase, then $C_1 \gg C_2$ and consequently the concentration gradient (ΔC) is nearly equal to C_1. Therefore, Equation 1.1 may be rewritten as

$$\frac{dC}{dt} \simeq -kC_1, \tag{1.2a}$$

which is the familiar form of a first order rate equation.

The concentration gradient can be replaced by the quantity of drug administered (A) and Equation 1.2a may then be written as

$$\frac{dA}{dt} = -k_a A, \tag{1.2b}$$

where k_a is the rate constant for absorption and represents the fraction of the amount administered that is absorbed in unit time. Integration of this equation· gives

$$A_t = A_0 e^{-tka}, \tag{1.3}$$

where A_0 is the amount of drug administered (dose), A_t is the amount remaining unabsorbed at time t after the commencement of absorption and e is the base of natural logarithms. Assuming no losses of drug occur before or during absorption, the quantity of drug absorbed in time t, (Q_t) is the difference between A_0 and A_t, i.e.

$$Q_t = A_0 - A_t. \tag{1.4}$$

Substituting for A_t in Equation 1.3 gives

$$Q_t = A_0(1 - e^{-tka}). \tag{1.5}$$

In other words, the quantity of drug absorbed rises rapidly initially and then more slowly, approaching exponentially a plateau level. As $t \to \infty$, $Q_\infty \to A_0$ since $e^{-\infty} \to 0$.

Replacing A_0 in Equations 1.3 and 1.5 by fD, where f is the fraction of the dose available to the body and D is the dose administered, gives

$$A_t = fD e^{-tka}, \tag{1.6}$$

$$Q_t = fD(1 - e^{-tka}). \tag{1.7}$$

As already stated, the rate of diffusion of a drug is a function of the surface area over which the transfer occurs, the permeability of the cell membrane and the concentration gradient across the membrane, i.e.

$$\text{rate of diffusion} = \left(\begin{array}{c}\text{permeability}\\\text{constant}\end{array}\right) \times \left(\begin{array}{c}\text{surface}\\\text{area}\end{array}\right) \times \left(\begin{array}{c}\text{concentration}\\\text{difference}\end{array}\right).$$

Thus a doubling of surface area of the membrane doubles the probability that drug molecules will collide with the membrane and, as a result, the rate of absorption will be increased by a factor of two. Similarly, the greater the concentration gradient, the greater will be the rate of diffusion of a drug across a membrane. However, many drugs pass rapidly through a membrane while others pass slowly. This difference in the ease of passage across a membrane may be expressed in terms of the permeability constant which is a characteristic of both the drug molecule and the cell membrane, i.e.

$$\left(\begin{array}{c}\text{permeability}\\ \text{constant}\end{array}\right) = \frac{(\text{diffusion coefficient}) \times (\text{partition coefficient})}{(\text{membrane thickness})}.$$

The major source of variation in this equation is the partition coefficient of a drug between the lipid membrane and the aqueous environment. Lipid-soluble drugs have high permeability constants and consequently penetrate membranes with ease. In contrast, ionized compounds partition poorly into lipids. Whilst the long hydrocarbon ester chains of the phospholipid membrane promote the solubility of drug molecules incorporating hydrocarbon and aryl groups (van der Waals' and hydrophobic forces are relevant) it must also be realized that natural phosphatidyl esters also possess dipolar characteristics due to C—O and C=O groups. These give rise to bond dipoles due to unequal distribution of electrons. Such features facilitate the lipid solubility of covalent molecules also possessing dipolar characteristics but which are still non-ionic in character. This explains why increased lipid solubility and hence penetration of cell membranes may be effected by incorporating electronegative substituents into neutral molecules. Thus, C—O, C—S and C—halogen groups promote dipole–dipole attraction with cell membrane structures, which aids passive diffusion into the cell.

(a) Lipid solubility   As previously stated, cell membranes can be considered to be a double layer of protein–lipid material studded with water-filled pores. It is therefore to be expected that lipid-soluble substances will cross such a membrane by simply dissolving in, and diffusing across, the lipid layers. The ability of a substance to dissolve in lipid can be measured in terms of its partition coefficient between an aqueous and immiscible non-aqueous phase such as *n*-octanol, or chloroform. The influence of a drug's partition coefficient on its ability to pass through biological membranes can be demonstrated by comparing the partition coefficients of a number of different members of a homologous series of lipid-soluble compounds with their ability to cross cell membranes. It is found that the permeability of the membranes to each member of the series is directly proportional to the partition coefficient. The increasing molecular weight as the series is ascended exerts only a negligible effect. This is in contrast to substances that diffuse through aqueous channels, where molecular size is important. In general, the higher the value of the partition coefficient the more rapidly will the drug be transferred across cell membranes (*see* Table 1.1).

(b) Influence of pK$_a$ and pH   Many drugs are weak electrolytes and as such are partly dissociated in solution. In general, only the undissociated molecule is soluble in the lipid, the ions are not. For this reason, the dissociation constant of a drug plays a vital part in determining the ability of a drug to cross cell membranes and this in turn is influenced by the pH of the environment. The interrelationship between the dissociation constant, pH of the medium and lipid solubility of a drug often dictates its absorption characteristics and constitutes the pH-partition theory of drug absorption. The dissociation constant is often expressed for both acids and

Table 1.1   Relationship between chloroform/water partition coefficient and the absorption of barbiturates from the rat colon[a]

Barbiturate	Partition coefficient	Percentage absorbed
Barbitone	0·7	12
Phenobarbitone	4·8	20
Cyclobarbitone	13·9	24
Pentobarbitone	28·0	30
Secobarbitone	50·7	40

[a] Data from Schanker L. S. (1959) Absorption of drugs from the rat colon. *J. Pharmacol. Exp. Ther.* **126**, 283–90.

bases as a pK_a value (the negative logarithm of the acid dissociation constant). The pK_a values of several drugs and their relative strengths as acids or bases are given in Fig. 1.1.

The relationship between pK_a and pH and the extent of ionization is given by the Henderson–Hasselbach equation, i.e.

$$\text{for an acid, } pK_a - pH = \log (f_u/f_i), \tag{1.8}$$

$$\text{for a base, } pK_a - pH = \log (f_i/f_u), \tag{1.9}$$

where f_u and f_i are the fractions of the drug present in the un-ionized and ionized forms, respectively (*see also* Section 3.1.1.1). Thus, a solution of the weak acid aspirin (pK_a 3·5) in the stomach at pH 1 will have more than 99% of the drug in the un-ionized form. Since the un-ionized form of aspirin is lipid soluble, the drug is rapidly absorbed in the stomach. Most weakly acidic drugs are absorbed in the stomach since they exist largely in the un-ionized state at low pH values.

In contrast, poor absorption of basic drugs in the stomach can be explained by Equation 1.9. For example, a solution of codeine (pK_a 8) in the stomach will have only one molecule in a million in the un-ionized form. Indeed, most basic drugs are so highly ionized in the acid fluids of the stomach that absorption is negligible. However, weak bases ($pK_a < 2·5$) such as antipyrine may be absorbed to some extent in the stomach because they are significantly un-ionized even in this strongly acidic environment. Absorption of most weakly basic drugs is rapid in the near neutral fluids of the small intestine (*see* Equation 1.9). Thus, the passage of a weakly acidic drug across a membrane is favoured by its presentation in an acid medium such as stomach fluids, while the transfer of a weakly basic drug is increased if the pH of the solution is increased. Nevertheless, the absorption of all orally administered drugs, weak acids as well as weak bases, probably takes place more rapidly in the proximal intestine than in the stomach. Whilst this may initially appear contrary to the pH-partition theory, the large surface area offered by the small intestine reduces the necessity for a large fraction of the drug to be in its un-ionized state. For example, at pH 7, only 0·1% of aspirin is in the un-ionized form but, despite this fact, aspirin is well absorbed from the small intestine when

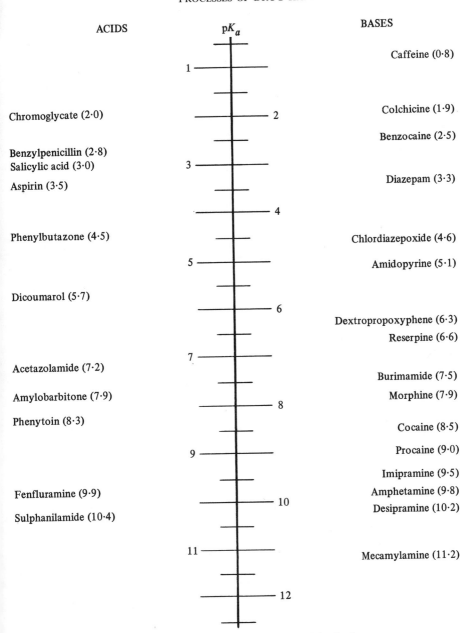

ACIDS

pK$_a$

BASES

Caffeine (0·8)

Chromoglycate (2·0)

Colchicine (1·9)

Benzocaine (2·5)

Benzylpenicillin (2·8)
Salicylic acid (3·0)

Aspirin (3·5)

Diazepam (3·3)

Phenylbutazone (4·5)

Chlordiazepoxide (4·6)

Amidopyrine (5·1)

Dicoumarol (5·7)

Dextropropoxyphene (6·3)

Reserpine (6·6)

Acetazolamide (7·2)

Burimamide (7·5)

Amylobarbitone (7·9)

Morphine (7·9)

Phenytoin (8·3)

Cocaine (8·5)

Procaine (9·0)

Imipramine (9·5)

Fenfluramine (9·9)

Amphetamine (9·8)

Desipramine (10·2)

Sulphanilamide (10·4)

Mecamylamine (11·2)

Fig. 1.1   Some pK$_a$ values of acidic and basic drugs.

administered orally to man. Certain strong organic acids and bases, such as sulphonic acid derivatives and quaternary ammonium bases, are ionized over a wide range of pH values and have low lipid solubility. Therefore, their passage across cell membranes is rather poor and this is reflected in their poor absorption from the gastrointestinal tract.

1.2.2.2   *Carrier-aided transfer*

Some substances, though polar and of low lipid solubility, penetrate membranes much faster than anticipated, assuming that only passive diffusion through an inert lipoidal barrier occurs. Here a specialized carrier-mediated transport system is involved.

A carrier can be considered as a membrane component capable of forming a complex with the substance to be transported. The complex moves across the membrane and releases the substrate on the other side. A characteristic of a carrier-aided transport system is that high concentrations of the transported substance saturate the carrier. The effect of this is to limit the amount of substrate that can be transported. This is in contrast to the process of passive diffusion across lipid membranes, or through pores, where the amount conveyed increases proportionately with its concentration.

Of the two types of carrier-aided transport which have been proposed, facilitated diffusion accounts for the transfer of very few drugs and is not further discussed here.

Although few drugs undergo active transport, it is an important mechanism for the transfer of their metabolites. In active transport, the substrate is carried through the membrane against a concentration gradient and expenditure of metabolic energy is involved. The carrier can be saturated and since it has group specificity it can be inhibited competitively by other substrates. Because active transport requires the expenditure of energy, this process will also be affected by metabolic inhibitors such as 2,4-dinitrophenol or reduced temperatures.

Active transport mechanisms occur in the gastrointestinal tract (e.g. amino acids and possibly methyldopa), in the renal tubule and across membranes dividing extracellular from intracellular fluid compartments at the blood–brain and placental barriers.

1.2.2.3   *Pinocytosis*

Pinocytosis is a term which describes the active uptake of substances by a process similar to phagocytosis. Microscopic invaginations of a cell membrane engulf drops of extracellular fluid and solute molecules are carried through in the resulting vacuoles. Although important in the absorption of large molecules such as proteins and nucleic acids, this process is of little importance in the transport of drug molecules across cell membranes, except perhaps in the case of oral vaccines. However, efforts are currently being directed towards incorporating drugs into liposomes, which may then be taken up selectively by cells that are capable of pinocytosis.

1.2.2.4   *Persorption*

It has been recognized recently that particles in the micrometer range (e.g. starch grains) pass through the intestinal wall directly, entering either the lymph or the portal circulation. Entry appears to be via loose junctions around intestinal goblet cells. The importance of this process for drug absorption from the gastrointestinal tract remains to be evaluated.

1.2.2.5 *Filtration or aqueous diffusion*

Water-soluble substances are able readily to diffuse through the aqueous channels or 'pores' in the cell membrane providing they are not of too large a molecular weight. This is essentially a process of solvent drag, the rate of diffusion being governed by Fick's first law.

1.2.2.6 *Diffusion of ions*

Ions are not soluble in lipids but, like water-soluble non-polar molecules, can diffuse across a membrane down a concentration gradient provided that their molecular weight is not too large. In instances where a cell membrane is polarized, one side being positively charged and the other negatively charged, a positive charged ion (cation) in aqueous solution will be driven across the membrane from the positive to the negative side. The extent to which this process will take place will be dependent on the potential difference across the membrane. Likewise, an anion in contact with the negative face will be driven across the membrane to the positive side. The passage of ions by this latter process does not require a concentration difference of the diffusing ion on the two sides of the membrane.

1.2.3 Routes of administration

Drugs are seldom, if ever, applied directly to their sites of action but are administered at regions remote from these sites. They subsequently have to be absorbed from the point of entry (e.g. stomach or intestine) into the bloodstream. When administering any drug, a route of administration, as well as a suitable dose and dosage form (e.g. tablet, capsule) must be selected in order to ensure that the drug will reach its site of action in a pharmacologically effective concentration and be maintained at this concentration for an adequate period of time. There is often a choice of route by which a drug may be given, so a knowledge of the advantages and disadvantages of the possible routes of administration is particularly important. Possible routes of drug administration are divided into two major classes: enteral, whereby drugs are absorbed from the alimentary canal and parenteral, in which drugs enter the bloodstream directly (intravenous injection) or by some other non-enteral absorptive route (intramuscular or subcutaneous injection).

1.2.3.1 *Enteral*

The enteral route of administration can be subdivided into three classes. Firstly, the oral route, where a drug is swallowed and is subsequently absorbed through the mucous membrane of the small intestine or, to a limited extent, from the stomach. Secondly, sublingual, where a drug is placed under the tongue and absorbed through the buccal cavity (e.g. glyceryl trinitrate in the treatment of angina pectoris). Thirdly, the rectal route, where a drug is given either in a solid form as a suppository (e.g. aminophylline for the relief of bronchial asthma), or in solution as an enema (e.g. paraldehyde for sedation) with absorption taking place through the rectal and colonic mucosa. In each case, passage of drug across the membranes dividing the absorption site from the blood is a prerequisite for absorption and, for this to occur, the drug must be in solution.

(a) Oral route   The most common method of drug administration is by swallowing. In such cases, the gastrointestinal tract plays a major role in determining the rate and extent of drug absorption. Oral ingestion is convenient, relatively safe and economical and is the route preferred by patients, providing the drug is presented in a palatable and suitable dosage form. However, this route has a number of disadvantages. The drug may cause irritation of the gastrointestinal mucosa, resulting in nausea and vomiting. It may become mixed with food, destroyed by digestive enzymes or low gastric pH, pass too rapidly down the gastrointestinal tract or interact with other drugs being administered concurrently. The small intestine is the most important site for drug absorption in the gastrointestinal tract. This is largely due to its structure, which offers a far greater epithelial surface area for drug absorption than other parts of the gastrointestinal tract.

Apart from the above, many other factors influence the rate and extent of drug absorption such as the physico-chemical properties of the drug, its concentration at the site of absorption, the surface area for absorption and blood flow to the site of absorption.

The great majority of drugs which are swallowed are weak organic bases or acids and, as previously stated, are absorbed from the gastrointestinal lumen by lipid diffusion of the un-ionized form. Since the fraction of ionized to un-ionized form is pH-dependent, the pH at the absorption site is an important factor in determining the rate and extent of absorption. Thus, absorption will be maximal where ionization is suppressed to the greatest extent. However, absorption is often complicated by other factors. Thus, despite the fact that aspirin is largely in the un-ionized form in the secretions of the stomach, its solubility is low. In fact, it is more soluble at the pH of the intestinal contents although it is then predominantly in its ionized form. This fact, together with the greater absorbing surface area of the small intestine, results in up to two-thirds of an orally administered dose of aspirin being absorbed from the intestine.

For very strong organic bases such as quaternary ammonium compounds, the concentration of un-ionized drug is so low that absorption by diffusion is slow and incomplete at any physiological pH. However, sufficient may be absorbed, possibly by aqueous diffusion, to produce a pharmacological effect (e.g. hexamethonium). In addition, a few drugs with low molecular weight are rapidly absorbed by the process of aqueous diffusion (e.g. ethanol).

Other mechanisms of drug absorption in the gastrointestinal tract include active transport, pinocytosis and co-absorption with lipids. Some drugs that are chemically related to nutrients are absorbed by the same active transport mechanism (e.g. methyldopa and L-dopa with amino acids; methotrexate with pyrimidines). Drugs with large molecular weights, or which exist in solution in molecular aggregates, are probably taken up by pinocytosis (e.g. the complex of intrinsic factor with vitamin B_{12}). A few drugs with very high lipid solubility are absorbed from the intestinal tract together with long-chain fatty acids and their monoglycerides, cholesterol and fat-soluble vitamins (e.g. digitoxin and griseofulvin).

In theory, weakly acidic drugs should be better absorbed from the stomach than the intestine because a large fraction of the dose would be in an un-ionized, lipid-soluble form. However, the limited time for which the drug is present in the stomach and the limited surface area of the stomach more than balance the influence of the pH in determining the optimal site for absorption. Thus, any factor that promotes gastric emptying increases the rate of absorption of nearly all drugs. Prompt gastric emptying is also important for drugs that are unstable in stomach fluids (e.g. benzylpenicillin). Gastric emptying is promoted by fasting or hunger, alkaline buffer solutions, anxiety, diseases such as hyperthyroidism and some drugs such as the anti-emetic metoclopramide. Generally gastric emptying of liquids is much faster than that of solid food or solid dosage forms.

Slow gastric emptying can seriously delay the onset of effects of drugs such as analgesics or sedatives. Gastric emptying can be retarded by fats and fatty acids in the diet, bulky or viscous foods, mental depression, diseases such as gastroenteritis, pyloric stenosis, gastric ulcer and hypothyroidism, and by many drugs including tricyclic antidepressants (imipramine, amitriptyline), anticholinergics (atropine, propantheline) and the antacid, aluminium hydroxide. Differences in gastric emptying among subjects is a major contributory factor in the variability of the rate of absorption of drugs from conventional dosage forms, although the overall extent or completeness of drug absorption is usually similar.

Motility of the intestine also plays its part in determining the duration of contact of a drug with absorbing surfaces. This is particularly important for drugs that are poorly absorbed from the intestine, where a prolonged intestinal transit time, brought about by atropine-like spasmolytics and morphine-like analgesics, may result in increased absorption. Conversely, a decrease in transit time, such as is produced by laxatives, may decrease absorption.

In general, gastrointestinal absorption is favoured by an empty stomach. Food will not only have the effect of reducing the concentration of drug in the gastrointestinal tract which will limit its rate of absorption (but not amount absorbed) but will also delay gastric emptying. This explains why drugs are frequently recommended to be taken on an empty stomach when a rapid onset of action is desired. Only when a drug is irritating to the gastric mucosa is it reasonable to administer it with or after a meal. In this instance, there may be a significant decrease in the rate of absorption although the total amount absorbed may be expected to be unchanged.

The absorption of a few drugs is promoted if taken after food. For example, the absorption of griseofulvin can be doubled following postprandial administration.

The intestine has an excellent blood supply which ensures that an absorbed drug is rapidly removed as soon as it passes through the intestinal membrane. In this way, the concentration gradient across the membrane is continuously maintained. For highly lipid-soluble drugs, or those that pass freely through the aqueous-filled pores, passage across a membrane may be so rapid that equilibrium is established between the drug in the blood and that at the absorption site by the time the blood is removed from the membrane. In this instance, the rate-limiting step controlling drug absorption is blood flow and not penetration of the intestinal membrane.

The binding of a drug to plasma proteins lowers the concentration of free drug after absorption and this results in the maintenance of a high concentration gradient which aids absorption.

Drug decomposition is an important factor in gastrointestinal absorption. Acid-labile drugs, such as the penicillins, are unstable at the low pH of the gastric contents. Likewise, a number of esteric drugs (e.g. procaine, acetylcholine and succinylcholine) are hydrolysed by gastric acid and are consequently relatively inactive when taken orally. Polypeptide drugs (e.g. insulin, oxytocin, vasopressin) are destroyed by the proteolytic digestive enzymes of the gastrointestinal tract. In addition to decomposition by host enzymes, drugs may be metabolized or undergo chemical changes by enzymes secreted by bacteria which live as commensal organisms in the large intestine. For example, by hydrolysing glucuronide conjugates, they allow the reabsorption of the parent drug molecule which may then be engaged in enterohepatic cycling (see pp. 35–6). Succinyl- and phthalylsulphathiazole have to be hydrolysed by bacterial enzymes to yield the active sulphonamide before they are effective as intestinal sterilizers.

The intestinal mucosa contains sulphate-conjugating enzymes which may inactivate certain drugs during absorption (e.g. isoprenaline). Similarly, the pharmacological activity of chlorpromazine may be decreased by sulphate conjugation while other drugs are only partly conjugated during absorption (e.g. oestrogens, methyldopa, L-dopa and salicylamide).

An amino acid decarboxylase present in the gastrointestinal mucosa inactivates part of the administered dose of L-dopa during its absorption. Since this decarboxylation takes place mainly in the gastric mucosa, the absorption of L-dopa is increased if gastric emptying is increased.

Hydrolytic enzymes in the gastrointestinal mucosa inactivate glyceryl trinitrate, and are the reason for this drug being administered by the sublingual route rather than being swallowed. These enzymes also partially inactivate analgesic drugs (e.g. pethidine, methadone, dextropropoxyphene and pentazocine). However, hydrolysis of aspirin and dexamethasone phosphate lead to breakdown products which retain pharmacological activity.

Drugs absorbed from the gastrointestinal tract are immediately carried away from their site of absorption by the portal circulation to the liver, where they may be subjected to rapid metabolism. In some instances almost total destruction of the drug results, while in others an active metabolite may be formed (e.g. propranolol, alprenolol; see Chapter 7). Loss of drug from the blood circulation on passage through the liver is termed a presystemic or first-pass effect (see p. 27). Oral administration is obviously inappropriate for drugs which undergo an extensive first-pass effect. Lignocaine, for example, cannot be administered by mouth, despite rapid absorption from the gastrointestinal tract, because it is extensively degraded by the hepatic microsomal enzyme system (*see* p. 21), leading to drug levels in the peripheral blood circulation which are inadequate to exercise a therapeutic effect.

Many drugs are converted to glucuronides in the liver and are then secreted as such into the bile. In the intestine the glucuronides may be hydrolysed to liberate the unconjugated drug which is then reabsorbed, passing directly to the liver where the glucuronide is again formed and secreted into the bile. This phenomenon is known as enterohepatic cycling and its effect is to prolong the duration of action of the drug (e.g. phenolphthalein, chloramphenicol and stilboestrol).

A number of drugs interact with concurrently administered drugs resulting in interference with drug absorption. In most instances of drug interactions there is a reduction of absorption. Tetracyclines form insoluble chelate complexes with polyvalent metal ions (*see also* Section 5.1.7) and will therefore interact with iron preparations; with antacids which contain aluminium, calcium or magnesium ions; or with food which contains polyvalent ions, when administered concurrently. The result will be decreased absorption of tetracycline with the possibility that this drug may cease to be therapeutically effective.

It is generally to be expected that drug absorption will be affected by gastrointestinal pathology. For example, patients with Crohn's disease exhibit decreased absorption of trimethoprim and lincomycin while patients with coeliac disease show increased absorption of trimethoprim, fucidin, erythromycin and cephalexin. However, problems of absorption where gastrointestinal pathology exists tend to be complex, and consequently whether drug absorption is accelerated or slowed is often considerably variable from patient to patient.

(b) Sublingual administration   A drug may be absorbed through the mucosa of the buccal cavity when it is given in lozenges or tablets which are placed under the tongue and allowed to dissolve. After absorption, the drug enters the blood circulation without first having to pass through the liver. The drug therefore avoids first-pass inactivation by hepatic microsomal enzymes. Since the drug does not have to enter the intestine, absorption is generally more rapid than after swallowing and the drug is likely to be effective at a lower dose. In addition, drug action can be terminated once therapeutic relief has been achieved simply by spitting out the tablet.

The sublingual route is useful for the administration of glyceryl trinitrate or isoprenaline at the first signs of an acute attack of angina pectoris or asthma, respectively.

(c) Rectal administration   Some drugs cause nausea and vomiting when given by mouth and these may be formulated as suppositories or enemas and be given rectally to be absorbed by the rectal mucous membrane. Drugs administered rectally are not subject to first-pass elimination by the liver, and include

ergotamine for migraine, aminophylline for bronchial asthma, and indomethacin for inflammatory disorders.

1.2.3.2 *Parenteral*

The term parenteral (par – beyond, enteral – intestinal) implies that a drug is given by a route which takes it directly into body fluids thus by-passing the preliminary process of passage across gastrointestinal membranes.

(a) Intravenous injection   The most common method of introducing a drug directly into the systemic circulation is to inject it into a vein. This route is employed when a rapid therapeutic response is required, such as in status asthmaticus, cardiac arrhythmias, epileptic seizures and induction of anaesthesia. When administered, the drug is rapidly removed from the injection site, being diluted in the venous blood as it is carried firstly to the heart and then to other tissues. Since the total circulation time in man is of the order of 15 seconds, the onset of drug effects is almost immediate. Indeed, great care is needed when administering a drug intravenously to ensure that overdosage is avoided, since time may not permit reversal of any drug-induced toxicity.

Drugs administered intravenously may be given as a single rapid injection lasting 1–2 minutes and known as a 'bolus' injection, or as a slow infusion over a period of several hours or even longer. This latter choice is preferred when a sustained level of drug in the bloodstream is required over a relatively long period of time (e.g. lignocaine and many antibiotics).

(b) Intramuscular injection   The delivery of an exact quantity of drug is assured by intramuscular administration, although the rate of drug absorption may vary considerably. Factors influencing the rate of absorption include the vascularity of the site, the degree of ionization and lipid solubility of the drug, the volume of injection, and the osmolarity of the solution.

The site of injection appears to be a critical factor in determining the absorption rate of drugs after intramuscular administration. Drugs are usually injected into the arm (deltoid), thigh (vastus lateralis) or buttocks (gluteus maximus). The injection spreads out between the sheaths of muscle bundles. This spread may be facilitated by adding hyaluronidase to the administered drug. This enzyme breaks down the hyaluronic acid of the connective tissue matrix, allowing the drug solution to spread over a wider area. In the resting patient, drug absorption is generally most rapid from the deltoid where the vascularity is greatest, and least rapid from the buttocks where there is poor blood circulation. In this way, relatively large volumes of drug may be administered.

Increasing the blood supply to the site of injection by heating or by massage hastens the rate of dissemination.

The intramuscular route is often used in patients who are unable to receive oral medication, or for drugs that are poorly absorbed from the gastrointestinal tract. Drugs with molecular weights above about 20 000 daltons are taken up principally into the lymphatics while those with molecular weights below 3000 are taken up mainly by the blood capillaries. In general, drugs administered by intramuscular injections are absorbed and exert their pharmacological effect more rapidly than after oral dosing.

(c) Subcutaneous injection   Drugs administered by this route spread out through the loose connective tissue of the subcutaneous layer. Since the skin is rich in sensory nerves, subcutaneous injections are more painful than intramuscular injection. This route is suitable only for small dose volumes and probably the most important drug that is routinely administered this way is insulin. Absorption of drugs from subcutaneous tissues is influenced by the same factors that determine the rate of absorption from intramuscular sites. However, the blood supply in this region is poorer than that in muscle tissues and in consequence absorption may be slower. In both cases, the local action of an injected drug can be prolonged by decreasing its rate of removal from the site of injection. This can be achieved by including a vasoconstrictor drug such as adrenaline in the injection. The action of subcutaneously administered drugs can also be sustained if drugs are injected as solutions in oil, the drug diffusing out only slowly from the vehicle. Steroid hormones are often administered in the form of solid pellets which are implanted under the skin, the active hormone slowly dissolving in the tissue fluid before diffusing through the capillary walls. Implants of deoxycortone acetate may remain effective for up to 6 months.

Other parenteral routes include intra-arterial, intraperitoneal, intrathecal, intradermal and intracutaneous injection.

(d) Pulmonary absorption   Gaseous and volatile anaesthetics may be inhaled and absorbed through the pulmonary epithelium and mucous membranes of the respiratory tract. Due to the large surface area, absorption into pulmonary blood is very rapid. Absorption is dependent on the concentration of the drug in the alveolar gas, the blood/gas partition coefficient and the rate of pulmonary blood flow.

Other drugs may also be administered by inhalation (e.g. aerosol preparations) either to produce a local effect in the respiratory tract, or to act systemically after absorption. In this instance, particle size determines its penetration into the respiratory tract. Particles of less than 2 μm diameter enter the alveoli while particles 2–10 μm diameter are trapped in the bronchioles and small bronchi. Particles of 10 μm or greater are trapped in the upper respiratory tract. This route is widely used for administering drugs in the treatment of bronchial asthma (e.g. isoprenaline, salbutamol, disodium chromoglycate).

(e) Topical application   Drug application to the skin or to mucous membranes such as the conjunctiva, nasopharynx or vagina is used primarily for local effects, although efforts are now being concentrated on developing new dosage forms where passage through the skin into the systemic circulation is the goal.

Few drugs readily penetrate the intact healthy skin, absorption of those that do being proportional to their lipid solubility since the epidermis acts as a lipid barrier. In contrast, the dermis is freely permeable to many solutes and therefore systemic absorption occurs more readily through broken skin. Absorption through the skin is increased by occlusive dressings which retain moisture and 'macerate' the epidermis. Recently introduced dosage forms of glyceryl trinitrate depend upon percutaneous absorption for therapeutic activity.

1.3   DISTRIBUTION

Once in the circulation most drugs are distributed throughout the body's fluids and tissues with relative ease and at a faster rate than that of drug elimination. In contrast to elimination, distribution represents a reversible transfer of drug between tissue sites and plasma. The pattern of distribution reflects the interplay of a number of factors relating to permeability, lipid solubility and binding to macromolecules.

1.3.1   Fluid compartments

Drugs distribute in the body's fluids and it is convenient to consider these as compartments. Total body water in the adult is about 60% of body weight and this may be divided into that which is: (a) inside cells (intracellular, 35%); (b) outside cells (extracellular: partly as the plasma volume, 4%; partly interstitial fluid that bathes tissues, 12%; and partly as inaccessible water in bone and dense connective tissue, 4%); and (c) as transcellular water present in secretions and lumena, 1·5%.

1.3.2   Capillary structure

For drugs of molecular weight up to about 600 daltons existing free in solution in plasma water, penetration into interstitial fluid is rapid. The reason appears to be that generally the capillary wall behaves like a leaky sieve. The lining endothelial cells of the capillary have junctions with each other that are discontinuous (loose) and these allow the passage of molecules of up to 600 daltons. This is an important route for polar compounds. However, for lipid-soluble compounds, both this route and diffusion through the actual capillary wall are available pathways.

There is a high permeability of capillaries in the kidney and liver. In the latter organ this is due to the capillaries (sinusoids) lacking a complete lining and blood making direct contact with the hepatic parenchymal cells.

For some drugs, where their receptors lie on the exterior aspect of cell membranes, diffusion into the interstitial fluid is sufficient for their effectiveness. Thus the highly polar bisquaternary, hexamethonium, can cause a profound hypotension within seconds of its intravenous administration because it is readily accessible to the interstitial fluid via the loose capillary junctions. Here it combines with the superficial receptors of the sympathetic ganglia. For drugs with an intracellular site of action, passage not only across the capillary wall is required for pharmacological activity, but also through the cell membranes of the tissue. As with absorption, uptake by tissues at this site is mostly passive and therefore lipophilicity is important. Polar compounds penetrate these cell membranes poorly and are thus likely to exhibit a restricted distribution. This in turn may reduce the potential sites of action of such compounds.

A drug like heparin, that cannot pass through the capillary walls, distributes within the plasma. Drugs traversing the capillaries but not capable of penetrating cell membranes (e.g. streptomycin) distribute in the extracellular volume. Drugs which penetrate all membranes (e.g. antipyrine and ethanol) distribute in total body water. In these cases, the volumes represent real volumes of body water in which the drug is distributed. However, it is more usual to utilize another parameter, the apparent volume of distribution, as a guide to the pattern of a drug's distribution in the body. This is the volume in which the drug appears to be dissolved and it is a proportionality constant relating plasma concentration of the drug to the total amount of that drug in the body ($V =$ amount/plasma level). An apparent volume of distribution of 0.04 litre kg^{-1} (plasma volume) would be compatible with the restriction of a drug to the plasma compartment (V for heparin, 0.05 litre kg^{-1}). Values in excess of total body water (about 0.6 litre kg^{-1}) indicate that a drug is being accumulated or stored in extravascular sites (e.g. nortriptyline 22–27 litre kg^{-1}).

1.3.3   Tissue perfusion

Blood perfusion of different tissues and organs varies widely, highly perfused areas being the lung (10 ml min^{-1} ml^{-1}), heart, liver, kidney and brain and areas with low perfusion being fat (0.03 ml min^{-1} ml^{-1}) and bone. The perfusion of muscle and skin occupies an intermediate position.

The concentration of a drug rises rapidly in well-perfused tissues and its equilibrium between blood and these sites is achieved within minutes after absorption. Delivery of a drug to muscle, skin and fat is slower, in some cases equilibrium being attained only after several hours.

The volume of the tissue is also important and some organs, such as thyroid and adrenal – having a small size together with a high blood perfusion, would be expected to achieve high drug concentrations. Changes in blood flow arising from, for example, heart disease may alter the perfusion of organs such as liver and kidney and greatly affect the rate of drug elimination.

1.3.4   Gradients of pH and binding

The penetration of a drug will depend to a large extent on the concentration gradient of the freely diffusible form and factors such as pH gradient and relative binding to intracellular and extracellular constituents will influence the accumulation in a tissue.

1.3.4.1   pH

Intracellular pH is slightly lower than extracellular pH (approx. pH 7.0 and 7.4 respectively) and this may in part account for the occurrence of relatively higher intracellular concentrations of basic compounds. The magnitude of the influence of pH will depend on the pK_a of the drug. It has been observed that several basic drugs and endogenous amines achieved high concentrations in pulmonary tissue and part of the explanation may be related to the low intracellular pH (6·8–6·5) reported for this organ. Alteration of pH gradients could occur as the result of disease where acidosis or alkalosis is a consequence. In the early stages of such pathophysiological changes, the pH of extracellular fluid is more responsive to change than is the pH of intracellular fluid. Thus in acidosis, the tissue uptake and efficacy of lignocaine are reduced. At sites of inflammation, changes of pH gradient occur, the extracellular value dropping to pH 6·8, while that of the intracellular fluid rises to pH 7·2. Such alterations are sufficient to influence the distribution of an acid, such as a non-steroidal anti-inflammatory drug ($pK_a \simeq 4$), leading to higher concentrations of the drug in the cells and membranes of the inflamed area.

1.3.4.2 Binding

An important factor in the distribution of drugs is their binding to macromolecules (largely proteins). This is usually a reversible process and it affects the concentration of freely diffusible drug available because the high molecular weight complex cannot cross the cell membrane. Although most study has been made of the extracellular binding, drugs also bind intracellularly and it is the binding gradient that is the important parameter affecting the distribution equilibrium. Cerebrospinal fluid possesses a very low level of protein compared to plasma and this limits the possibility for binding. This virtual binding gradient influences the distribution of drugs such as phenytoin and nortriptyline which achieve concentrations in the CSF that are not more than 12% of the concurrent steady state plasma levels.

In plasma, the main protein for drug binding is albumin and the binding forces involved may be ionic, van der Waals', hydrogen and/or hydrophobic bonds. As binding is mostly reversible, there is an equilibrium between bound and unbound drug and the interaction follows the Law of Mass Action. Thus,

$$D_F + nP \underset{k_2}{\overset{k_1}{\rightleftharpoons}} D_B, \tag{1.10}$$

where D_F is the molar concentration of unbound drug, D_B is the molar concentration of bound drug, P is the molar concentration of protein and n is the number of binding sites per mole of protein; and

$$K = k_1/k_2, \tag{1.11}$$

where k_1 is the rate constant for association, k_2 is the rate constant for dissociation and K is the equilibrium association constant. At equilibrium

$$D_B = \frac{1}{(1/KnP) + (D_F/nP)}, \tag{1.12}$$

so that

$$K = D_B/D_F(nP - D_B). \tag{1.13}$$

It is clear that binding of a drug in the plasma depends upon the association constant, the number of binding sites, and the concentrations of protein and of drug. As the plasma level of a drug $(D_F + D_B)$ is gradually increased after absorption the fraction of drug in the free form rises slowly at first, but as the binding sites become saturated this fraction rises very sharply. In practice, however, the fraction of free drug in the plasma is essentially constant over the range of therapeutic plasma concentrations for most drugs. Saturation is most likely to occur with drugs possessing high association constants that are administered in high dose (e.g. some sulphonamides).

It is important to view the degree of binding to plasma in relation to a drug's extravascular binding and this may be done by means of the apparent volume of distribution. Thus, while nortriptyline is 93% plasma bound under steady state conditions, the total amount in plasma is less than 1% of that in the remainder of the body because of its large apparent distribution volume.

The intracellular binding of drugs has received less attention, although a number of documented examples are available. Thus acridines (e.g. mepacrine) reach tissue concentrations that may be a thousand-fold or more higher than in plasma on chronic administration. This results from the binding of these drugs by DNA. Chloroquine has an affinity for melanin and accumulates in the retina where it may cause a retinopathy. Tetracyclines accumulate in bone by incorporation into the crystal lattice. The relatively high uptake of the antihypertensive, indapamide, into arterial walls has been associated with its ability to bind to elastin.

1.3.5 Partition into fat

Lipid-soluble drugs may achieve high concentrations in adipose tissue, being stored by physical solution in the neutral fat. Since fat is normally 15% of body weight (in grossly obese subjects as high as 50%), it can serve as an important reservoir for such drugs. It also has a role in terminating the effects of highly lipid-soluble compounds by acting as an acceptor of the drug during a redistribution phase. Thus thiopentone, after intravenous injection, enters the brain rapidly, but also leaves it rapidly because of falling plasma levels and this terminates the action. There follows a slow redistribution into fatty tissues where as much as 70% of the drug may be found, 3 hours after administration.

1.3.6 Active transport

Uptake into tissues may also occur (though less commonly) by a process of active transport. Guanethidine owes its high concentration in cardiac tissue to being taken up into adrenergic nerve endings by the re-uptake mechanism for noradrenaline. It has also been found that bases such as methadone, propranolol and amphetamine are transported into lung tissue by an active process. This may be an important mechanism for the high pulmonary uptake of such drugs.

1.3.7   Blood–brain barrier

Penetration of drugs from the circulation into the CNS extracellular space and CSF is restricted by the nature of the absorption surface presented. The endothelial cells of the brain capillaries possess tight junctions. In addition, layers of glial cells closely surround the capillaries. Thus, a markedly lipid barrier (that probably constitutes the blood–brain barrier) must be traversed by a drug in order to gain access to central neurones. While highly lipid-soluble compounds reach the brain rapidly after administration, more polar compounds penetrate at a much slower rate (e.g. thiopentone and barbitone respectively). As the rate of penetration of a drug will depend on its degree of ionization in plasma and on its lipid solubility, it is possible to consider exploiting these variables to influence distribution. Although atropine is extensively ionized in the plasma, its un-ionized form is extremely lipophilic and it enters the brain where it may produce pharmacological effects (*see also* Section 3.3.3). Its quaternized derivative, methyl atropine, is highly polar and penetrates the blood-brain barrier with difficulty (*see also* p. 66). As a consequence it has essentially no central actions unless administered directly into the brain. Such possibilities have been applied to the development of dopa decarboxylase (A.A.A.D.) inhibitors that are excluded from the CNS (e.g. carbidopa, benzserazide, *see* Section 4.3.5). They are administered in combination with L-dopa in the treatment of Parkinson's disease. This allows the decarboxylation of dopa to dopamine to take place in the CNS and not peripherally. In Parkinson's disease there is a deficiency of dopamine in the brain. However, dopamine is unable to cross the blood–brain barrier, while its precursor dopa can. Preventing the peripheral metabolism of dopa leads to a more efficient utilization of the administered dose.

Removal of drugs from the CNS may be by back-diffusion through the blood–brain barrier. In addition, drugs may be removed via the CSF, with which the extracellular fluid of many parts of the brain shows ready diffusional exchange. Thus, drugs may be removed with the CSF as it flows through the arachnoid villi into the venous sinus below the skull. Alternatively, a drug in the CSF may be actively secreted through the epithelial lining of the choroid plexus into the bloodstream. At this location, there are transport mechanisms for both cationic and anionic molecules.

1.3.8   Placental barrier

The placenta is a complex barrier well developed for the exchange of materials between the maternal and foetal circulations. Foetal blood is separated from maternal blood by a cellular barrier composed of the trophoblastic layer, mesenchymal tissue and foetal capillary endothelium. The thickness of this composite barrier is greater (25 μm) in early pregnancy than in late pregnancy

(2μm). Although specific transport systems for endogenous materials are present in the placenta and may be a means of transport for some drugs (e.g. α-methyl dopa, 5-fluorouracil), it appears that most drugs cross the placenta by passive diffusion. Penetration is therefore rapid with lipid-soluble un-ionized drugs and least with very polar compounds. However, some degree of foetal exposure is likely to occur with virtually all drugs and, in view of the uncertain effects of such drugs on the foetus, caution is required in drug administration during pregnancy.

1.4   METABOLISM

Most drugs, prior to removal from the body, are subjected to biotransformation (metabolism). The enzymic reactions leading to such changes are classified as Phase I reactions (asynthetic changes) and Phase II reactions (conjugations). As the original compound is chemically altered by these means, metabolism may be considered as a drug elimination mechanism although the problem of excreting the metabolites remains. In most instances, the metabolites have a markedly different partition character from the parent compound, in that lipophilicity is decreased. Such products tend to be well excreted as they are not readily reabsorbed from the renal tubular fluid. Drug metabolites also often have a smaller apparent volume of distribution than their precursors.

Metabolism influences the biological activity of a drug in a number of ways (see Table 1.2). In many instances, pharmacological activity is reduced or lost by metabolism and for such drugs this may be an important determinant of duration of effect and even intensity of action. Occasionally a drug may be transformed into a metabolite possessing a pharmacological effect of comparable intensity (see Chapter 7). For a relatively small number of drugs (pro-drugs), biologically inactive per se, metabolic activation is a prerequisite for therapeutic utility (see Chapter 7). Finally, a growing list of drugs and other xenobiotic compounds is metabolized to intermediates that may subsequently react with tissue macro-molecules leading to toxic effects.

The main site of drug metabolism is the liver, followed by the gastrointestinal tract. However, metabolism also occurs in the kidney, lung, skin and blood but, quantitatively, these sites are less important.

1.4.1   Phase I metabolism

The Phase I reactions are oxidation, reduction and hydrolysis.

1.4.1.1   Oxidations

Many of the oxidation reactions, such as aliphatic and aromatic hydroxylation, epoxidation, dealkylation, deamination, N-oxidation and S-oxidation (see Table 1.3), are catalysed by enzymes (mixed function oxidases) bound to the endoplasmic reticulum. This latter is a branching tubular system within cells, that is also involved in protein synthesis and lipid metabolism. When a tissue such as liver is

Table 1.2   Examples of effect of drug metabolism on pharmacological activity

Effect	*Drug*	*Metabolic reaction*
Deactivation		
Drug metabolite less active than parent molecule or inactive	Aminoglutethimide	Conjugation (with acetic acid)
	Amphetamine	Oxidation
	Barbiturates	Oxidation
	Chloramphenicol	Conjugation (with glucuronic acid)
	Procaine	Hydrolysis
	Tolbutamide	Oxidation
Co-activation		
Drug metabolite possessing equivalent activity to parent molecule	Diazepam	Oxidation (to nordiazepam)
	Methsuximide	Oxidation (to 2-methyl-2-phenyl succinimide)
	Phenylbutazone	Oxidation (to oxyphenyl-butazone)
	Propranolol	Oxidation (to 4-hydroxy-propranolol)
	Procainamide	Conjugation (to *N*-acetyl procainamide)
Activation		
Metabolite is responsible for (pro-) drug activity	Chloral hydrate	Reduction (to trichloroethanol)
	Chlorazepate	Oxidation (to nordiazepam)
	Palmitic ester of chloramphenicol	Hydrolysis (to chloramphenicol)
	Proguanil	Oxidation (to cycloguanyl)
	Prontosil red	Reduction (to sulphanilamide)
Toxification		
Drug metabolite possessing toxic effects	Malathion	Oxidation (to malaoxon)
	Methanol	Oxidation (to formaldehyde and formic acid)
	Paracetamol	Oxidation (to an electrophilic imido-quinone)

homogenized, this reticulum fragments into rounded bodies (microsomes) sedimenting at 10–100 S. Many metabolic oxidations have been studied using this microsomal enzyme fraction. The terminal oxygen transferase of the system is cytochrome P450. This is coupled to the flavoprotein enzyme, cytochrome P450-reductase, and linked to NADPH as a source of electrons. Under the influence of cytochrome P450, an oxygen atom from molecular oxygen is transferred to a drug molecule (DH→DOH). The remaining oxygen atom combines with two protons to yield a molecule of water. Cytochrome P450 is so named because its reduced carbon monoxide-ligand spectrum has a maximum absorption at 450 nm. It is now known that cytochrome P450 and its reductase both exist in multiple forms and the cytochrome P450 variants appear to possess overlapping substrate specificities.

Table 1.3   Some microsomal oxidations

Aromatic oxidation

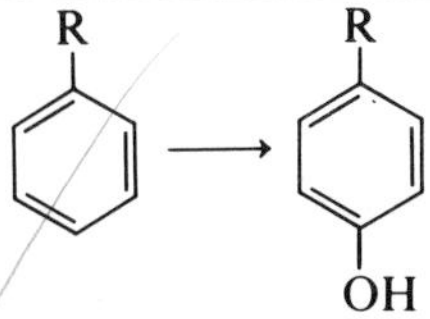

(phenobarbitone→5-ethyl-5(4-hydroxyphenyl) barbituric acid)

Aliphatic (side-chain) oxidation

$$R—CH_3 \longrightarrow RCH_2OH$$

(pentobarbitone $\longrightarrow$ 5-ethyl-5(3-hydroxy-1-methylbutyl) barbituric acid)

Epoxidation

$$R—CH=CH_2 \longrightarrow RCH \overset{O}{\overset{\diagup\diagdown}{—}} CH_2$$

(carbamazepine $\longrightarrow$ carbamazepine 10,11 epoxide)

Dealkylation

$$R—X—CH_3 \longrightarrow R—X—CH_2OH \longrightarrow R—XH + HCHO$$

(X = NH or NCH$_3$, imipramine $\longrightarrow$ desmethylimipramine)

(X = O, phenacetin $\longrightarrow$ paracetamol)

(X = S, 6-methylthioprine $\longrightarrow$ 6-mercaptopurine)

Oxidative deamination

$$R—\underset{\underset{NH_2}{|}}{CH}—CH_3 \longrightarrow \left[R—\underset{\underset{NH_2}{|}}{C(OH)}—CH_3 \right] \longrightarrow R—COCH_3 + NH_3$$

(amphetamine $\longrightarrow$ phenylacetone)

N-hydroxylation

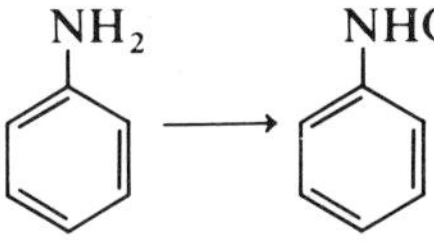

(aminoglutethimide $\longrightarrow$ N-hydroxyaminoglutethimide)

N-oxidation

$$R_3N \longrightarrow R_3N \to O$$

(trimethylamine $\longrightarrow$ trimethylamine N-oxide)

Sulphoxidation

$$R_2S \longrightarrow R_2S \to O$$

(chlorpromazine $\longrightarrow$ chlorpromazine sulphoxide)

Desulphuration

$$R_2C=S \longrightarrow R_2C=O$$

(thiopentone $\longrightarrow$ pentobarbitone)

In addition to an ability to bind to cytochrome P450, requirements of a substrate for metabolism by this system include: a molecular weight above 150 daltons (below this size, compounds are normally capable of ready excretion), a sufficient degree of lipophilicity to enter the endoplasmic reticulum and the appropriate chemical substituents. Chemical reactivity at sites on a molecule influence the site of oxidative enzyme attack. Thus, with nitrobenzene, the main oxidative metabolite is 3-hydroxynitrobenzene, while with aniline, 2- and 4-hydroxyaniline are the major ring-oxidized products.

A non-cytochrome P450-dependent microsomal flavoprotein oxidase has been described in liver that effects sulphoxidation of nucleophilic sulphur compounds (e.g. methimazole), hydroxylamine formation from secondary amines (e.g. desipramine, nortriptyline) and amine oxide formation from tertiary amines (e.g. brompheniramine, guanethidine).

Oxidations are also carried out by non-microsomal enzymes such as alcohol and aldehyde dehydrogenases and monamine and diamine oxidases. Although the oxidations are less varied than those of the microsomal enzymes, they are important pathways for several naturally occurring compounds as well as drugs.

1.4.1.2   Reductions

Only a small number of drugs is metabolized by reduction, the reductases being located at both microsomal and non-microsomal sites. Some reductases are also found in the micro-organisms of the gut. Aromatic azo and nitro compounds are reduced by microsomal flavoprotein enzymes. The nitro-reductase converts the substrate (e.g. chloramphenicol, nitrazepam) to the corresponding amine by the following sequential reactions, $ArNO_2 \rightarrow ArNO \rightarrow ArNHOH \rightarrow ArNH_2$. Azo-reductase effects a reductive cleavage of its substrate by the following sequence $Ar'N{=}NAr'' \rightarrow Ar'NH{-}NHAr'' \rightarrow Ar'NH_2 + Ar''NH_2$ (e.g. prontosil red $\rightarrow$ sulphanilamide + 1,2,4 triaminobenzene). There is a marked azo-reductase activity in the gut microflora. A hepatic microsomal enzyme, requiring NADPH and oxygen, is responsible for replacing halogen with hydrogen in aliphatic halogenated compounds such as halothane, methoxyflurane and carbon tetrachloride (e.g. $CCl_4 \rightarrow CHCl_3$). Examples of reductions carried out by non-microsomal enzymes, are the transformation in the blood of disulphiram $((C_2H_5)_2NCSS{-}SSCN(C_2H_5)_2)$ into diethyldithiocarbamate $((C_2H_5)_2NCSSH)$ and the reduction of chloral hydrate to trichloroethanol by alcohol dehydrogenase.

1.4.1.3   Hydrolyses

Drugs containing an ester group may be hydrolysed by esterases which have both microsomal and non-microsomal locations. The former tend to be more concentrated in the liver. Such an enzyme is responsible for the hydrolysis of pethidine. The non-microsomal esterases occur in blood and some tissues; procaine is metabolized by a plasma esterase. The esterases also hydrolyse amides (e.g.

procainamide), though more slowly than the corresponding esters. Epoxide hydrases, present in the microsomal fraction of many tissues, convert epoxides to the corresponding dihydrodiols.

1.4.2   Phase II metabolism

Phase II metabolism involves the coupling of a drug or its metabolites with various endogenous components. The reaction, which is carried out by a transferase enzyme, requires that either the endogenous or the exogenous component is activated prior to conjugation.

1.4.2.1   *Glucuronide formation*

Probably the most common conjugation pathway is that of glucuronide formation. The combination with glucuronic acid occurs readily with compounds possessing a functional group with a reactive proton, usually attached to a hetero-atom (e.g. hydroxyl, carboxyl, amino and sulphydryl). These functional groups may be already present in a drug molecule (e.g. paracetamol) or may be acquired by Phase I metabolism (e.g. phenytoin hydroxylation). Depending on the grouping through which conjugation takes place, these metabolites can be described as O-glucuronides (ether type – combination through a hydroxyl group, e.g. alcohol metabolites of barbiturates; ester type – combination through a carboxyl group, e.g. salicylic acid), N-glucuronides (via amino groups, e.g. meprobamate) and S-glucuronides (via sulphydryl groups, e.g. 2-mercaptobenzothiazole). Glucuronic acid is derived enzymically from glucose and its active form, uridine diphosphoglucuronic acid (UDP-GA), is utilized by the UDP-glucuronyl-transferase to effect the conjugation.

Glucuronides are very polar and relatively strong acids ($pK_a \simeq 3$). They are thus extensively ionized at the pH of blood and urine; this makes them good candidates for excretion.

Recently it has been found that, in mammals, phenolic and carboxylic compounds can be conjugated with glucose, the high energy glucose donor being UDP-glucose. The glucosides are more water-soluble than the free aglycones but less polar than the corresponding glucuronides.

1.4.2.2   *Sulphate formation*

Sulphate esters are formed by the soluble fraction (i.e. 100 S supernatant), the high energy sulphate being 3′-phosphoadenosine-5′-phosphosulphate (PAPS) and the other component substrate being either a phenol (e.g. paracetamol, salicylamide) or aliphatic and steroid alcohol (e.g. ethanol, androsterone). Sulphamates may also be formed in a similar manner from aromatic amines. The capacity to form sulphate conjugates is somewhat limited, and this appears to be related to the low availability of sulphate.

1.4.2.3 *Methylation*

Methylation is an important physiological process for the conversion of noradrenaline into adrenaline (N-methylation). Both of these catecholamines are also
metabolized by O-methylation under the influence of catechol-O-methyl transferase (COMT). The methyl group is derived from methionine, the active methyl
donor form of which is S-adenosylmethionine. Drugs or their metabolites
containing primary aliphatic amine, phenolic or sulphydryl group may be
N-, O- or S-methylated respectively, by methyltransferases. Thus the minor
catechol metabolite of phenytoin, 5-phenyl-5-(3,4-dihydroxyphenyl) hydantoin, is
conjugated to give the corresponding 3-O-methylcatechol.

1.4.2.4 *Acylation*

Several acylation conjugation reactions of importance may occur with some drugs.
This pathway involves the reaction between an amine and a carboxylic acid to yield
an amide, the high energy molecule required being a coenzyme A derivative of the
carboxylic acid. The drug, or its metabolite, can be either of the conjugating
molecules. Thus, aromatic primary amines (e.g. sulphonamides, aminoglutethimide) and hydrazine derivatives (e.g. isoniazid) are acetylated, utilizing acetyl
coenzyme A. It should be noted that acetylation has little influence on the polarity
of a drug, in fact it decreases the basicity of the amino group. The acetylated
metabolite of sulphathiazole is some fourteen times less soluble in water (37 °C)
than its parent molecule. Because of this property, and a lowered solubility at acid
pH, there is the danger of injury to the kidney resulting from precipitation of the
conjugated sulphonamide in the renal tubular fluid as the kidney concentrates
urine and lowers its pH (*see also* Section 4.3.1). The acetyltransferase appears to be
located in the soluble fraction of reticulo-endothelial cells present in the liver and
kidney.

Benzoic acid and its derivatives are activated by combination with acetyl
coenzyme A and conjugated with glycine to form hippurates (e.g. salicylic acid
metabolized to salicyluric acid). This takes place in the mitochondria of the liver
and kidney.

1.4.2.5 *Glutathione conjugation*

The tripeptide, glutathione (cysteine-glycine-glutamate), may be coupled via its
sulphydryl group to various compounds possessing an electrophilic centre. In the
case of paracetamol, such a site is introduced as a result of oxidative metabolism.
This conjugation reaction is an important mechanism for the effective disposal of
electrophiles (e.g. reactive epoxides) before they are able to react with nucleophilic
centres of nucleic acids and enzymes to initiate toxic responses. Myleran
(busulphan), azathioprine and urethane are examples of drugs conjugated by this
pathway. Glutathione conjugates are polar and of high molecular weight (above
300 daltons) and are eliminated as such in the bile. However, the glutathione
portion of the conjugate may be further metabolized (via the peptide bonds) to

mercapturic acids that are the normal urinary products of this conjugation pathway.

1.4.3 Factors influencing metabolism

It will be evident from the foregoing that even the simplest of drugs may be subjected to several types of metabolic transformation. Thus, propranolol is conjugated directly with glucuronic acid, ring-hydroxylated and oxidized in the side chain. A complex molecule like chlorpromazine may give rise to an extremely large number of different metabolites.

1.4.3.1 *Stereoisomerism*

Where a drug exists in stereoisomeric forms, the rate and routes of metabolism may differ between the enantiomers. Thus (−)-hexobarbitone and (−)-warfarin are metabolized faster than the (+)-isomers. While the (+)-isomer of glutethimide is hydroxylated in the 4-position of the glutarimide ring, the (−)-isomer undergoes oxidation of the ethyl substituent on the 2-position of the ring structure.

1.4.3.2 *Presystemic metabolism*

For drugs administered orally, there is the possibility of their metabolism as they pass through the wall of the small intestine and (via the portal circulation) through the liver before they reach the heart for distribution systemically. This first-pass or presystemic metabolism has a profound influence on the bioavailability of drugs such as isoprenaline, terbutaline, propranolol, alprenolol, imipramine, dextropropoxyphene and lignocaine.

1.4.3.3 *Dose-dependent metabolism*

In most cases, the metabolism of a drug is a first order process which means that a constant fraction of the drug is metabolized in unit time. However, the therapeutic doses of some drugs (e.g. phenytoin 300–350 mg daily) result in concentrations able to saturate the metabolizing enzymes and zero order kinetics operate (i.e. a constant amount of drug is metabolized per unit of time). In this situation, steady state concentrations of the drug rise very sharply with relatively small increments of daily dose and toxicity may arise. Saturation of one metabolic pathway may allow for a shift in the metabolic pattern of a drug. Thus, after paracetamol overdosage (e.g. 20 g), the glucuronide and sulphate conjugation pathways become saturated, making available a greater fraction of the dose for oxidation to a reactive and potentially toxic metabolite.

1.4.3.4 *Inter-species variation*

Differences in drug metabolism may occur between species and this is of great importance in drug development investigations. The differences may be associated with the rate of drug metabolism, e.g. hexobarbitone is oxidized by the following species in order of decreasing rate: mouse > rat > dog > man. For the mixed function oxidases, there is direct correlation with their activity and the tissue oxygen concentration in a species. The route of metabolism may also be influenced by species. Thus bethanidine is mainly *N*-demethylated by the dog, ring-hydroxylated by the rat and excreted unchanged by man. Well-documented examples of species differences include the poor acetylation of aromatic amines in the dog, the deficiency of glucuronide formation in the cat and the absence of atropinesterase in man.

1.4.3.5   *Intra-species variation*

Different rates and extents of drug metabolism also occur within a species (including man). After a dose of imipramine to human subjects, the plasma levels of the drug 12 h later show a twelve-fold variation between individuals. Similar ranges of variations have been found with desipramine and chlorpromazine. The plasma half-lives of certain drugs oxidized by hepatic microsomal enzymes (e.g. antipyrine, phenylbutazone) show much more marked differences between pairs of fraternal twins than between pairs of identical twins. This indicates that genetic rather than environmental causes give rise to such inter-subject variability. A notable example is the hydrolysis of suxamethonium. In some patients, the normal dose gives rise to prolonged muscle relaxation and apnoea. These individuals possess an atypical pseudocholinesterase with a low affinity for suxamethonium. Drug metabolism defects may sometimes be clearly associated with certain congenital abnormalities, e.g. in Down's syndrome, glycine conjugation is deficient and in Gilbert's syndrome, glucuronide formation is impaired. Wide variation in the extent of acetylation of isoniazid, hydrallazine, phenelzine, dapsone and some sulphonamides exists and distinct sub-populations of fast or slow acetylators can be defined. Rapid acetylation is inherited as a dominant character which determines the presence of large amounts of the N-acetyltransferase. The relative proportions of rapid and slow acetylators has been shown to vary between ethnic groups (e.g. proportion of slow acetylators in Canadian Eskimos 0%, Swedes 50%, British 60%, Egyptians 72%). Slow acetylators are more susceptible to adverse effects from ioniazid, hydrallazine and phenelzine.

1.4.3.6   *Age*

A newborn child is deficient in microsomal enzymes including cytochrome P450 and UDP-glucuronyl-transferase, although this may be modified (induction, *see* p. 29) by drugs taken by the mother during the latter part of gestation. As a result, the half-lives of several drugs are prolonged in the neonate compared to the adult (e.g. $t_{\frac{1}{2}}$ for tolbutamide, 40 h at birth, 8 h in adult). Drugs may therefore have more prolonged or intense effects and adverse reactions may arise. For example, chloramphenicol, requiring conjugation with glucuronic acid, is much more toxic to a newborn infant than to an adult. In general, enzyme activity increases to maximum levels over the first 8 weeks of life. There is some evidence that drug metabolism (of e.g. theophylline, phenobarbitone, diazoxide) in children, prior to puberty, may be faster than in adults. A decrease in drug metabolism may occur with advancing years as is shown by the slower oxidation of amylobarbitone in individuals over 65 years of age. However, the influence of old age appears to be obscured in many cases by environmental factors (inducers) such as cigarette smoking.

1.4.3.7 *Inhibition of metabolism*

Inhibition of drug-metabolizing enzymes may arise from a competitive interaction of two substrates for the enzyme. The overall effect depends on the relative concentrations of the two substrates and their affinities for the active sites. Novobiocin has been reported to cause jaundice in the newborn, arising from its inhibition of bilirubin conjugation with glucuronic acid. In the late stages of pregnancy, the high maternal levels of progesterone and pregnanediol inhibit the metabolism of drugs such as pethidine, barbiturates and coumarins.

1.4.3.8 *Induction of metabolism*

A number of drugs and other compounds, when repeatedly administered, can bring about an increase (induction) in the activity of the hepatic microsomal mixed function oxidases and other enzymes (e.g. UDP-glucuronyl-transferase, epoxide hydrase) as well as at other sites as a result of increased enzyme synthesis. Drugs such as phenobarbitone increase the level of cytochrome P450 and its associated reductase. Other examples of inducing agents in man are dichloralphenazone, phenylbutazone, griseofulvin, phenytoin, glutethimide, aminoglutethimide and rifampicin. Their effect is maximal after 2–3 weeks of repeated dosing. On stopping administration, enzyme levels revert to normal within 3–4 weeks. It is thought that these inducers, because of a high concentration or a slow metabolism, occupy the active sites of the enzyme to be induced for a prolonged period. This leads to derepression of gene function, followed by increased synthesis of the enzyme protein, and hence results in enhanced enzyme activity. The consequences of induction upon drug effects depend on the biological activity of the metabolites that are formed in increased amounts.

1.5   EXCRETION

The most important route of excretion for a drug or a drug metabolite is through the kidneys. The major alternative is elimination through the biliary system into the small intestine, the drug or its metabolites being available either for reabsorption (enterohepatic cycling) or for elimination with the faeces. Minor pathways of excretion include saliva and milk, this latter route often posing problems for breast-fed infants. Elimination of volatile substances such as anaesthetic gases takes place via the pulmonary epithelium.

1.5.1   Renal elimination of drugs

The renal handling of drugs is a rather complex phenomenon, involving one or more of the following processes, glomerular filtration, active tubular secretion and passive reabsorption (*see* Fig. 1.2). The removal of drugs or drug metabolites from the body by the kidneys is termed renal clearance.

1.5.1.1   *Glomerular filtration*

The kidneys receive about 20–25% of the cardiac output or 1·2–1·5 litres of blood per minute. Of this volume, approximately 10% is filtered at the glomerulus. Although the pores of the glomerular capillaries are sufficiently large to permit the passage of most drug molecules, they restrict the passage of blood cells and plasma proteins. Thus, only drug in plasma water is filtered, drugs bound to plasma proteins being retained in the bloodstream. The rate at which plasma water is filtered ($120-150$ ml min^{-1}) is conventionally called the 'glomerular filtration rate' (GFR). If a drug is only filtered and all filtered drug is excreted in the urine, then its rate of elimination or clearance will depend on the GFR and the concentration of drug in plasma water. In fact, renal clearance (by filtration) will be equal to: GFR $\times (f_u)$ where f_u is the fraction of non-protein bound drug to total plasma drug concentration. The renal clearance values of creatinine and inulin for individual persons are a close measure of GFR, since neither substance is bound to plasma protein nor secreted, and all the filtered load is excreted into the urine.

1.5.1.2   *Active tubular secretion*

The proximal convoluted tubules actively transport a wide range of substances from plasma into the tubular urine. Secretion of a drug is indicated when the rate of urinary elimination exceeds the rate of glomerular filtration. Apart from specific transport mechanisms (e.g. for amino acids and glucose) there are two relatively non-specific transport systems, one for secreting acids (anions) and the other for bases (cations). Both systems are energy-dependent, the energy being derived from tubular cell metabolism. Many drugs and drug metabolites are actively secreted into the proximal tubules and some of these are presented in Table 1.4. As with other carrier processes, substances transported by the same system will of course compete with each other. In contrast to glomerular filtration, the extent to which a drug is actively secreted into the urine is not necessarily related to the degree of binding to plasma protein. This is because the affinity of many substances for the active transport systems is greater than the affinity of binding to plasma proteins. For example, secretion of *p*-aminohippuric acid (PAH) is so extensive that it is almost completely cleared from the plasma in one passage through the kidney, despite the fact that it is about 90% bound to plasma protein. Since PAH is not reabsorbed in the proximal tubule, its renal clearance is a measure of renal plasma flow. It would appear that most of the blood supply to the kidney is in contact with the proximal tubule for a sufficient period of time to allow the dissociation of the drug–protein complex to take place, thus making the drug available for active secretion.

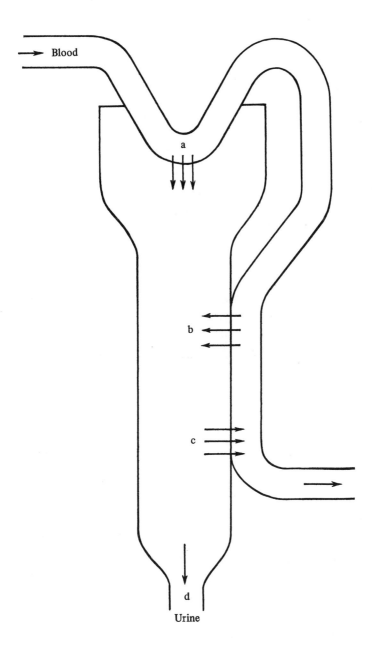

Fig. 1.2   Schematic representation of drug elimination by the kidneys. a, glomerular filtration of the non-protein bound fraction of most drugs and plasma water. b, active tubular secretion of organic acids and bases. c, passive reabsorption of lipid-soluble drugs. d, urinary excretion.

Table 1.4 Some drugs and drug metabolites actively secreted into the proximal renal tubules

Acids	Bases
Chlorpropamide	Amiloride
Ethacrynic acid	Dihydrocodeine
Frusemide	Dihydromorphinone
Glucuronic acid conjugates	Dopamine
Glycine conjugates	Guanidine derivatives
Indomethacin	Mecamylamine
Penicillins	Mepacrine
Phenylbutazone	Morphine
Probenecid	Pempidine
Salicylic acid	Pethidine
Sulphate conjugates	Procaine
Sulphathiazole	Quaternary ammonium compounds
Thiazide diuretics	Quinine
	Thiamine
	Tolazoline
	Triamterene

1.5.1.3 *Passive reabsorption*

Perhaps the most important factor controlling the renal handling of drugs is reabsorption. For the majority of drugs, reabsorption is a passive process although specific transport mechanisms occur for many substances including vitamins, electrolytes, glucose and amino acids. The degree of passive reabsorption depends on the physico-chemical characteristics of the drug or metabolite. Since the tubular epithelium has the properties of a lipid membrane, lipophilic molecules tend to be extensively reabsorbed while polar molecules are not. Reabsorption also depends on physiological variables like the rate of urine flow and the pH of the urine.

Although some 180 litres of protein-free filtrate pass through the glomerulus each day, only about 1·8 litres are eliminated as urine. Of the remainder, 80–90% is reabsorbed in the proximal tubule, with some reabsorption taking place in the distal tubule and collecting ducts. Consequently, with water reabsorption, drugs concentrate in the glomerular filtrate. If a drug is neither reabsorbed (generally polar) nor secreted, the concentration of drug in the urine will be about 100 times as great as that of unbound drug in the plasma.

Strong acids ($pK_a < 2$) and strong bases ($pK_a > 12$) are almost completely ionized over the physiological range of urinary pH (4·8–7·5) and their clearance is therefore unaffected by pH changes in urine. On the other hand, weak organic acids and bases may well be affected by urinary pH, their renal clearance being in accordance with the pH-partition hypothesis (*see* p. 5). When the urine is more acid, the degree of ionization of basic drugs is increased and consequently reabsorption is depressed, but the ionization of acidic drugs is decreased and their reabsorption is enhanced. The reverse occurs when the urine is more alkaline. For basic drugs, including amphetamine, antihistamines, morphine-like analgesics and tricyclic antidepressants, renal excretion may be increased by acidifying the urine with ammonium chloride, large doses of vitamin C, or a high protein diet. Phenobarbitone and salicylates are excreted, in part, in the unchanged form and (being weak organic acids) are ionized by alkaline pH. Their excretion rate may be increased by making the urine alkaline, by administering sodium bicarbonate, a diuretic of the carbonic anhydrase inhibitor type, or a vegetable diet. Clinically, manipulation of urinary pH can be useful for either prolonging the therapeutic action of drugs which tend to be excreted very rapidly, or for accelerating the excretion of ingested poisons.

1.5.1.4   *Renal clearance and half-life*

The efficiency of renal elimination of a drug can be expressed in terms of a hypothetical volume of plasma (ml) that is completely cleared of that substance by the kidney per unit time (min). The amount of drug cleared in unit time may be constant (e.g. linear clearance) but this is relatively uncommon. Most drugs are cleared from the body in an exponential fashion, the amount of drug cleared in unit time being proportional to the amount remaining in the body. For such drugs, clearance is theoretically never complete and in practice it is convenient to measure the time to clear one-half of the drug from the body, i.e. half-clearance time, or the elimination half-life of the drug ($t_{\frac{1}{2}}$). Knowledge of the half-life of a drug is clearly beneficial in deciding appropriate dosage regimens. Approximate values of the half-time for elimination of a number of drugs are presented in Table 1.5.

Estimates of renal clearance provide information with respect to excretion mechanisms although giving no direct data on the half-life of a drug. As previously stated, creatinine and inulin are eliminated by renal excretion with neither tubular secretion nor reabsorption occurring, and consequently they have a renal clearance rate of the order of $125 \, \text{ml} \, \text{min}^{-1}$. Clearance values for a drug which exceed $125 \, \text{ml} \, \text{min}^{-1}$ will indicate renal tubular secretion of the drug. Clearance values which fall below $125 \, \text{ml} \, \text{min}^{-1}$ even when calculated in terms of free (unbound) drug are indicative of tubular reabsorption. However, care should be taken in interpreting clearance values as secretion and reabsorption processes may be operative at the same time in the renal elimination of a drug.

The half-life of a drug in the body is a function of both its renal clearance and apparent volume of distribution. Renal clearance is equal to the ratio of a drug's urinary excretion rate ($\mathrm{d}U/\mathrm{d}t$) to its plasma concentration (C), i.e. renal clearance

$$Cl = \frac{\mathrm{d}U/\mathrm{d}t}{C}. \tag{1.14}$$

However, for a drug eliminated solely by the kidney

$$\mathrm{d}U/\mathrm{d}t = K_{\text{elim}}B = K_{\text{elim}}V_{\text{d}}C, \tag{1.15}$$

where K_{elim} is the elimination rate constant of the drug, B is the amount of drug in the body, V_{d} is the apparent volume of distribution and C is the plasma drug

Table 1.5 Approximate elimination half-life values (h) of a number of drugs

Drug	Half-life	Drug	Half-life	Drug	Half-life	Drug	Half-life
Suxamethonium	<0.5 h	Levodopa	2-3 h	Thiopentone	6-8 h	Pentobarbitone	30-40 h
Tubocurarine		Methyldopa		Theophylline		Pimozide	
Aminosalicylic acid	0.5-1 h	Oxprenolol		Tolbutamide		Amitriptyline	
Benzylpenicillin		Paracetamol		Vancomycin		Chlorpropamide	
Bupivacaine		Pentazocine		Bethanidine	8-10 h	Warfarin	
Cephalexin		Streptomycin		Indomethacin		Butobarbitone	40-50 h
Cephalothin		Triamterene		Oxytetracycline		Carbamazepine	
Ethacrynic acid		Alprenolol	3-4 h	Probenecid		Digoxin	
Inulin		Amidopyrine		Propantheline		Methaqualone	
Oxacillin		Aspirin		Sulphanilamide		Quinalbarbitone	
Amoxicillin	1-2 h	Azathioprine		Amantadine	10-15 h	Ethosuximide	50-60 h
Ampicillin		Chloramphenicol		Chlorpheniramine		Nortriptyline	
Bacitracin		Ephedrine		Glibenclamide		Oxyphenbutazone	
Cephaloridine		Pindolol		Imipramine		Flurazepam	60-80 h
Chlorothiazide		Terbutaline		Orphenadrine		Phenylbutazone	
Cloxacillin		Vinblastine		Phenformin		Dicoumarin	80-100 h
Cromoglycate		Acetazolamide	4-6 h	Quinidine		Phenobarbitone	
Heparin		Allopurinol		Carbenoxolone	15-20 h	Barbitone	100-120 h
Hexamethonium		Caffeine		Chlorpromazine		Chloroquine	
Lignocaine		Chlortetracycline		Clonidine		Digitoxin	
Methacillin		Hydrallazine		Griseofulvin		Mepacrine	
Oriprenaline		Metoprolol		Haloperidol	20-24 h	Reserpine	
Phenacetin		Pethidine		Ouabain			
Vincristine		Polymyxin B		Diazoxide	24-30 h		
Codeine	2-3 h	Propranolol		Lithium			
Erythromycin		Diphenhydramine	6-8 h	Pipradol			
Frusemide		Sulphacetamide					
Gentamicin		Sulphadimidine					
Insulin							

concentration. Accordingly

$$Cl = K_{\text{elim}} V_{\text{d}}. \tag{1.16}$$

Rearranging this equation and recognizing that half-life $(t_{\frac{1}{2}})$ is equal to $0.693/K_{\text{elim}}$, it follows that

$$t_{\frac{1}{2}} = \frac{0.693\,V_{\text{d}}}{Cl}. \tag{1.17}$$

Thus, a drug with a large clearance will have a short half-life unless it also has a large apparent volume of distribution.

1.5.1.5 Renal elimination in disease

Drugs which are largely cleared by renal excretion show a prolonged half-life in patients with age-dependent (newborn or elderly) or pathological impairment of renal function where renal clearance is reduced. In contrast, clearance of drugs eliminated mainly by a mechanism other than urinary elimination will be unaffected by renal impairment. Differences between anuric and normal subjects in eliminating a number of antibacterial drugs is presented in Table 1.6. When the

Table 1.6 Elimination half-lives (h) of some antibacterial drugs in patients with either normal or impaired renal function

Drug	Normals	Anurics
Benzylpenicillin	0.5	23.0
Cephalothin	0.5	12.0
Cephalexin	1.0	23.0
Erythromycin	1.4	5.5
Cephaloridine	1.7	23.0
Gentamicin	2.4	35.0
Streptomycin	2.5	70.0
Kanamycin	2.8	70.0
Lincomycin	4.7	12.0
Vancomycin	5.8	230.0
Tetracycline	8.5	87.0
Rifampicin	2.8	2.8
Doxycycline	23.0	23.0

half-life of a drug is prolonged in renal failure accumulation of the drug will occur, resulting in toxicity unless the dosage rate is reduced to correspond with the degree of decrease in elimination rate.

1.5.2 Biliary elimination

Many drugs are actively transported by the liver cells from blood into bile, which then passes into the intestine. If the drug is lipid-soluble then it may be reabsorbed by the intestine and undergo enterohepatic cycling. However, if it is highly water-soluble it will remain in the intestine and be excreted with the faeces. Biliary secretion and intestinal reabsorption may continue until metabolism, renal and faecal excretion ultimately eliminate the drug from the body. Enterohepatic cycling may thus result in greatly prolonging the lifetime of a drug in the body. Examples of drugs which undergo enterohepatic cycling include oestrogens, indomethacin, digitoxin and phenolphthalein. Formation of a glucuronide or other conjugate in the liver results in a metabolite which, although secreted into the bile, is highly polar and cannot be reabsorbed. In some instances deconjugation takes place in the intestine and the liberated parent drug is free to be reabsorbed.

Anions, cations and un-ionized molecules containing both polar and lipophilic groups may be excreted in bile provided that their molecular weights exceed about 300 daltons in rats or 400–500 daltons in man. Substances of lower molecular weight may undergo reabsorption during passage through the smaller canaliculi of the liver. Drugs which have significant biliary components to their excretion patterns include penicillin, ampicillin, rifampicin, streptomycin, tetracycline, steroid hormones, cardiac glycosides (e.g. digitoxin and digoxin), and quaternary atropine-like drugs. It is of interest that biliary excretion appears to be much more important for drug elimination in laboratory animals such as the rat and dog than in man.

1.5.3 Drugs in saliva

Some drugs appear in saliva, where they may cause a disagreeable taste or irritate the oral tissues. The transfer of a drug from blood to saliva appears to depend on its lipid solubility, pK_a and plasma protein binding. Since the average pH of saliva (6·5) is lower than the pH of plasma (7·4), it is most likely that for weak acids the concentration of drug in the saliva will be less than that of free drug in the plasma, whereas for weak bases it will be greater in saliva. Some drugs are actively transported from blood to saliva (e.g. lithium) and in these instances the concentration of drug in saliva may be two to three times higher than in plasma. In general, un-ionized drugs of high lipid solubility and low molecular weight are more likely to pass into saliva than drugs of low lipid solubility.

For several drugs the plasma-to-saliva drug concentration ratio has been shown to be relatively constant for an individual. This is the case for drugs such as tolbutamide, digoxin, lithium, theophylline, salicylate, phenacetin, phenytoin and antipyrine. This has created interest in the use of monitoring saliva drug concentrations as an indicator of plasma concentrations in pharmacokinetic-type studies.

1.5.4 Drugs in milk

Almost any drug present in a lactating mother's blood will appear in the milk, the concentration being dependent on the concentration of drug in maternal blood, its lipid solubility, degree of ionization and extent of plasma protein binding. While the amounts of most drugs in breast milk are relatively small, the immature hepatic and renal function of an infant may result in delayed metabolic inactivation and elimination of a drug, leading to unwanted effects in the infant (e.g. anthraquinone purgatives, diazepam, dichloralphenazone, phenindione, lithium). In general, drugs should be avoided whenever possible during lactation, since there is only limited information on the possible harmful effects of drugs transferred from mothers to their breast-fed infants.

1.5.5   Drugs in expired air

Volatile substances, such as the inhalation anaesthetics, nitrous oxide and halothane, diffuse readily across the lipoidal barriers of alveolar membranes and are eliminated in expired air. Once administration of the anaesthetic is ceased its concentration in the lungs drops below that in the blood. Since these drugs are extremely fat soluble, they readily and rapidly pass back into the lungs from the bloodstream and are then exhaled in expired air, thus eventually terminating anaesthesia.

1.5.6   Elimination in other secretions

Drugs and drug metabolites may appear in many other secretions although their concentrations are normally quite low. In general, un-ionized drugs of low molecular weight and high lipid solubility are more likely to cross cell membranes than drugs of low lipid solubility. One minor pathway of elimination is in gastric secretions. Owing to the great difference between the pH of plasma (7·4) and of gastric secretions (1·0–2·0) the excretion of weakly basic drug is favoured by this route. Some drugs such as mecamylamine pass readily from the blood into the stomach where they are 'trapped' as a result of ionization in the acid of the gastric secretions.

Another minor route of elimination is through the skin, in solution in sweat, or as bound material in skin cells and hair as they are sloughed off (e.g. lead). For the anti-leprosy drug diethyl dithioisophthalate, ditophal, the sweat is a major route of excretion.

FURTHER READING

1. Curry S. H. (1977) *Drug Disposition and Pharmacokinetics*, 2nd ed. Oxford, Blackwell Scientific.
2. La Du B. N., Mandel H. G. and Way E. L. (1971) *Fundamentals of Drug Metabolism and Drug Disposition*. Baltimore, Williams & Wilkins.
3. Parke D. V. (1968) *The Biochemistry of Foreign Compounds*. Oxford, Pergamon.
4. Rowland M. and Tozer T. N. (1980) *Clinical Pharmacokinetics*. Philadelphia, Lea & Febiger.
5. Williams R. T. (1959) *Detoxication Mechanisms*, 2nd ed. London, Chapman & Hall.

Chapter 2

The influence of formulation on drug availability

The influence of formulation on drug availability

2.1 INTRODUCTION

Drugs are rarely, if ever, administered to patients in an unformulated state. The vast majority of the available medicinal compounds which are potent at the milligram or microgram levels could not be presented in a form providing an accurate and reproducible dosage unless mixed with a variety of excipients and converted by controlled technological processes into medicines. Indeed, the primary skills of the pharmacist lie in the design, production and evaluation of a wide range of dosage forms, each providing an optimized delivery of drug by the selected route of administration. The aims therefore of this chapter are to outline mechanisms by which the onset, duration and magnitude of the therapeutic response can be controlled by the designer of the drug delivery system.

It has been appreciated for a considerable time that dosage forms possessing the same amount of an active compound (chemically equivalent) do not necessarily elicit the same therapeutic response. The rate at which the drug is liberated from the dosage form and the subsequent absorption, distribution, metabolism and excretion kinetics will determine the availability of the active species at the receptor site.

The majority of systemically acting drugs are administered by the oral route and therefore must traverse certain physiological barriers including one or more cell membranes. Pro-drugs may alter this part of the overall rate process (see Chapter 7) although generally, control of plasma levels is achieved by modulation of the drug liberation process from the dosage form. The critical drug activity at the receptor site is usually related to blood and other distribution fluid levels, as well as elimination rates. Other factors affecting activity include deposition sites, biotransformation processes, protein binding and the rate of appearance in the blood. Hence in order to obtain the desired response, the drug must be absorbed both in sufficient quantity and at a sufficient rate.

The term bioavailability is used to express the rate and extent of absorption from a drug delivery system into the systemic circulation. The crucial influence of rate as well as extent of absorption in considerations of bioavailability can be seen in Fig. 2.1.

The plasma levels are illustrated following a single oral administration of three chemically equivalent delivery systems (A, B and C) but with different drug liberation rates (A > B > C). Formulation A has a shorter duration of activity but results in a more rapid onset of activity compared with formulation B. The magnitude of the therapeutic response is also greater for A than B. Formulation C is therapeutically inactive, as the minimum effective plasma concentration (MEC)

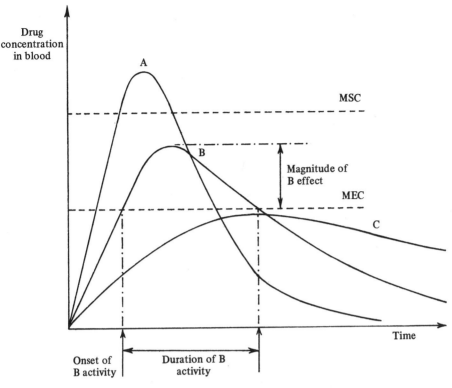

Fig. 2.1   The influence of drug release rate on the blood level–time profile following the oral administration of three chemically equivalent formulations. MSC = Maximum safe concentration; MEC = Minimum effective concentration.

is not achieved. Therefore, unless a multiple dosing regimen is to be considered, C has no clinical value.

It should also be noted that the plasma concentrations from A exceed the maximum safe concentration (MSC) and some toxic side-effects will be observed. Unless rapidity of action is of paramount importance and the toxic effects can be tolerated, B therefore becomes the formulation of choice. Generally, however, a rapid and complete absorption profile is required to eliminate variation in response due to physiological variables which include gastric emptying rate and gut motility. Bioavailability can also therefore be influenced by physiological and pathological factors, although in this chapter only the pharmaceutical or formulation aspects will be considered.

Bioavailability may be assessed by the determination of the induced clinical response which, because it often involves an element of subjective assessment, makes quantitation difficult. Measurement of drug concentrations at the receptor site is not feasible; therefore, the usual approach is the determination of plasma or blood levels as a function of time, making the implicit assumption that these concentrations correlate directly with the clinical response. Areas under the concentration–time profiles give the amount of drug absorbed and hence (if related to those of an intravenous solution of the same drug) permit an absolute bioavailability to be determined, whilst if related to a 'standard' formulation (often the original or formula of the patent holder) then the term 'relative bioavailability' is employed.

2.2 FORMULATION AIMS

Formulation aims, in the light of bioavailability considerations, are to produce a drug delivery system such that:

(i) A unit dose contains the intended quantity of drug. This is achieved by homogeneity during the manufacturing process and a suitable choice of excipients, stabilizers and manufacturing conditions to ensure both drug and product stability over the expected shelf-life.

(ii) The drug is usually totally released but always in a *controlled* manner, in order to achieve the required onset, intensity and duration of clinical response as previously outlined. Most dosage forms can be designed to give a rapid response; if however a long duration of response is required then it is easier to achieve sustained release using solid rather than liquid formulations.

2.3 PHYSICO-CHEMICAL FACTORS INFLUENCING DRUG BIOAVAILABILITY

Drug concentrations in the blood are controlled either by the rate of drug liberation from the dosage form or by the rate of absorption. In many cases it is the drug dissolution rate that is the rate-determining step in the process. Dissolution is encountered in all solid dosage forms, i.e. tablets, hard gelatin capsules as well as suspensions, whether intended for oral use or administration via the intramuscular or subcutaneous routes. If absorption is rapid, then it is almost inevitable that drug dissolution will be the rate-determining step in the overall process and hence any factor which affects the solution process will result in changes in the plasma–time profile. Hence the pharmacist has the opportunity of controlling the onset, duration and intensity of the clinical response by controlling the dissolution process.

2.3.1 Rates of solution

Dissolution of a drug from a primary particle in a non-reacting solvent can be described by the Noyes–Whitney equation

$$\mathrm{d}w/\mathrm{d}t = k(c_s - c) = DA/h(c_s - c),$$

where $\mathrm{d}w/\mathrm{d}t$ is the rate of increase of the amount of drug dissolved; k is the rate constant of dissolution; c_s the saturation solubility of the drug in the dissolution media; c the concentration of drug at time t; A is the surface area of drug undergoing dissolution; D the diffusion coefficient of the dissolved drug molecules and h, the thickness of the diffusion layer. Hence it can be readily appreciated that the dissolution rate is dependent on the diffusion of molecules through the diffusion layer of thickness h. Closer examination of this equation will demonstrate some of the mechanisms for controlling solution rate.

(1) $dw/dt \propto A$. Reduction in the particle size of the primary particle will result in an increase in surface area and hence more rapid dissolution will be achieved. A change in the shape of the plasma–time profile will result and it is possible also to increase the area under this curve, which of course means an increase in bioavailability. It is therefore possible to achieve a reduction in the time necessary for the attainment of maximum plasma levels, an increase in the intensity of the response and an increase in the percentage of the dose absorbed. Griseofulvin is one of the most widely studied drugs in relation to bioavailability, as this poorly water-soluble, antifungal drug exhibits a striking example of dissolution rate-limited absorption. Plasma levels have been shown to increase linearly with an increase in specific surface area and thus, despite the cost of micronization, griseofulvin is marketed as a preparation in this form because identical blood levels can be achieved by using half the amount of drug present in the unmicronized formulation. Micronization, however, is not the only solution to the griseofulvin bioavailability problem. For example, microcrystalline dispersions have been formed in a water-soluble solid matrix in which the dispersion state is determined by the preparative procedures, some of which result in true solid solutions. The two most widely accepted approaches are (a) crystallization of a melt, resulting from fusing of drug and carrier and (b) co-precipitation of drug and carrier from a common organic solvent. In the latter case a griseofulvin–polyvinylpyrrolidone dispersion resulted in a ten-fold increase in solution rate, compared with a micronized preparation. It should be emphasized however that griseofulvin is at the extreme end of the bioavailability spectrum! For drugs exhibiting good aqueous solubility, little is to be gained by reducing the particle size of the drug, as plasma levels are unlikely to be dissolution rate-limited. Indeed, if enzymatic or acid degradation of the drug occurs in the stomach, then increasing dissolution rates by reducing particle size can result in reduced bioavailability.

(2) $dw/dt \propto c_s$. Many drugs are weak acids or bases and hence exhibit pH-dependent solubility. It is therefore possible to increase c_s in the diffusion layer by adjustment of pH in either (a) the whole dissolution medium or (b) the microenvironment of the dissolving particle. The pH of the whole medium can be changed by the co-administration of an antacid. This raises the pH of the gastric juices and hence enhances the dissolution rate of a weak acid. However, this is rarely a practical proposition and therefore most pH adjustments are made within the very localized environment of the dissolving drug particles. Solid basic substances may be added to a weakly acidic drug, which raises the pH of the microenvironment. Probably the best known example is that of buffered aspirin products which use the basic substances sodium bicarbonate, sodium citrate or magnesium carbonate. Rather than employ another agent to alter the pH, a highly water-soluble salt of the drug can be equally, if not more, effective. The dissolving

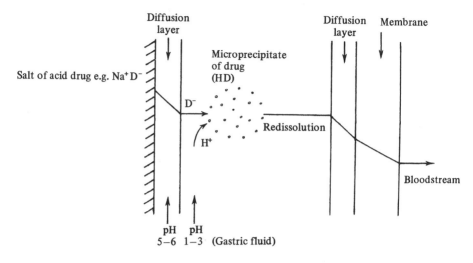

Fig. 2.2   The dissolution of a highly water-soluble salt of a weak acid in the stomach.

salt raises the pH of the gastric fluids immediately surrounding the dissolving particle. On mixing with the bulk of the gastric fluids the free acid form of the drug will be precipitated, but in a microdispersed state with a large surface area to volume ratio which will rapidly redissolve. The process is represented diagrammatically in Fig. 2.2.

Many examples exist to illustrate the importance of salt formation on bioavailability. One such example is provided by the antibiotic, novobiocin, where the bioavailability was found to decrease in the order, sodium salt > calcium salt > free acid. The dissolution rate of weak bases can be similarly changed by salt formation; however, dissolution rate-limited absorption is less important for bases than acids. This is because little absorption occurs in the stomach where the bases are ionized; most of the drug being absorbed post gastric emptying and this delay compensates any benefits accruing from more rapid solution rates. However, basic drugs are often administered as salts, e.g. phenothiazines and tetracyclines, to ensure that gastric emptying, and not dissolution, will be the rate-limiting factor in the absorption process.

A large number of drugs exhibit polymorphism, that is exist in more than one crystalline form. Polymorphs exhibit different physical properties including solubility, although only one polymorph will be stable at any given temperature and pressure. Others may exist in a metastable condition, reverting to the stable form at rates which may permit their use in drug delivery systems. The most desirable property of the metastable forms is their inherently higher solubility rates which arise from the lower crystal lattice energies.

Amorphous or non-crystalline drugs are always more soluble than the corresponding crystalline form because of the lower energy requirements in transference of a molecule from the solid to the solution phase. Crystalline novobiocin dissolves slowly *in vitro* compared with the amorphous form, kinetics which correlate well with bioavailability data. Amorphous chloramphenicol stearate is hydrolysed in the gastrointestinal tract to yield the absorbable acid, whilst the crystalline form is of such low solubility that insufficient is hydrolysed to give effective plasma levels.

Solvates are formed by some drugs; when the solvent is water, the hydrates dissolve more slowly in aqueous solutions than the anhydrous forms, e.g. caffeine and glutethimide. For ampicillin, greater bioavailability has been shown for the higher energy form anhydrate than the trihydrate, which illustrates the dependence of solubility and dissolution rates on the free energy of the molecules within the crystal lattice. Conversely, organic solvates such as alkanoates dissolve more rapidly in aqueous solvents than the desolvated forms.

2.3.2 Complexation

Increased solubility or protection against degradation may be achieved by complex formation between the drug and a suitable agent. Complexes may also arise unintentionally as a result of drug interaction with an excipient or with substances occurring in the body. Complex formation is a reversible process and the effect on bioavailability is often dependent on the magnitude of the association constant. As most complexes are non-absorbable, dissociation must therefore precede absorption.

The formation of lipid-soluble ion-pairs between a drug ion and an organic ion of opposite charge should result in greater drug bioavailability. Rarely have such results been achieved, presumably due to the dissociating influence of the mucosa and the poor membrane partitioning of the bulky ion-pair.

Surfactants are used in a wide range of dosage forms often to increase particle wetting, control the stability of dispersed particles, and to increase both solution rates and the equilibrium solubility by the process of solubilization. Bioavailability may however be enhanced or retarded and often exhibits surfactant concentration dependent effects. Below the critical micelle concentration (CMC), enhanced absorption may be encountered due to partition of the surfactant into the membrane, which results in increased membrane permeability. At post CMC levels, the dominant effect is the 'partitioning' of the drug into the micelle, a lower drug thermodynamic activity results and absorption is reduced. Micellar solubilization of membrane components with a loss of membrane integrity can also occur. Thus it is not easy to predict the effect of surfactants on bioavailability for, although dissolution rates will be increased by high concentrations of surfactant, the effect on the absorption phase may be complex.

2.3.3 Drug stability

Drug stability, in addition to being of paramount importance to product shelf-life, can also affect bioavailability. Some therapeutic substances are degraded by the acid conditions of the stomach or by enzymes encountered in the gastrointestinal tract. Reduced or zero therapeutic effectiveness will result. Penicillin G is an example of a drug rapidly degraded in the stomach and for which enteric coating is not a solution to the problem, as the drug is poorly absorbed from the small intestine. The semisynthetic penicillins such as ampicillin and amoxacillin show much greater acid stability. Improved bioavailability of acid-labile drugs can sometimes be achieved by reducing the rate of drug release from the dosage form.

2.4 INFLUENCE OF ROUTE OF ADMINISTRATION AND TYPE OF DOSAGE FORM

Although many routes exist for the administration of a systemically acting drug (including parenteral, rectal, vaginal, pulmonal, nasal, transdermal, etc.) by far the most popular is the oral route. Bioavailability, in addition to being dependent on the route of administration, will also be influenced by the dosage form selected. Although it is not possible to generalize completely regarding the relative drug release rates and hence bioavailabilities from different dosage forms, Table 2.1

Table 2.1 The ranking of dosage forms for oral administration with respect to the rate of drug release

Increasing release rates and bioavailablilty ↑	Aqueous solutions
	Emulsions
	Soft gelatin capsules
	Suspensions
	Powders
	Granules
	Hard gelatin capsules
	Tablets
	Coated tablets

attempts to provide guidelines. It is however possible, for example, to produce a tablet with bioavailability equivalent to an aqueous solution!

Aqueous solutions are rarely used due to solubility, stability, taste and non-unit dosing problems. The use of oils as drug carriers either as an emulsion, in which homogeneity and flavour masking are important, or in a soft gelatin capsule, provide efficient oral dosage forms. The release of the oil from the soft gelatin capsule shell is rapid but the surface area of the oil/water interface is lower than in an emulsion and hence partitioning of the drug is slower. Suspensions are suited to drugs of low solubility and high stability. Although a large surface area is provided, a dissolution stage nevertheless exists. On proceeding along the sequence from powders to hard gelatin capsules to tablets (*see* Table 2.1), the particles become more compacted and hence the deaggregation/dissolution phase becomes longer (*see* Fig. 2.3).

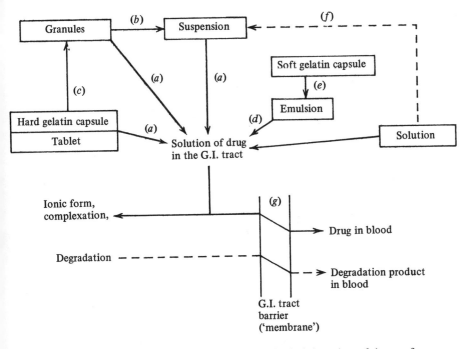

Fig. 2.3 Summary of the processes following oral administration of dosage forms. Processes: (a) dissolution; (b) deaggregation; (c) disintegration; (d) partitioning; (e) dispersion; (f) precipitation; (g) absorption.

2.5 FORMULATION FACTORS

It should by now be appreciated that, by design, it is possible to formulate a potent, well-absorbed drug in such a manner that it is essentially non-absorbable. Hence the pharmacist with his unique skills in designing drug delivery systems can significantly influence the therapeutic efficacy of a drug. In most cases, the formulator can only influence bioavailability if the drug release phase is the rate-controlling step in the overall process.

2.5.1 Solutions

As the drug is in a form readily available for absorption, few problems should exist. However, if the drug is a weak acid or a cosolvent is employed, then precipitation of the drug in the stomach may take place. Rapid redissolution of these 'micro-precipitates' normally occurs. Aqueous solutions will require the addition of a suitable selection of colours and flavours to minimize patient non-compliance, and preservatives and perhaps buffers to optimize stability. Such factors would be elucidated in preformulation studies.

2.5.2 Emulsions

The use of oral emulsions is on the decline. Most oils are unpalatable and an emulsion is an inherently unstable system. The choice of carrier oil dictates the extent and rate of drug partitioning between the oil and water. Emulsifying agents are either a mixture of surfactants or a polymer. Polymers may also be present to control the rheological properties of the emulsion and achieve an acceptable rate of creaming. The effect of surfactants on bioavailability has been previously discussed. Polymers can form non-absorbable complexes with drugs and an increase in viscosity brought about by 'thickening agents' can delay gastric emptying which in turn may affect absorption. Viscosity effects, however, are not likely to be encountered with small dose volumes (5–10 ml).

2.5.3 Soft gelatin capsules

After rupture of the glycero-gelatin shell, a crude emulsion is formed when the oil containing the drug is dispersed in the aqueous contents of the gastrointestinal tract. Oils are not always used to fill soft gelatin capsules, indeed occasionally water-miscible compounds such as polyethylene glycol 400 are used as vehicles. Soft gelatin capsules are a convenient unit dosage form generally exhibiting good bioavailability.

2.5.4 Suspensions

A high surface area of the dispersed particles ensures that the dissolution process begins immediately the administered dose is diluted with the fluids of the gastrointestinal tract. Most pharmaceutical suspensions may be described as coarse, that is they have particles in the size range 1–50 µm. Colloidal dispersions are expensive to produce and the theoretically faster solution rates arising from increased surface area are often offset by the spontaneous aggregation of the particles due to the possession of high surface energy. Particles > 50 µm result in poor suspensions with rapid sedimentation, slower solution rates and poor reproducibility of the unit dose. In order to achieve desirable settling rates and ease of redispersion of the resulting sediments, controlled flocculation of the suspension is necessary. This is normally achieved by the use of surfactant or polymers, both of which may significantly influence drug bioavailability for reasons previously discussed. Polymers are also used, as with emulsions, as thickening agents to achieve the desired bulk rheological properties. On storage, the particle size distribution of suspensions may change with the growth of large particles at the expense of small. Hence solution properties and bioavailability may well be altered on storage.

2.5.5 Hard gelatin capsules

It might be assumed that powders distributed into loosely packed beds within a rapidly dissolving hard gelatin capsule would not provide bioavailability problems.

However, in practice, this is not true. One of the classic bioavailability cases in the pharmaceutical literature arose when the primary excipient in phenytoin capsules, calcium sulphate dihydrate, was substituted (by the manufacturing company in Australia) by lactose. Minor adjustments were also made to the magnesium silicate and magnesium stearate levels. The overall effect was that previously stabilized epileptic patients suddenly developed the symptoms associated with phenytoin overdose. It is now generally accepted that the calcium ions form a poorly absorbable complex with phenytoin.

Another study demonstrated the reduced bioavailability of tetracycline from capsules in which calcium sulphate and dicalcium phosphate were used as fillers. The calcium–tetracycline complex formed in such formulations is poorly absorbed from the gastrointestinal tract.

The choice and quantity of lubricant employed can greatly influence bioavailability. Even with a water-soluble drug it is possible to vary the drug release patterns from rapid and complete to slow and incomplete. With hydrophobic drugs, the problems can be even more acute. Hence, hydrophilic diluents should be employed to aid the permeation of aqueous fluids throughout the powder mass, reduce particle clumping and hence increase solution rates.

2.5.6 Tablets

For economic reasons as well as for the convenience of the patient, the compressed tablet is the most widely used dosage form. However, by virtue of the relatively high compression forces used in tablet manufacture, together with the inevitable need of a range of excipients (including fillers, disintegrants, lubricants, glidants and binders), tabletting of drugs can give rise to serious bioavailability problems. As was seen in Fig. 2.3, the active ingredient is released from the tablet by the processes of disintegration, deaggregation and dissolution; the latter occurring, however, at all stages in the overall liberation process. The rate-limiting step is normally dissolution, although by the use of insufficient or an inappropriate type of disintegrant, disintegration may become the all-important rate-limiting step. Division of the disintegrant between the granule interior and the intragranular void spaces can accelerate the disintegration process. Several interdependent factors determine disintegration rates, including concentration and type of drug, the nature of diluent, binder and disintegrant as well as the compaction force. High compression forces will often result in the retardation of disintegration due to reduced fluid penetration and extensive interparticulate bonding. Soluble drugs and excipients may lead to a decrease in disintegration due to the local formation of viscous solutions.

The effect of hydrophobic lubricants is similar to that observed for capsules. The method by which the lubricant is incorporated, as well as the efficiency of mixing, have also been shown to influence drug dissolution rate from tablets.

When the excipient–drug ratio is increased, thus increasing tablet size, solution rates of poorly water-soluble drugs also increase.

2.5.7   Coated tablets

The application of an outer coat to a tablet presents a further barrier between the fluids of the gastrointestinal tract and the drug particles and one which is the first to be dissolved/ruptured prior to the fluid penetration of the tablet mass. Film coats are usually thin and readily soluble and hence would be expected to have but a negligible effect on bioavailability. The more traditional sugar coat is similarly water-soluble.

Enteric coatings can give rise to considerable variations in drug plasma levels due primarily to variation in stomach residence times, which, for non-disintegrating tablets, can vary between 1·5 and 6 hours. As a single enteric coated tablet or capsule empties from the stomach in an all or none manner, better control of the plasma concentration–time profile is obtained by the use of individually enteric-coated granules either packed into a capsule or compressed into a rapidly disintegrating tablet.

2.6   SUSTAINED RELEASE DOSAGE FORMS

Fig. 2.4 illustrates the differences between three distinct drug release profiles achieved by the use of (A) the usual single dose preparation, (B) a sustained release preparation and (C) a prolonged release preparation. Sustained release products are rarely achieved in practice although in many respects they represent an ideal delivery system. Initially a loading dose is rapidly released from the sustained action delivery system to provide the necessary blood levels to elicit the desired pharmacological response. The remaining fraction of the dose (maintenance dose) is then released from the preparation at rates which ensure the maintenance of a constant blood level. Prolonged action delivery systems merely

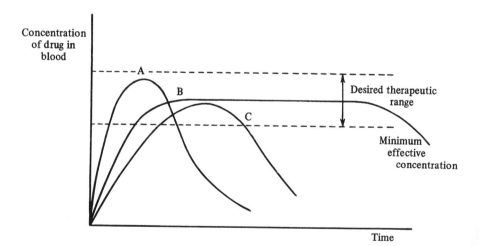

Fig. 2.4   The difference between sustained and prolonged release dosage forms as illustrated by the blood concentration–time profiles.

extend the duration of the pharmacological response compared with the usual single dose preparation. Not all drugs are suitable candidates for prolonged action medication as (*a*) the drug must be absorbed efficiently over a substantial portion of the gastrointestinal tract (*b*) the drug must possess a reasonably short biological half-life and (*c*) the size of the prolonged action dosage form must not be too large for ease of swallowing, i.e. the drug must be effective at a 'reasonable' dose level.

Prolongation of action may be achieved by a variety of techniques which include various encapsulation procedures, dispersion in hydrophobic vehicles or porous polymer materials, binding of drug to macromolecules or polymers and the formation of drug–carrier complexes.

2.7   BIOEQUIVALENCE

There are many instances reported in the pharmaceutical literature of chemically equivalent products which have been shown to be bioinequivalent. Any change in a formulation can potentially change the bioavailability. Even with identical formulae, changes in the many process variables can occur in the production of a generic product undertaken by different manufacturers giving rise to bioinequivalent products. In a granulation process, for example, the nature, quantity and method of addition of the granulating fluid; the drying process; the ageing and storage conditions of the granules prior to tabletting; can all influence the drug release characteristics of the final product. The choice of granulating agent can lead to differences in tablet hardness upon storage, which of course in turn will lead to prolonged disintegration and dissolution times. However, some drugs are known to provide greater bioinequivalence problems than others. The Food and Drug Administration (U.S.A.), in response to this situation, published a list of 115 drug substances for which *in vitro* or *in vivo* bioequivalence data are required.

When a patient is being successfully treated or stabilized on a branded product, it is therefore undesirable to change to a chemically equivalent product from an alternative manufacturer unless bioequivalence has been proven. Economic pressures advocating change of product should be resisted – at least until bioequivalence data are presented.

FURTHER READING

General
1. Blanchard J., Sawchuk R. J. and Brodie B. B. (ed.) (1979) *Principles and Perspectives in Drug Bioavailability*. Basel, S. Karger.
2. Notari R. E. (ed.) (1975) *Biopharmaceutics and Pharmacokinetics: An Introduction*, 2nd ed. New York, Dekker.

Sustained release
3. Robinson J. R. (ed.) (1978) *Sustained and Controlled Release Drug Delivery Systems*. New York, Dekker.

Chapter 3

Molecular size, shape and ionization in drug action

Molecular size, shape and ionization in drug action

3.1 INTRODUCTION

The size and shape of a molecule can be a significant feature in its biological action. Some types of activity are dependent on a flat structure whilst other types of activity require a bulky three-dimensional molecule. Such structural features enable important groups, essential for activity, to be suitably orientated in space so that drug–receptor interaction takes place.

The receptor with which a drug interacts may be visualized as a relatively small region of a macromolecule such as an enzyme, a polypeptide or a nucleic acid present in the living cell. The conformation of the macromolecule enables specific regions to be spatially orientated so that interaction may occur with complementary groupings on the drug molecule thereby initiating a biological response. The identity of the target molecule and the ultimate interaction mechanism at the cellular level are known only for a few drugs. Some of these will be described later.

3.1.1 Factors involved in drug–receptor binding

The forces involved in binding a small molecule (drug, metabolite or substrate) to a macromolecule (receptor, or enzymic active site) are manyfold:

3.1.1.1 *Electrostatic interaction*

Electrostatic interaction may occur between drug and receptor and involves the following sources of binding:

(*a*) *Ionic*   Many drugs are bases whose ionization may be expressed as

$$BH^+ \rightleftharpoons B + H^+.$$

An acidic ionization constant is usually employed so that the ionization of both bases and acids may be recorded on the same scale

$$K_a = [B][H^+]/[BH^+].$$

The small and inconvenient values obtained for these constants are overcome by employing their negative logarithms, $-\log K_a$, expressed as pK_a values. The relationship between pK_a, pH and ionization may be derived from the above equilibrium expression and formulated as the Henderson equation

$$pK_a = pH + \log[BH^+]/[B].$$

This may be further transposed to a form which enables the percentage ionization of the base to be calculated at a particular pH

$$\% \text{ ionized} = 100/1 + \text{antilog} (\text{pH} - pK_a).$$

Several basic drugs are appreciably ionized at physiological pH and are thus capable of interacting with anionic regions, such as ionized carboxyl and phosphate groups, of a macromolecular structure.

(b) Ion–dipole/dipole–dipole Differences in electronegativity between carbon and other atoms such as oxygen and nitrogen lead to an unsymmetrical distribution of electrons, giving rise to bond dipoles. These are capable of forming weak bonds with regions of high or low electron density, such as ions or other dipoles. Dipolar functions such as carbonyl, ester, amide and ether are often located in drugs, metabolites and biological macromolecules.

3.1.1.2 Hydrogen bonding

The high concentration of positive charge on a uniquely small atomic volume enables hydrogen to act as a 'bond' between two electronegative atoms, provided that the three atoms can assume a linear orientation, e.g. —O—H- - -N—, —O—H- - -O. Hydrogen bond formation is important both in drug–receptor interactions and in maintaining the structure of macromolecules such as proteins and DNA.

3.1.1.3 van der Waals' forces

These arise from the fact that molecules possess energy leading to internal vibrations. These vibrations set up dipoles in constituent atoms which induce dipoles in neighbouring atoms of other molecules. This process causes a net attraction which is distance-specific, being significant only when parts of the molecules concerned are in close proximity.

van der Waals' forces between atoms increase with increasing atomic weight, being negligible for hydrogen atoms but having a strength of about 2 kJ mol^{-1} between atoms of atomic weight 12–16 (e.g. C, O, N) such as are involved in drug–receptor interactions. When two molecules are able to fit sufficiently close together, enabling many atoms in both molecules to make contact (e.g. two phenyl rings), strong binding (20 kJ mol^{-1}) comparable with ionic forces between cation and anion can be attained.

3.1.1.4 Hydrophobic binding

The contribution of this type of receptor binding has been increasingly recognized over the years. The majority of peptide structures constituting receptor macromolecules have a high proportion of amino acid residues with non-polar side chains such as the isopropyl group of valine, the secondary and isobutyl groups of leucines and the benzyl group of phenylalanine.

When a drug is present in the aqueous phase, in the vicinity of a receptor, its hydrocarbon framework disturbs the degree of randomness of the water molecules. Since water molecules cannot solvate non-polar hydrocarbon structures, they will associate by hydrogen bonding to form quasi-crystalline clusters or 'ice-bergs'. This localized increase in the ordered structure of water would result in a loss of entropy, acccompaned by an increase in the free energy of the system. Thus, a driving force operates to reject the hydrocarbon region of the drug from the aqueous phase so that binding to a similar hydrocarbon chain on the receptor is facilitated. The consequential reduction in the overall hydrophobic area exposed to water results in a decrease in the structured component of water, with a regain in entropy and decrease in the free energy of the system.

The contribution of a single —CH_2— group to the strength of hydrophobic binding, although quite small ($3\cdot4\,kJ\,mol^{-1}$), becomes considerable when a large number of such interactions occur.

3.1.2 Optical isomerism and biological activity

The complementarity required between receptor and drug molecule may extend to distinguishing between enantiomorphic forms of a compound. Thus, *penicillium glaucum* has long been known to selectively oxidize (+)-lactic, (+)-mandelic and (−)-glyceric acids rather than their enantiomorphic forms. Further, the broncho-dilating effect of (−)-isopropylnoradrenaline (isoprenaline) is 800 times more potent than that of its (+)-isomer, whilst the (+)-form of acetyl-β-methylcholine is 200 times as effective in promoting intestinal tone than its (−)-form.

Something of the nature of a receptor may be learnt from such observations, provided that the absolute configuration of the active isomer can be elucidated. Fischer had earlier assigned relative configurations by advocating the use of plane projection diagrams. Thus, the two optical isomers of lactic acid **(3.1)** may be distinguished as follows:

(3.1)   (3.2)

The atoms to the right and left (—H and —OH) are attached to the central carbon by bonds which project towards the reader, whilst the bonds attaching the —CH_3 and —COOH groups project below the plane of the paper **(3.2)**. However, prior to modern techniques of X-ray crystallography, there was no means of telling which of the two structures represented the (+)- and (−)-enantiomorphs, respectively. Nevertheless, their relative configurations may be correlated with arbitrarily assigned configurations for (+)- or (−)-glyceraldehyde, nominated as D and L respectively. This kind of correlation requires a particular enantiomorph to be chemically related, via a series of reactions precluding racemization, to either D(+)- or L(−)-glyceraldehyde. Thus, (−)-lactic acid has been shown to have the D configuration (3.3) and is designated as D(−).

$$
\begin{array}{ccc}
\text{CHO} & \text{CHO} & \text{COOH} \\
\text{H}-\!\!\!-\text{OH} & \text{HO}-\!\!\!-\text{H} & \text{H}-\!\!\!-\text{OH} \\
\text{CH}_2\text{OH} & \text{CH}_2\text{OH} & \text{Me}
\end{array}
$$

D(+)-glyceraldehyde   L(−)-glyceraldehyde   (3.3)

In 1951, X-ray crystallography revealed the absolute configuration of salts of (+)-tartaric acid which had been previously related to L(−)-glyceraldehyde. It was also shown that D(+)-glyceraldehyde had the configuration previously arbitrarily assigned to it. This enabled the absolute configuration of molecules, whose stereochemistry had been established by the glyceraldehyde system, to be ascertained. Thus, (+)-glucose, (−)-deoxyribose and (−)-fructose, having the terminal configuration of D(+)-glyceraldehyde, are related to the D- series. Proteins are formed exclusively from amino acids of the L- series and are related to L(−)-serine (3.4).

$$
\begin{array}{cc}
\text{COOH} & \text{COOH} \\
\text{H}_2\text{N}-\!\!\!-\text{H} & \text{H}-\!\!\!-\text{OH} \\
\text{CH}_2\text{OH} & \text{C}_6\text{H}_5
\end{array}
$$

(3.4)   (3.5)

Naturally occurring laevorotatory (−)-adrenaline and (−)-noradrenaline have been related by degradation studies to D(−)-mandelic acid (3.5). The increased pressor activity of D(−)-adrenaline over L(+)-adrenaline has been attributed to the ability of the former to establish a three-point contact with its receptor involving (*a*) the basic group, (*b*) the benzene ring with its two phenolic groups and (*c*) the alcoholic hydroxyl group. L(+)-adrenaline can only attain a two-point contact with relevant complementary groups (A, B and C) on the receptor (*see* Fig. 3.1).

The use of the D-, L- convention in assigning absolute configurations has some disadvantages. The degradative or synthetic steps involved in converting one compound to another may induce racemization, resulting in incorrect assignment of configuration. A further difficulty arises when there is more than one centre of asymmetry in the molecule. Thus, (−)-ephedrine (3.6) is sterically related to D-mandelic acid (3.5) and L-alanine (3.7). In order to overcome these difficulties Cahn, Ingold and Prelog evolved their Sequence Rule. This requires the four substituents around each chiral centre to be considered in order of descending atomic number of the connecting atoms – a, b, c, d. The asymmetric centre is then viewed from the side opposite the substituent with the lowest priority, d. If the sequence of the remaining three substituents, in descending order of priority,

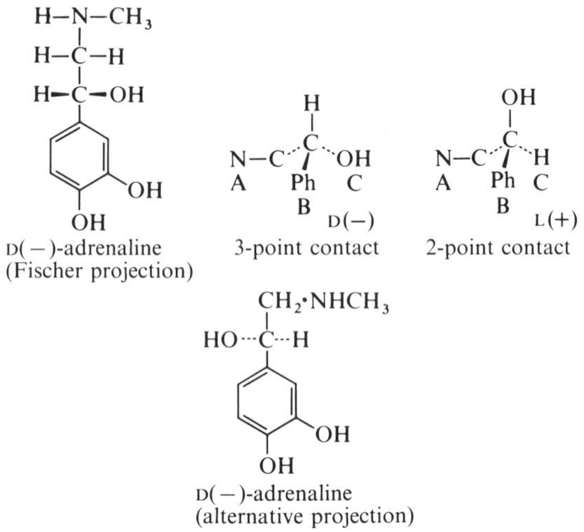

$$H-N-CH_3$$
$$H-C-H$$
$$H-C-OH$$

D(−)-adrenaline
(Fischer projection)

N−C $\overset{H}{\underset{Ph}{\overset{C}{\diagup}}}$ OH
A   Ph   C
B   D(−)
3-point contact

N−C $\overset{OH}{\underset{Ph}{\overset{C}{\diagup}}}$ H
A   Ph   C
B   L(+)
2-point contact

$$CH_2 \cdot NHCH_3$$
$$HO \cdots C \cdots H$$

D(−)-adrenaline
(alternative projection)

Fig. 3.1   Stereoselective binding to receptor.

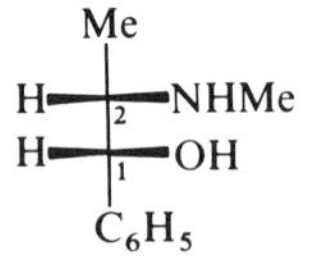

Me

H━━NHMe
    2
H━━OH
    1
C_6H_5

(3.6)

COOH

H_2N━━H

Me

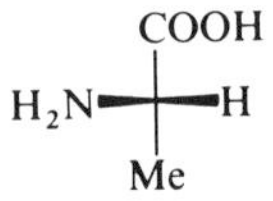

(3.7)

appears clockwise then the configuration is designated as R (rectus). Conversely if the substitutents, in descending order of priority, appear anticlockwise in sequence the configuration is referred to as S (sinister). Where the connecting atoms of two

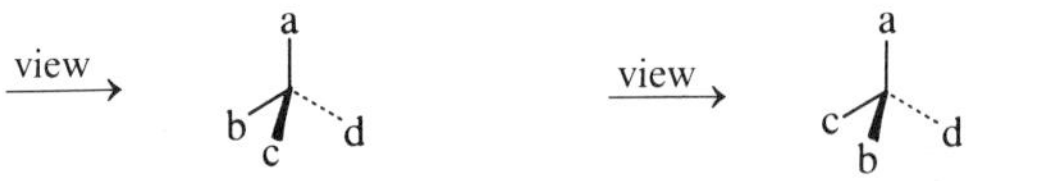

$\xrightarrow{\text{view}}$ S-configuration

$\xrightarrow{\text{view}}$ R-configuration

or more substitutents are identical, priority is given to the substituent whose second atom has the highest atomic number. Thus, L(−)-alanine (3.7) has an S-configuration, D(−)-adrenaline (Fig. 3.1) is R and (−)-ephedrine (3.6) is 1R, 2S.

The remaining part of this chapter illustrates the importance of steric factors in the biological activity of several groups of drugs and in some instances indicates how such considerations have revealed the nature of some receptor targets.

3.2   OPIATE ANALGESICS

3.2.1   Development

Once the major alkaloidal component of opium (morphine) had been isolated, the elucidation of its structure became possible. This was achieved by Gulland and

Robinson in 1925. Subsequently, this led to the development of a large number of derivatives of morphine, both semisynthetic and synthetic, with the aim of separating the analgesic effects from the undesirable effects of respiratory depression, constipation, nausea and dependence liability. Such a trail of events has been repeated in the elaboration of many types of drugs. Thus, a natural product is found to possess properties of medicinal benefit, the active principle is extracted and its chemical structure elucidated. Synthetic analogues are then developed in order to seek improved therapeutic effects.

Semisynthetic derivatives of morphine (3.8a) include codeine (3.8b) and pholcodine (3.8c) which are mild analgesics and cough sedatives, free from respiratory depression and much less addictive. Diacetylmorphine (heroin) (3.8d) has fewer side effects (e.g. constipation and nausea) than morphine so that dependence is more readily acquired. Dihydromorphine (3.8e) and dihydrocodeine (3.8f) are employed in the relief of mild to moderate pain.

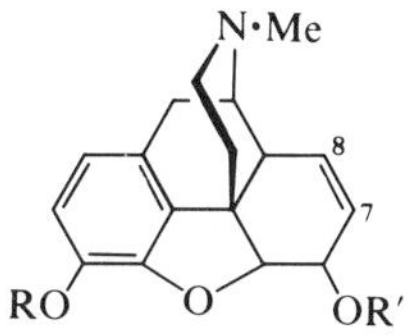

(a) R = R′ = H
(b) R = Me, R′ = H
(c) R = O—N·CH$_2$·CH$_2$·, R′ = H
(d) R = R′ = MeCO·
(e) R = R′ = H; 7,8—dihydro
(f) R = Me, R′ = H; 7,8—dihydro

(3.8)

Synthetic analogues such as pethidine, meperidine (3.9) and methadone (3.10), representing 'fragments' of the morphine molecule, indicate that a simplified analogue of the natural product retains activity. Dextropropoxyphene (3.11) has

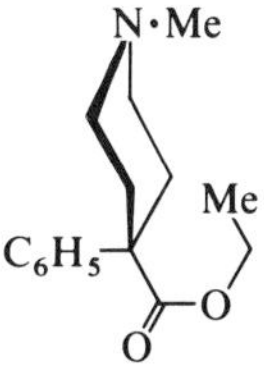

(3.9) 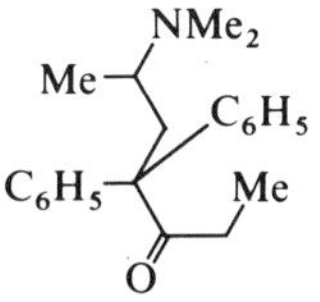   (3.10) 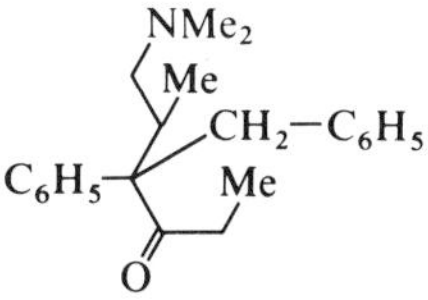   (3.11)

been widely used, in conjunction with paracetamol, but is less potent than methadone and has some side-effects, e.g. dizziness, in common with morphine.

The morphinans (3.12) and benzomorphans (3.13) are synthetic analogues which more closely resemble morphine. Phenazocine (3.13a) is a particularly potent derivative.

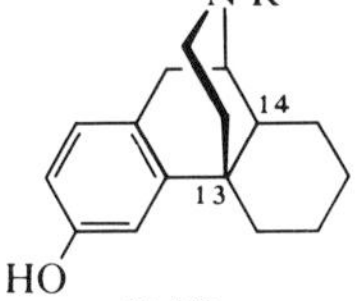

(a) R = Me, levorphanol
(b) R = CH$_2$—CH=CH$_2$, levallorphan

(3.12)

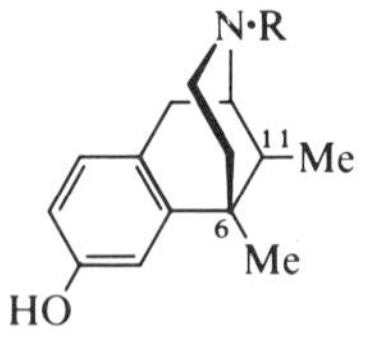

(a) R = $CH_2 \cdot CH_2 \cdot C_6H_5$
(b) R = $CH_2 \cdot CH = CMe_2$

(3.13)

3.2.2 Morphine antagonists

Morphine antagonists are obtained by replacing the *N*-methyl group by *N*-allyl. *N*-allyl normorphine (nalorphine) and levallorphan (**3.12b**) antagonize most of the effects of a previously administered narcotic. Hypotension, respiratory depression and nausea are considerably reduced whilst, in a drug addict, abstinence symptoms appear. In addition to antagonizing the undesirable effect of morphine, nalorphine also has a weak, though effective, analgesic property in man. Unfortunately, psychotomimetic phenomena (hallucinations) precluded its clinical use as an analgesic free from unwanted side-effects. Nevertheless, this proved to be an important discovery for the development of opiates with decreased dependence liability. A subsequent search for analgesics with both agonist and antagonist effects (this apparent contradiction in activity will be discussed later) resulted in the discovery, in 1967, of pentazocine (**3.13b**) which proved a moderately effective analgesic. Its prolonged use could, however, still lead to dependence.

Naloxone (**3.14a**) is an example of a pure narcotic antagonist: it abolishes respiratory depression, nausea, hypotension *and* analgesia. It does not relieve pain and has no potential for addiction. The observation that naloxone is almost totally free from side-effects led to the synthesis of related compounds. Thus, nalbuphine (**3.14b**) and naltrexone (**3.14c**) were prepared and found to possess good analgesic

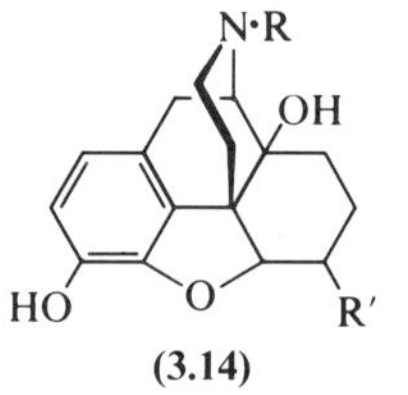

(a) R = $CH_2 - CH = CH_2$, R' = =O
(b) R = $CH_2 -$◁, R' = OH
(c) R = $CH_2 -$◁, R' = =O

(3.14)

activity with low abuse potential. Further variations in structure led to butorphanol (**3.15**) which proved more potent than morphine and phenazocine. It is an extremely safe drug, free from respiratory depression and psychotomimetic

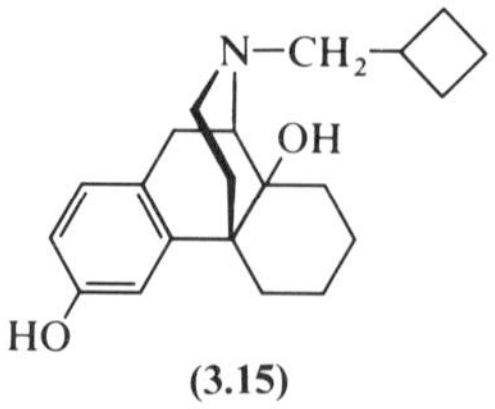

(3.15)

effects. Only in habitual narcotic users does it produce discomfort, inducing abstinence symptoms attributed to its antagonist action. Butorphanol represents some considerable progress towards the ideal non-addictive powerful analgesic. It is effective both orally and by injection.

Another recent derivative with similar properties to butorphanol owes its origin to the early work of D. K. Bentley and Robert Robinson at Oxford on the chemistry of thebaine which occurs in opium. Those workers felt that a more rigid and more elaborate structure, built up from thebaine, could yield a greater separation of analgesic and addictive properties by interacting in a more selective manner with a pain-blocking centre. A large number of Diels–Alder products of thebaine were prepared with the subsequent discovery of buprenorphine (*see* Fig. 3.2) in 1978. Early clinical studies reveal it to be as effective as diamorphine, diacetylmorphine, in relieving the pain of myocardial infarction.

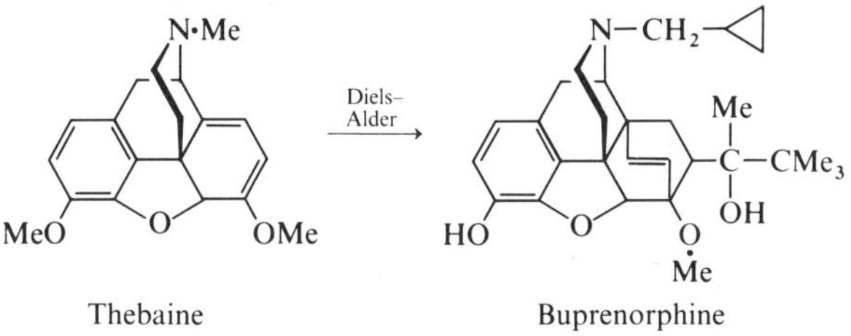

Fig. 3.2   Diels–Alder product from thebaine.

3.2.3   Stereochemical studies

One of the significant features in the action of opiates is that whenever an analgesically active compound is resolved into its enantiomeric forms, one isomer has greater activity than the other. Morphine occurs naturally as its (−)-isomer, whose relative configurations at five asymmetric centres ((**3.16**) positions 5, 6, 9, 13,

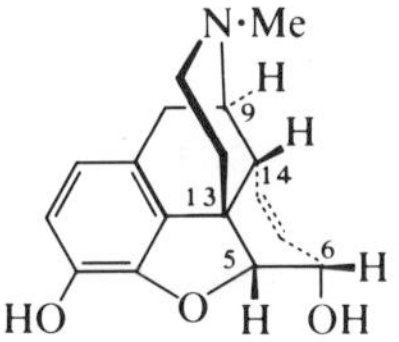

(3.16)

14) have been established by X-ray crystallographic studies. The absolute configurations of C-13 and C-14 have been confirmed by degradation of the related thebaine to a dicarboxylic acid of known stereochemistry (D-series). The absolute geometry (5R, 6S, 9R, 13S, 14R) of the entire molecule (essentially two planes at right-angles) has been solved by optical rotatory dispersion (ORD) measurements. L(+)-morphine, synthesized from sinomenine, has inverted configurations at C-9 and C-13 and is analgesically inactive.

Within the morphinan series, antagonism of (−)-levorphanol **(3.12a)** is shown only by the *N*-allyl derivative in its (−)-form, levallorphan **(3.12b)**. More significantly, chemical and ORD studies have revealed that the absolute configurations of the C-13 and C-14 centres are identical in (−)-levorphanol, (−)-levallorphan, (−)-morphine and (−)-nalorphine. Further, within the benzomorphan series **(3.13)**, two pairs of enantiomers are possible since the methyl groups can be *cis*- (α) or *trans*- (β) orientated. Activity resides mainly in the (−)-form of each and these have been shown by ORD and Cotton effects to possess absolute configurations at C-6 and C-11, identical with C-13 and C-14 centres of (−)-morphine and (−)-levorphanol.

The acyclic analogue methadone **(3.10)** has one chiral centre which has been shown, by chemical and ORD studies, to have an R configuration **(3.17)**

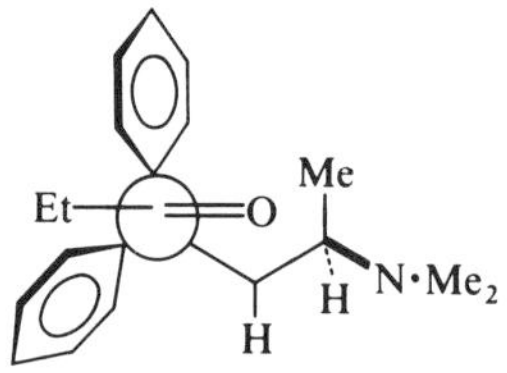

(3.17)

comparable with C-9 of (−)-morphine. Further, spectroscopic and X-ray crystallographic studies on methadone and pethidine **(3.9)** have indicated similar conformations, although the latter does not possess a chiral centre.

These considerations have led to the concept of analgesic (opiate) receptors which must be stereospecific. Beckett, in 1960, proposed that the structural features of the receptor macromolecule were so orientated that they were complementary only to isomers of optimal configuration which, as a result of binding, produced either an agonist or an antagonist response. A proposed model (*see* Fig. 3.3) suggests that the active configuration of morphine, a morphinan or benzomorphan allows the piperidine ring to be accommodated in a fold or depression in the receptor biopolymer so that

    (i) the ionized basic group may bind electrostatically with a complementary anionic group (e.g. carboxyl or phosphate anion) and

    (ii) the flat benzene ring may bind by van der Waals' forces to a complementary flat chemical structure on the biopolymer.

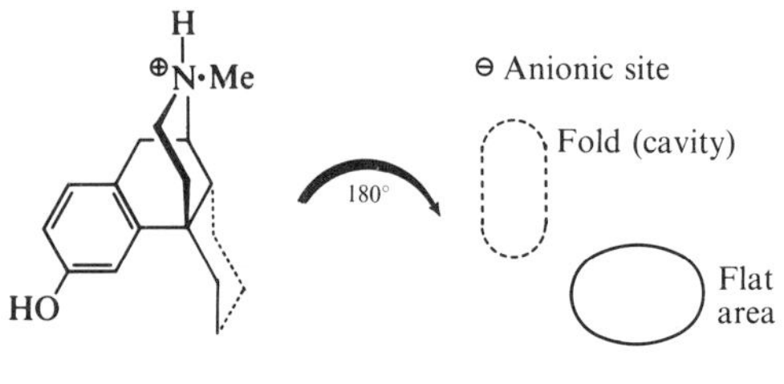

Fig. 3.3   Analgesic receptor.

In more recent years this 'rigid' receptor theory has been questioned, as it does not take into account the total profile of opioid activity. Studies involving X-ray diffraction, nuclear magnetic resonance and ORD have suggested that the steric relationship of the phenyl ring is unimportant to activity. Thus, it is axially orientated to the piperidine ring in morphine, morphinans and benzomorphans but equatorially disposed in pethidine. The mixed agonist–antagonist activity of more recent opioids also requires further rationalization. In order to overcome some of these difficulties Snyder, in 1976, proposed a flexible receptor. This hypothesis was based on the recognized ability of enzymes and other macro-molecules to undergo conformational changes on interaction with small molecules such as substrates or drugs. It was suggested that the opiate receptor could exist in either an 'antagonist' or an 'agonist' conformation, dependent on sodium ion concentration. Sodium ions increased the number of sites available for antagonists, thus reversing a conformation favoured by agonists. The uniquely high potency of opiates possessing an additional phenyl ring (such as phenazocine **(3.13a)** and fentanyl **(5.33)** was thought to be due to binding at an additional lipophilic site on the receptor, thus stabilizing an agonist conformation. (Molecular models indicated that the additional phenyl ring in these compounds had a common conformational location.) Other analgesics with additional phenyl rings, e.g. methadone, are less potent since the two rings cannot assume the necessary critical orientation in relationship to the basic nitrogen. The moderate potency of morphine was associated with the lack of a second phenyl ring.

Analogues possessing N-allyl, N-cyclopropyl or the N-cyclobutyl group are believed, by Snyder, to interact with a specific antagonist binding site on the receptor. The presence of a 14-hydroxy group, as in naloxone **(3.14a)**, reduces the free rotation of the piperidyl N-allyl group fixing it in an equatorial, rather than axial, position which is regarded as optimal for interacting with an antagonist binding site. Subsequent binding to this site stabilizes the receptor in the antagonist conformation. Other drugs lacking a 14-OH group, such as nalorphine and pentazocine **(3.13b)**, possess mixed agonist–antagonist activity since the N-allyl or related groups may adopt equatorial or axial positions.

Another theory, of increasing acceptance, postulates the existence of three receptor populations (μ, κ and σ) to account for the total profile of opioid activity. Morphine is seen as the prototype, at μ receptors producing analgesia, euphoria and physical dependence. At κ receptors, nalorphine is the prototype producing analgesia. Dysphoria and hallucinations of the nalorphine type are produced at σ receptors. Thus nalorphine possesses agonist effects at κ and σ receptors and antagonist effects at μ receptors.

In recent years, a further receptor population, δ, for binding endogenous opioid peptides has been recognized.

3.2.4 Enkephalins and endorphins

Biochemical evidence for the existence of opiate receptors was first obtained in 1973. Use of the highly potent tritium (^{3}H) labelled etorphine demonstrated that areas of the brain such as the periaqueductal grey (PAG) contained a high proportion of receptors. Later, electrical stimulation of the PAG was shown to produce powerful analgesia which was reversed by naloxone. This suggested the existence of a powerful endogenous opioid-like neurological process. Since none of the recognized neurotransmitter substances (such as acetylcholine, catecholamines, γ-aminobutyric acid and 5-hydroxytryptamine) appears to interact with opiate receptors, it was suggested in 1975 that the endogenous ligand might be a peptide. Two such pentapeptides, characterized as met-enkephalin, H-tyr-gly-gly-phe-met-OH, and leu-enkephalin, H-tyr-gly-gly-phe-leu-OH, were isolated from pig-brain in a 3 : 1 ratio. Their opioid activity was first demonstrated in isolated tissues (guinea-pig ileum and mouse vas deferens) known to have opiate receptors. Enkephalins, like morphine, blocked the electrically induced contraction of these tissues and this blockade could be reversed by naloxone. Further, the stereospecific nature of met-enkephalin was shown by replacement of natural L-tyrosine by D-tyrosine, which resulted in an inactive peptide. Snyder has suggested that met-enkephalin may interact with the opioid receptor by utilization of the phenyl rings of tyrosine and phenylalanine.

The precursor of met-enkephalin is believed to be the pituitary hormone – β-lipoprotein – which contains 91 amino acid residues. From pig hypothalamus, three fragments containing the met-enkephalin sequence have been isolated. These are called endorphins and possess powerful opioid activity. β-Endorphin, containing 31 amino acid units, is 20–30 times as potent as morphine.

The in vivo analgesic activity of enkephalins is difficult to demonstrate, after introducing directly into the brain, since rapid hydrolysis of the tyr–gly peptide link by amidase enzymes occurs. Resistance, to aminopeptidases of the brain and plasma and inactivating enzymes of the kidney and liver, has been achieved by substitution of the unnatural D-alanine for glycine at position 2 together with alkylation of the phenylalanine residue. Such modifications are believed to effect conformational changes in the molecule so that enzymic cleavage is resisted. Further modifications to the methionine residue have resulted in a pentapeptide (FK 33-824) which is considerably more potent than morphine and capable of

$$\text{H—tyr—(D-ala)—gly—(Me·phe)—NH—CH·CH}_2\text{OH}$$
$$\text{CH}_2\text{·CH}_2\text{·S} \diagup^{\text{O}}_{\diagdown\text{Me}}$$

(FK 33-824)

penetrating the CNS after injection. Its effectiveness in combating post-operative pain is, however, offset by side-effects which include face flushes and heaviness of muscles.

Evidence is mounting to suggest that the endogenous opioid pentapeptides function as neurotransmitters in the CNS. This requires a specific inactivation mechanism to operate in the vicinity of opioid receptors to turn off rapidly the enkephalin signal. Recently (1978) a high affinity peptidase enzyme has been identified as capable of splitting the pentapeptide to a tripeptide (tyr-gly-gly) following enkephalinergic transmission.

3.3   ACETYLCHOLINE AT THE MUSCARINIC RECEPTOR

Acetylcholine is a neurotransmitter at several sites including (*a*) the neuromuscular junction of nerve and voluntary muscle, (*b*) the junction of parasympathetic nerves and involuntary muscle and (*c*) the ganglionic synapses of both parasympathetic and sympathetic nerve fibres. The arrival of a nerve action potential at the junction of parasympathetic nerves and involuntary muscle liberates acetylcholine from storage depots. This combines with receptors on the muscle end plates, which results in contraction of the muscle. The binding of acetylcholine induces a change in the macromolecular conformation of the membrane, resulting in increased permeability to K^+, Na^+ and Ca^{2+} during the short excitation period. Such changes are manifested in miotic activity and gastrointestinal peristaltic activity. Lachrymal and salivary secretions are also increased.

3.3.1   Stereochemical studies

Considerable progress has been made in the isolation of acetylcholine receptors but, up to the present, most of the knowledge has been indirectly derived from structure–activity studies involving agonists. At the junction of parasympathetic nerves with involuntary muscles, the action of acetylcholine is mimicked by the alkaloid (+)-muscarine. The muscarinic receptor for acetylcholine is highly stereospecific. Thus, of the eight possible stereoisomeric forms of muscarine, only the natural L(+)-isomer **(3.18)** is active. The 5-CH_3 and 2-$CH_2N^+(CH_3)_3$ groups are *cis* to one another and *trans* orientated to the 4-OH group. L(+)-muscarine possesses the 2S, 4R, 5S configuration.

Synthetic acetyl-β-methylcholine, methacholine, in its L(+)-form **(3.19)**, is at

(3.18)   (3.19)

least 200 times more active than its D(−)-enantiomer. L(+)-methacholine also has an S configuration, thus establishing the orientation of groups to be identical with C-2 of L(+)-muscarine.

There has been much speculation about the favoured conformation of acetylcholine at the muscarinic receptor. It has been suggested that L(+)-muscarine is a rigid analogue of acetylcholine and that the corresponding groups of acetylcholine assume a similar conformation at the receptor. Evidence for this comes from X-ray diffraction studies on crystalline acetylcholine bromide and L(+)-muscarine. Thus, in acetylcholine, the cationic head and acyloxy function have a gauche arrangement **(3.20)** which also characterizes the $^+$NCCO sequence in (+)-muscarine. However, it must be recognized that the conformation of acetylcholine could be very different in aqueous media where it would not be constrained by similar neighbouring molecules. Further examination of the conformation by ^{1}H nuclear magnetic resonance (n.m.r.) studies in deuterium oxide solution, employing vicinal coupling constants, provided support for the X-ray studies.

In the above compounds, binding of the quaternary head to a receptor anion is facilitated by the partial delocalization of the positive charge on the nitrogen over three methyl carbon atoms (3.21).

(3.20)   (3.21)

3.3.2 Antagonists at the muscarinic receptor

At the postganglionic nerve endings with involuntary muscles, the effect of acetylcholine is antagonized by an alkaloid extracted from the roots and leaves of *Atropa belladona*, Deadly nightshade. As a result of this antagonism, atropine produces both a mydriatic and antispasmodic (spasmolytic) effect accompanied by a reduction in the secretion of gastric acid. Secretions in the mouth, trachea and bronchioles are also decreased which explains why atropine may be administered before general anaesthesia.

Although not a quaternary ammonium compound, the high pK_a of the basic group indicates that atropine is largely ionized at physiological pH. This facilitates binding to an anionic site on the muscarinic receptor, whilst the presence of a phenyl ring and several methylene groups ensures that the molecule dissociates from the receptor, at a lesser rate than acetylcholine.

Activity resides only in the naturally occurring (−)-form of the alkaloid. Stereochemical investigations have established the asymmetric centre to be S-orientated and the 3-acyloxy function to be *trans* to the basic group (3.22a). The piperidine ring is assigned the chair conformation as a result of ^{1}H n.m.r. studies on atropine base in deuterio-chloroform and the hydrochloride salt in deuterium oxide. Some investigators have drawn attention to the similarity in distances separating the $>\overset{+}{N}$ H Me group, the ether oxygen and carbonyl oxygen of atropine when these are compared with analogous groups in the preferred conformation of acetylcholine.

3.3.3 Synthetic analogues of atropine

Some unpleasant side-effects (mental confusion, hallucinations) have been reported with atropine, due to penetration of the CNS. This has been overcome by quaternization of the basic group to give analogues which cannot penetrate the lipophilic blood–brain barrier. Thus, atropine methonitrate is used in a spray solution for the relief of bronchial asthma. Similar analogues which have been developed more recently are the ethobromide and isopropobromide.

Further development of synthetic analogues revealed that the intact tropane ring was not required for activity. This recognizes that the strength (pK_a) of a tertiary basic group in a heterocyclic ring compares with a similar group bound by open alkyl chains. Hence, simplification of the structure followed similar lines of development as those used in the elaboration of synthetic local anaesthetics related to cocaine **(3.22b)**. Thus, the structure of the natural product was simplified with

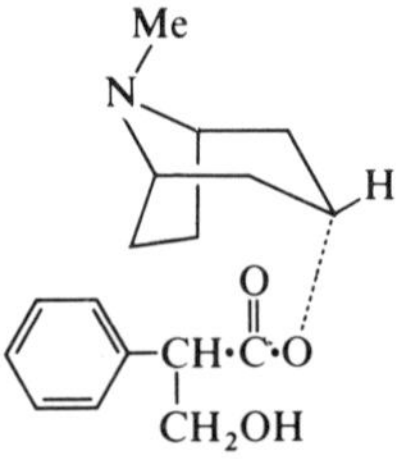

(3.22a) 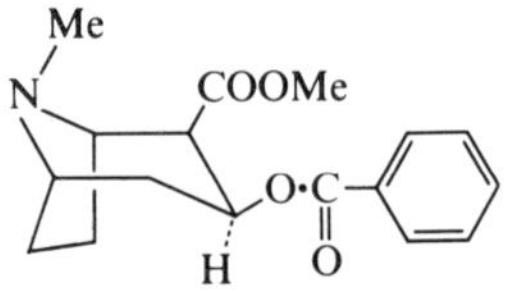   (3.22b)

the preparation of dialkylaminoalkyl esters of the type: $R_2N \cdot CH_2 \cdot CH_2 \cdot O \cdot CO \cdot R$. This led to the availability of drugs which were more specific in action than atropine, in that they were either mainly mydriatic or mainly spasmolytic. The latter drugs give relief in treating peptic ulcer. Gastric hydrochloric acid and pepsin secretion is also decreased since acetylcholine has a direct effect on the secretory cells.

It was soon realized that an esterifying acid residue of greater bulk was important for spasmolytic activity. One of the earlier successes, trasentin **(3.23a)**, produced considerable local anaesthetic effects. Further improvements came only very slowly by (*a*) increasing the size of the ester group still further, (*b*) quaternizing the basic group or (*c*) restoring a basic ring structure. Examples include propantheline **(3.23b)**, oxyphenonium **(3.23c)**. oxyphencyclimine **(3.23d)**

$$R \cdot (CH_2)_n \cdot O \cdot \overset{\text{O}}{\underset{||}{C}} \cdot R'$$

(3.23)

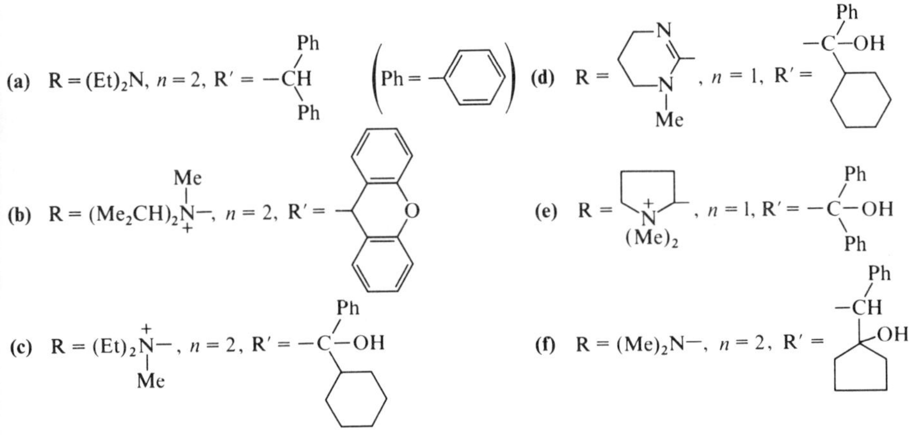

and poldine (3.23e). Other derivatives, such as cyclopentolate (3.23f), retain the mydriatic effect of atropine and are used in optometry as an alternative to atropine when an effect of shorter duration is desirable.

Atropine analogues were the first drugs to be established in the control of the symptoms of Parkinsonism. It was discovered rather empirically that anticholinergic drugs reduce the tremor and rigidity associated with this condition. Several synthetic preparations (e.g. benzhexol (3.24a), biperidine (3.24b) were developed in

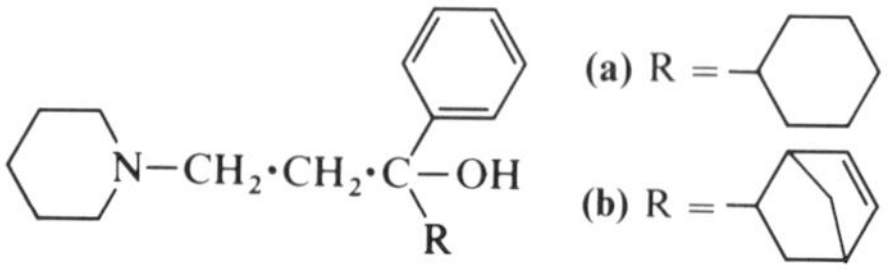

(a) R =

(b) R =

$$N-CH_2 \cdot CH_2 \cdot C-OH$$
     $$|$$
     $$R$$

(3.24)

an effort to enhance these properties. Although the mechanism of action of these drugs is obscure, activity is confined to those which pass the blood–brain barrier, i.e. tertiary amines but not quaternary ammonium compounds. There is some evidence that acetylcholine is a neurohumoural agent in the CNS, as well as peripherally, and that anticholinergics block its action.

3.4   HISTAMINE H_2-RECEPTOR ANTAGONISM

The secretion of hydrochloric acid from acid-secreting glands in the stomach is not only cholinergically mediated but also mediated by the action of histamine (3.25) on smooth muscle in the gut wall. These H_2-receptors are distinct from H_1-receptors in the nose, bronchi and skin. Antihistamines controlling the symptoms seen in allergy (see Section 5.2) block the action of histamine only at H_1-receptors.

In an attempt to elucidate the distinguishing features of these two receptors Kier, in 1968, employed molecular orbital calculations to determine the preferred conformations of the basic side chain of histamine. He concluded that there were two conformations of nearly equal preference (3.26).

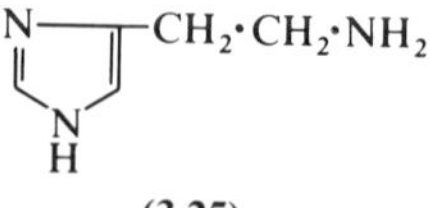

$$N-CH_2 \cdot CH_2 \cdot NH_2$$

(3.25)

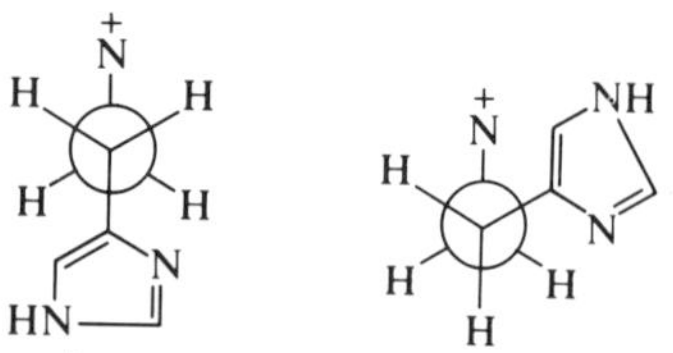

trans

cis (gauche)

(3.26)

Since the distance separating the two basic centres in the trans form, compared with a similar inter-nitrogen dimension in the potent antihistamine triprolidine (3.49), it was concluded that histamine adopted the trans conformation at H_1-receptors. However, this assertion may be unlikely since more recent ^{1}H n.m.r.

studies indicate that the proportion of *trans* isomer increases with decreasing pH, such as prevails in the gastric environment, due to repulsive forces arising in the di-cation. This would suggest that histamine invokes a H_2-receptor response in the *trans*, rather than the *cis*, conformation.

Whilst antagonists of histamine at H_1-receptors have been available for many years, antagonism of H_2-receptor activity is of much more recent origin. This discovery has enabled the clinical control of gastric secretion and the subsequent healing of gastric ulcers without recourse to surgery. In 1972, workers at the Smith, Kline and French laboratories characterized two histamine receptors by showing that, whilst H_1-receptors were selectively stimulated by 2-methylhistamine, H_2-receptors were responsive to 5-methylhistamine. This action at H_2-receptors was later shown to be selectively antagonized by burimamide (3.27).

$$N \underset{\underset{H}{N}}{\overset{}{\rule{0pt}{0pt}}} - CH_2 \cdot CH_2 \cdot CH_2 \cdot CH_2 \cdot NH \cdot \underset{\underset{S}{\|}}{C} \cdot NHMe$$

(3.27)

3.4.1 Ionization studies

The poor absorption characteristics and low activity of burimamide were subsequently improved by modifying its structure so as to more closely resemble histamine. This was accomplished as a result of ionization studies which recognized that, in burimamide, the imidazole ring (pK_a 7·25) was 40% ionized at physiological pH whilst in histamine it was only 4·0% ionized (pK_a 6·0). These respective pK_a values are a consequence of the alkyl side chain in burimamide possessing an electron-repelling ($+I$) inductive effect whilst the highly ionized basic side-chain (pK_a 9·8) of histamine (3.25) has an electron-withdrawing ($-I$) influence on the imidazole nucleus. These two contrasting inductive effects of the side-chains will also result in differing tautomeric structures, A and B, for the un-ionized forms of the respective imidazole rings. Thus, in histamine, the electron-withdrawing $-CH_2 \cdot CH_2 \cdot \overset{+}{N}H_3$ group facilitates dissociation of a proton from the nearest NH-3 group (3.28) whilst in burimamide the electron-repelling alkyl group consolidates binding of this proton so that dissociation occurs from the other NH-1 group (3.29).

$$N \underset{\underset{H}{N}}{\overset{}{\rule{0pt}{0pt}}} - CH_2 \cdot CH_2 \cdot NH_2 \quad \overset{2H^+}{\longrightarrow} \quad \overset{3}{H}N \underset{\underset{H}{\overset{+}{2}N_1}}{\overset{}{\rule{0pt}{0pt}}} - CH_2 \cdot CH_2 \cdot \overset{+}{N}H_3 \quad \rightleftharpoons \quad \overset{3}{N} \underset{\underset{H}{N_1}}{\overset{}{\rule{0pt}{0pt}}} - CH_2 \cdot CH_2 \cdot \overset{+}{N}H_3 + H^+$$

(3.28) ($-I$)   A

$$N \underset{\underset{H}{N}}{\overset{}{\rule{0pt}{0pt}}} - (CH_2)_4 - NHCSNHMe \quad \overset{H^+}{\longrightarrow} \quad \overset{3}{H}N \underset{\underset{H}{\overset{+}{2}N_1}}{\overset{}{\rule{0pt}{0pt}}} - (CH_2)_4 - \quad \rightleftharpoons \quad HN \underset{\underset{}{N}}{\overset{}{\rule{0pt}{0pt}}} - (CH_2)_4 - + H^+$$

(3.29) (+I)   B

In an attempt to increase the proportion of tautomer A, so as to more closely resemble the predominating imidazole species of histamine at physiological pH, the electron-repelling ($+I$) side-chain of burimamide was converted to an electron-withdrawing ($-I$) group by incorporating an electronegative sulphur atom at a position near to the ring. To compensate for the lesser ($-I$) effect, compared with $-CH_2\cdot CH_2\cdot \overset{+}{N}H_3$, an electron-releasing ($+I$) methyl group was substituted at position 5 of the imidazole ring so as to consolidate the proton on the adjacent NH group. This produced metiamide (**3.30a**) which possessed greater potency, selectivity and absorption (cf. burimamide) after oral administration. Unfortunately, side-effects involving agranulocytosis, previously noted in drugs containing a thiourea unit, marred the activity of metiamide. This led to its replacement by a guanidino, $-NH\cdot C(=NH)\cdot NH-$, structure since H_2-receptor antagonism had been previously observed in certain guanidine derivatives. The undesirably high degree of ionization of the guanidine residue caused absorption problems which were subsequently corrected by substitution of an electron-withdrawing ($-I$) cyanide group to give the cyanoguanidino derivative, cimetidine (**3.30b**). This

$$^3N\underset{\underset{H}{N}}{\overset{\qquad\qquad}{\bigg|}}\!\!\!-CH_2\cdot S\cdot CH_2\cdot CH_2-R$$
$$Me \quad ^5$$

(**3.30**)

(a) R = $-NH\cdot \underset{\parallel}{C}\cdot NHMe$
       S

(b) R = $-NH\cdot \underset{\parallel}{C}\cdot NHMe$
       N·CN

proved twice as active as metiamide in inhibiting gastric secretion and, since its introduction in 1976, over 11 000 000 patients, world-wide, have benefited from its use.

Doubts concerning the safety of cimetidine appeared early in 1979 when it was reported that patients subjected to long term treatment showed signs of stomach cancer. This could arise as a result of lowered gastric activity increasing the production of nitrosamine-producing bacteria. It has been suggested that, due to its chemical structure, cimetidine could undergo conversion to a nitrosoderivative bearing a close similarity to *N*-methyl-*N'*-nitro-*N*-nitrosoguanidine (known to be carcinogenic). Although there is no proof that cimetidine is carcinogenic, it has been recommended that the drug be used in long term therapy only with patients in whom the recurrence of an ulcer might necessitate surgery (*see also* ranitidine, p. 155).

3.4.2 Conformational studies

Studies reported in 1980 on the conformation of cimetidine may have a biological significance. It was shown that metiamide and cimetidine in the crystalline state adopt a 10-membered ring conformation in which a basic imidazole nitrogen, N-3 (**3.30a, b**), is intramolecularly hydrogen bonded to the NH furthest from the imidazole ring. Burimamide, which does not contain sulphur in the side-chain, adopts an open chain configuration. Infra-red studies on solutions of metiamide and cimetidine indicate that metiamide adopts an 8-membered ring conformation in which the basic imidazole nitrogen, N-3, is hydrogen bonded to the NH nearest to the ring. Cimetidine, as a result of intramolecular hydrogen bonding, adopts either an 8-membered or a 10-membered cyclic configuration in solution.

The compact, folded, ring structure will be more lipophilic than the extended form and, consequently, will influence membrane permeability and distribution of the antagonist. It is also possible that the folded conformation is the preferred structure for interaction at the H_2-receptor site. Replacement of a side-chain —CH_2— by —S— could, therefore, have the added bonus of enabling the intramolecular hydrogen bonded ring formation necessary for biological activity to occur.

3.5 ACTIVITY RELATED TO INTERCALATION

3.5.1 Antibacterial aminoacridines

Paul Ehrlich, a pioneer in chemotherapy, discovered trypanocidal activity in the dye, acridine yellow (3.31a) and, as a result of earlier work on organic arsenicals, assumed that the methyl groups did not assist activity. Consequently, he requested his associates to synthesize (3.31b), which was presented as the quaternary

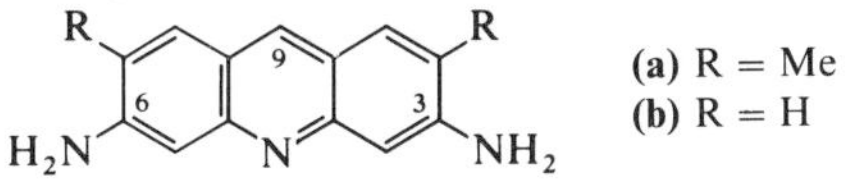

(a) R = Me
(b) R = H

(3.31)

methochloride, acriflavine. It was with this compound that Browning, a pupil of Ehrlich, subsequently discovered antiseptic properties. Later he showed that the commercial product contained proflavine (3.31b). Both proflavine and acriflavine were extensively used for the topical treatment of wounds during the Great War of 1914–18.

Acridine itself is a planar, feebly basic molecule but when an amino group is substituted at position 3, 6 or 9 strong bases are obtained as a result of a resonance effect which delocalizes the positive charge on the cation (3.32).

Studies, by Albert in 1939, involving a considerable number of acridine derivatives and several species of bacteria, revealed that only those capable of high ionization at physiological pH were active as antibacterials. Thus, proflavine and aminacrine, 9-aminoacridine, became widely adopted as antiseptics. When the magnitude of the antibacterial effect was determined, over a restricted pH range

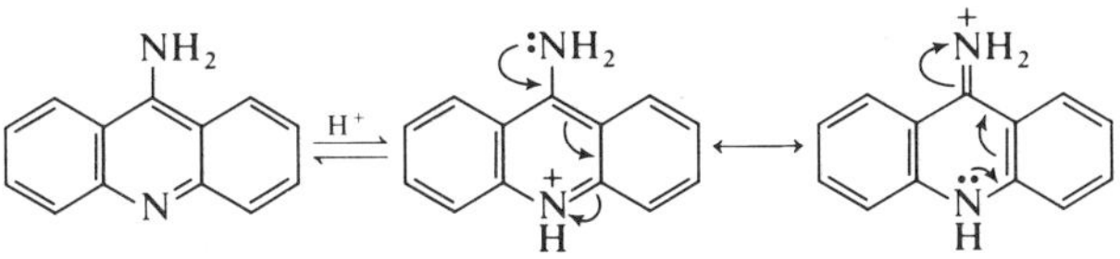

(3.32)

(5·5–8·5), where proflavine and aminacrine are fully ionized, it was found that with increasing pH a progressively decreasing concentration of aminoacridine (expressed as the cation) was required for a given bacteriostatic effect. This suggested that acridine cations competed with hydrogen ions for a vitally important anionic group in the micro-organism. This could be an acidic function which, at a higher pH, increasingly dissociates. In addition to providing the first clue to the mode of action of aminoacridines, this led to instructions recommending sodium bicarbonate irrigation of wounds prior to their treatment.

A second clue to the mode of action of aminoacridines was provided by the discovery that a critical minimum area of flatness of the molecule was essential for antibacterial activity. Thus, in a series of aminobenzoquinolines, whose structures represent a rearrangement of the rings in aminoacridine, the same relationship between ionization and antibacterial activity prevailed. However, when compounds (3.33) representing the successive removal of one or two rings from

(3.33)

aminoacridine were examined, antibacterial activity was lost even though high ionization was retained. The loss of bacteriostasis with decreasing area of flatness was further illustrated by the reduced activity of 1,2,3,4-tetrahydro-9-aminoacridine. This led to the suggestion that the large flat area facilitated binding of the aminoacridine to a complementary flat surface on a receptor. Lerman, in 1961, further elaborated this view by producing evidence for intercalation of 3,6-diaminoacridine between two layers of base pairs of the bacterial DNA – which occurs as a single chromosome attached to the cytoplasmic membrane of the cell. The flat acridine ring is believed to be held by van der Waals' forces to correspondingly flat purine (e.g. adenine) and pyrimidine (e.g. thymine) rings. Since acridine is π-electron-deficient and both adenine and thymine are π-electron-excessive, charge-transfer complex formation resulting from orbital overlap also consolidates this binding. The acridine cation, bound in this manner, will also be suitably positioned for two positively charged amino groups to ionically bind with two phosphate anions of the twin-helical DNA structure. Interaction of proflavine with DNA was shown to increase the viscosity and decrease the sedimentation coefficient of the complex in solution. These changes were attributed to the helix being stiffened and extended by the intercalated molecules. X-ray diffraction studies indicated that one molecule of aminoacridine was stacked parallel to the base pairs in a 1:3 ratio.

Acridines probably inhibit the synthesis of DNA by combining with the small amount of DNA required as 'starter' material for a DNA polymerase enzyme which builds up mononucleotides into DNA. The importance of aminoacridines in providing a pointer towards the mode of action of other drugs has by now exceeded their prominence as antibacterial agents.

3.5.2   Antimalarials

The increasing incidence of malaria presents a major problem due to the decreasing sensitivity of the parasite to existing drugs. The first synthetic antimalarials to be introduced were mepacrine (3.34) and pamaquine (3.35). Their discoveries followed the observation, by Ehrlich in 1891, that methylene blue (3.36) possessed weak antimalarial activity. Investigations were held up whilst awaiting the discovery of suitably infected laboratory test animals. When birds were found to be adequate, progress was more rapid. The simplification of mepacrine led to chloroquine (3.37).

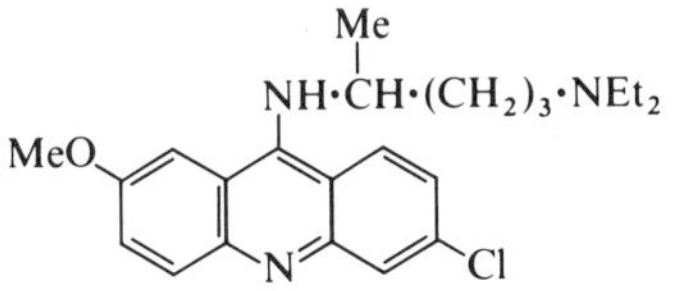

MeO

NH·CH·(CH$_2$)$_3$·NEt$_2$ / Me

Cl

(3.34)

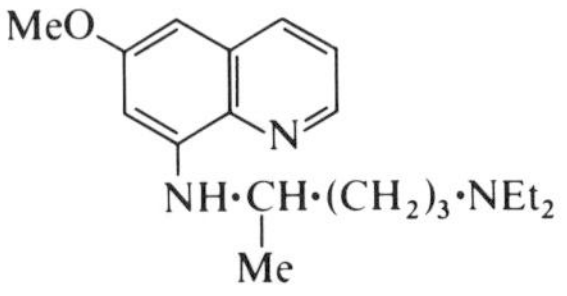

MeO

NH·CH·(CH$_2$)$_3$·NEt$_2$ / Me

(3.35)

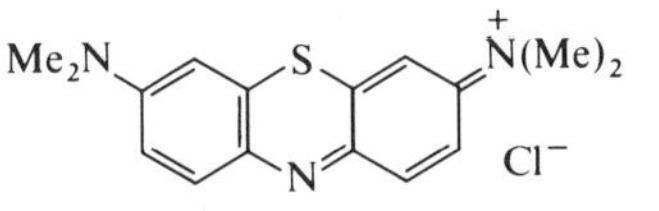

Me$_2$N — S — N(Me)$_2$$^+$

Cl$^-$

(3.36)

Me

NH·CH·(CH$_2$)$_3$·NEt$_2$

Cl

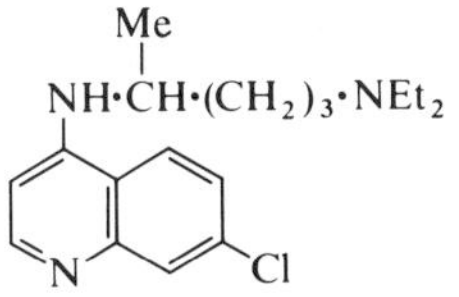

(3.37)

It has been shown, by Lerman in 1963, that both mepacrine and chloroquine became intercalated into DNA when van der Waals' forces and charge-transfer interactions stabilize the resultant complex. The two basic groups of the side-chain are highly ionized at physiological pH and are thought to bind two vertically adjacent phosphate anions on the same strand of DNA. Combination of the drug with DNA 'starter' material results in the inhibition of protozoal DNA polymerase.

The earlier mainstay in treating malaria (quinine) is, by comparison, an inefficient drug since much of the dose is oxidized in the 2-position by liver microsomes. The bulky quinuclidine ring may also interfere with binding to DNA sites. Microsomal oxidation may be overcome by insertion of a non-oxidizable substituent in the 2-position. Mefloquine (3.38) is such an example where the 2-trifluoromethyl also increases lipophilic properties essential for concentrating the

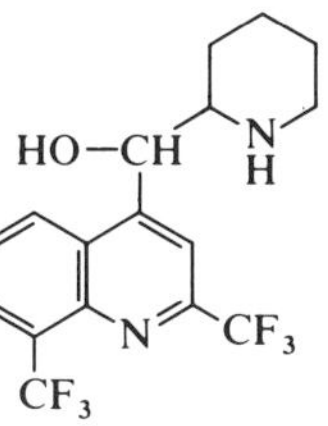

HO—CH   N / H

CF$_3$

CF$_3$

(3.38)

drug in mammalian erythrocytes (which bear the schizonts). The therapeutic importance of (3.38) lies in its activity against chloroquinine-resistant protozoal strains.

The stereochemistry of the fragment CH(OH)—CH—N has been examined in both mefloquine- and quinine-type compounds. Quinine and quinidine have configurations corresponding to R–S and S–R respectively, whereas epiquinine and epiquinidine are S–S and R–R respectively. The latter enantiomeric pair are not antimalarial since the hydroxy group and the nitrogen atom are prevented, by the bulkiness of the quinucludine moiety, from attaining the correct juxtaposition required for activity. However, when the rigid quinuclidine nucleus is substituted by the more flexible piperidine ring, all four enantiomers are found to be active. Mefloquine consists of equal parts of R–S and S–R forms. There is evidence to suggest that the bulky CF_3 groups interfere with DNA intercalation, so that further investigations are needed to explain the exceptional properties of this agent.

3.5.3 Carcinostatic antibiotics

These anticancer agents are termed antibiotics since they are derived from fungal species, usually *Streptomyces*, and have antibacterial activity. One of the first to be used for treating cancer was actinomycin D. It has been particularly useful in treating Wilm's tumour of the kidney, choriocarcinoma and testicular tumours. Actinomycin D (3.39) has an aminophenoxazine nucleus, bearing two identical

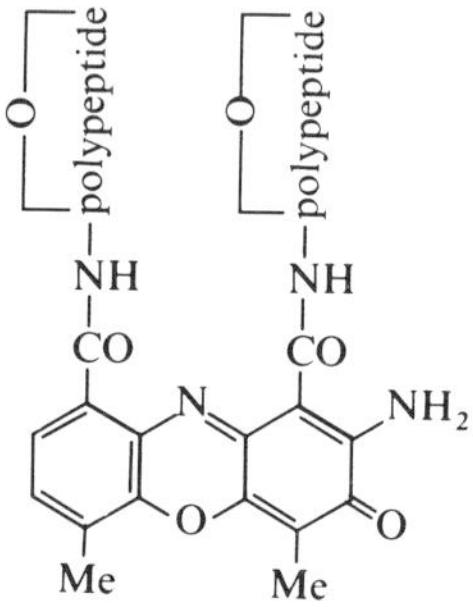

(3.39)

polypeptide side-chains consisting of threonine, D-valine, L-proline, sarcosine and, terminally, N-methylvaline. The first and last amino acids are linked by a lactone ring. It has been shown by X-ray diffraction data that the phenoxazine ring intercalates between adjacent guanine–cytosine base pairs of the DNA twin-helix. The complex is further stabilized by hydrogen bonding between a D-valyl NH group and a phosphate O atom of the DNA chain. As a result, DNA-dependent RNA synthesis is inhibited.

By far the most clinically useful of the cytotoxic antibiotics, owing their activity to intercalation with DNA, are the anthracyclines daunorubicin (3.40a) and doxorubicin (adriamycin (3.40b)). The DNA-intercalated complex is also con-

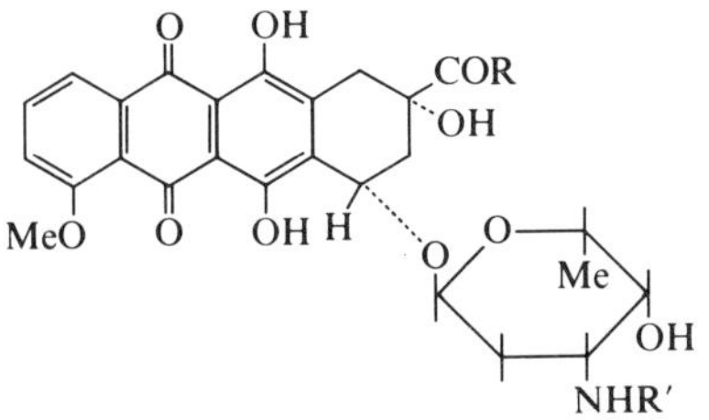

(a) R = Me
    R′ = H
(b) R = CH$_2$OH
    R′ = H
(c) R = CH$_2$O·COnBu
    R′ = COCF$_3$
(d) R = Me
    R′ = COMe

(3.40)

solidated by ionic binding of the ionized basic amino group with a phosphate anion. As a consequence DNA and RNA polymerases are inhibited.

Doxorubicin has a wider range of activity than daunorubicin since it is effective against a number of solid tumours as well as lymphomas and leukaemias. The clinical usefulness of the anthracyclines has led to the synthesis of analogues e.g. (3.40c, d), with fewer of the toxic side-effects (e.g. cardiac myopathy, bone marrow- and lung-damage) which mar the activity of the parent compounds. In a more recent derivative, the cyclohexyloxyaminopyranose moeity has been replaced by two hydroxyethylaminoethylamino side-chains (—NHCH$_2$·CH$_2$·NH·CH$_2$·CH$_2$·OH) substituted at positions 5 and 8, respectively, of a 1,4-dihydroxyanthraquinone nucleus. Molecular models have revealed that the nitrogen atom at the centre of the side-chain and the nitrogen of the aminosugar of adriamycin are superimposable. The antileukaemic activity of this compound is undergoing clinical evaluation.

3.6 TRICYCLIC PSYCHOTHERAPEUTIC DRUGS

3.6.1 Development

Dramatically useful drugs for the treatment of psychiatric disorders such as mania and schizophrenia began to be discovered in the 1950s. These constitute the major tranquillizers and antidepressants. One of the most important major tranquillizers, chlorpromazine (3.41a), was discovered as a result of a search for antihistaminic compounds based on the clinically successful phenothiazine derivative, promethazine (3.41b). The tranquillizing properties (strong sedation, state of indifference and disinterest without effecting sleep) of chlorpromazine were observed during its clinical evaluation as an antihistamine. Since its introduction in 1952, the population size in our mental institutions has been almost halved. The success of chlorpromazine resulted in another variant (3.42) of the ring skeleton being synthesized and evaluated as a tranquillizer. When compared with chlorpromazine

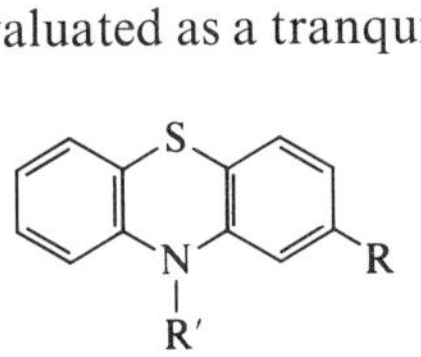

(a) R = Cl,
    R′ = CH$_2$·CH$_2$·CH$_2$·NMe$_2$
(b) R = H
    R′ = CH$_2$·CH(Me)·NMe$_2$

(3.41)

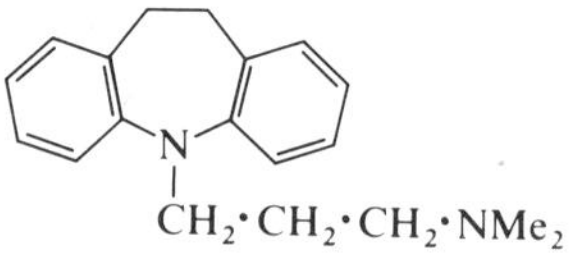

$$CH_2 \cdot CH_2 \cdot CH_2 \cdot NMe_2$$
(3.42)

for treating schizophrenia, it proved to have little effect in controlling hallucinations but was found to counteract the depressed component of the symptom
complex. The antidepressant properties of **(3.42)** were finally established by re-
evaluating the drug (later to be called imipramine) in patients who were primarily
depressed. The discovery of an animal model for depression was aided by
imipramine. It was found that the tranquillizer reserpine could induce clinical
depression and, in animals, could also invoke a pattern of observable and
reproducible pharmacological responses such as eyelid closing and hypothermia. It
was then thought that the capacity of a drug such as imipramine to reverse those
effects could indicate clinical antidepressant properties.

Many different kinds of psychotherapeutic drugs, isosterically related (*see*
Section 5.2) to these two essential frameworks (chlorpromazine and imipramine),
have by now been synthesized and introduced clinically. Thus, derivatives of
phenothiazine (e.g. chlorpromazine **(3.41a)** and thioxanthene (e.g. chlorprothixene
(3.43)) have major tranquillizing, neuroleptic activity, whilst derivatives of dibenzazepine (e.g. imipramine) and dicycloheptadiene (e.g. amitryptyline **(3.44)**)
are primarily antidepressant, thymoleptic drugs.

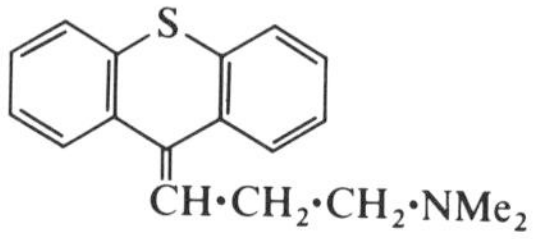

$$CH \cdot CH_2 \cdot CH_2 \cdot NMe_2$$
(3.43)

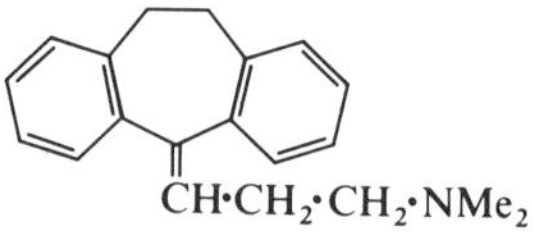

$$CH \cdot CH_2 \cdot CH_2 \cdot NMe_2$$
(3.44)

3.6.2   Steric considerations

It proved difficult, at first, to understand why apparently minor modifications in
structure produced different activity – neuroleptic or antidepressant. An attempt to
elucidate the relationship of structure to activity was developed by Wilhelm and
Kuhn in 1970. They suggested that the site of action of the molecule and its precise
pharmacological effect depended on the particular type of steric configuration
which the tricylic ring system adopted.

The shape of the tricyclic system depends on three steric parameters:

(1) The angle of flexure or bending (α). This is the angle which the planes of the
two lateral aromatic rings make when projected towards one another (*see* Fig. 3.4).
The bending angle (α) is believed to be most responsible for the pharmacological
activity. Thus, phenothiazine and thioxanthene are relatively flat molecules
($\alpha = 25°$) having mainly neuroleptic properties, whilst dibenzazepine ($\alpha = 65°$) and

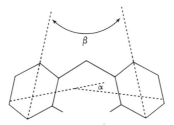

Fig. 3.4   Angles of flexure (α) and annellation (β).

dibenzocycloheptadiene ($\alpha = 55°$) are prominently bent molecules possessing mainly antidepressant activity.

(2) The angle of annellation (β). This is the extent of rotation of the two lateral aromatic rings away from a straight line or, alternatively, the angle at which the two lateral aromatic rings are attached to the central ring (*see* Fig. 3.4). This is 60° for dihydrophenanthrene, 10° for phenothiazine and thioxanthene and 40° for dibenzazepine.

(3) The angle of torsion (γ). This measures any twisting of the planes of the two lateral aromatic rings relative to one another. It is 0° for phenothiazine and thioxanthene and up to 20° when a 7-membered central ring is present.

These measurements are based on the assumption that the shape of the molecules approximate to molecular models constructed on the principle of minimal angular strain. The values are also closely in agreement with those calculated from X-ray structural analysis. Thus, relatively flat tricyclic conformations show mainly neuroleptic activity whilst skeletons which are bent ($\alpha \simeq 60°$) show mainly antidepressant activity.

The basic side-chain of the structure may also modify activity, in that shortening or branching renders the neuroleptics more sedative and hypnotic whilst antidepressants become less antidepressant and more sedative. X-ray crystallographic and electron spin resonance studies indicate that for neuroleptic action the three carbon side-chain adopts a configuration where the terminal basic group is near a benzene ring whilst in antidepressants the terminal basic group overlaps a benzene ring. Such correlations have been checked by referring to derivatives of dibenzo[b,e]bicyclo[2,2,2]octadiene which has a rigid ring structure with a precisely defined angle of flexure (60°) (*see* Fig. 3.5). Thus, benzoctamine

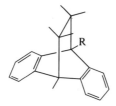

Fig. 3.5   Dibenzo[b,e]bicyclo[2,2,2]-octadiene derivatives.

(R = CH$_2$·NHCH$_3$) has a short basic side-chain at the bridgehead position so that the basic group cannot overlap a benzene ring. This does not possess anti-depressant activity. However, maprotiline (R = CH$_2$·CH$_2$·CH$_2$·NHCH$_3$) which has a longer side-chain, enabling the basic nitrogen to overlap a benzene ring, has pronounced antidepressant activity.

The view that the above rationalization of structure–action relationships provides a basis for designing new drugs is supported by the introduction of maprotiline into clinical use.

3.6.3 Other structural modifications

Although chlorpromazine is still one of the most widely used neuroleptics (prescribers have confidence in its efficacy) several structural modifications have come into clinical use. The replacement of —Cl by —CF$_3$ in ring position 2 and the modification of the basic side-chain to include a piperazine moiety is thought to enhance neuroleptic potency by increasing lipophilicity so that entry into the CNS is more readily facilitated. Fluphenazine **(3.45)** is an example of a modification

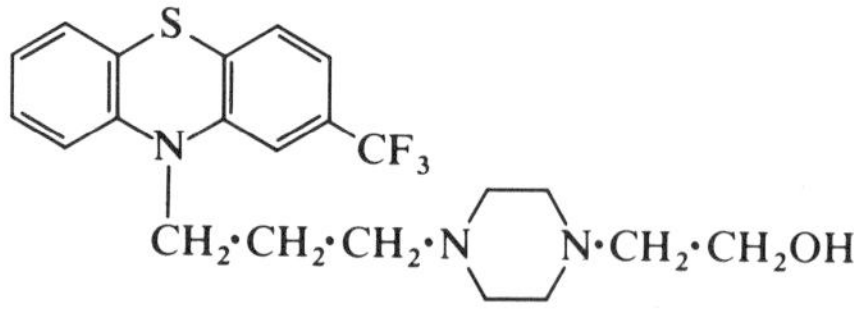

(3.45)

which has also been esterified with long-chain acids such as decanoic and heptanoic (enanthate) to give a product suitable for, once monthly, intramuscular (depot) injection in treating schizophrenia.

Similarly, piperazine side-chains have been substituted in the dibenzazepines whilst the antidepressant dibenzocylcoheptadienes have been isosterically modified (*see* Section 5.2) to novel bridged-ring ether derivatives **(3.46)** possessing powerful

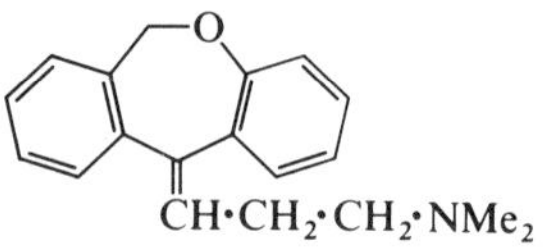

(3.46)

activity. Further modifications include the replacement of —O— by —S—, —SO—, —SO$_2$— and —NH—. The alkene linkage introduces the possibility of *cis–trans* isomerism into the structure where, in some instances, one form is more active than the other.

Novelty abounds in the search for tricyclic structures with antidepressant activity. Thus, mianserin **(3.47)** possesses a basic side-chain which has been incorporated into an additional fused ring. This has recently been clinically

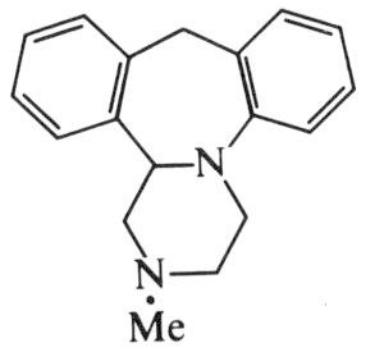

(3.47)

adopted for treating endogenous depression where it has been found to be free from the cardiotoxicity which accompanies many tricyclic antidepressants.

3.6.4   Mode of action

Phenothiazine neuroleptics appear to effect their action by blocking dopamine, 2-(3′,4′-dihydroxyphenyl)ethylamine, receptors. Schizophrenia is believed to be associated with an increased accumulation of dopamine in the striatum and other brain regions where it results in overfiring of neurones (monoamine oxidase levels are known to be low in chronic schizophrenics). Since Parkinson's disease is associated with a deficiency of dopamine, neuroleptic therapy may invoke Parkinson-like symptoms. More recent evidence points to prostaglandin (PGE_1) deficiency in schizophrenics. A low PGE_1/dopamine ratio may be due to an abnormality in the biosynthesis of the former. Direct therapy to raise the level of PGE_1 may, in future, prove clinically beneficial.

The tricyclic antidepressants appear to act by increasing the amount of transmitter amines at adrenergic neurones in the brain. Whilst monoamine oxidase inhibitors act by inhibiting the destruction of noradrenaline within nerve endings, the tricyclic agents are believed to inhibit the 'pump' which returns noradrenaline into the neurones. Thus, they increase the concentration of noradrenaline in the synaptic area.

A recently introduced tricyclic antidepressant, iprindole (3.48), in which a

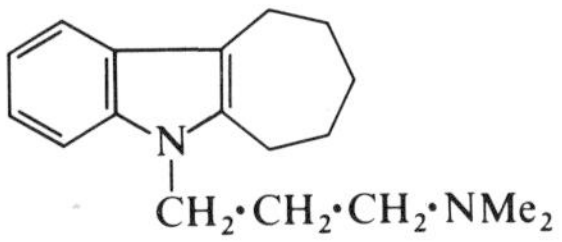

$CH_2 \cdot CH_2 \cdot CH_2 \cdot NMe_2$

(3.48)

central indole nucleus is bound by phenyl and a saturated 7-membered ring, appears to have a different mode of action. Instead of inhibiting neuronal uptake of noradrenaline it may potentiate the central actions of adrenergic amines by inhibiting their metabolism.

3.7   GEOMETRICAL ISOMERISM ABOUT AN ALKENYLIC BOND

Geometrical isomers become possible when rotation of atoms in a molecule is restricted by a double bond arising from plane-trigonal carbon atoms. Selective biological action has previously been noted (*see* p. 78) in 7-membered ring substituted dibenzocycloheptadienes, with *cis* or *trans* orientated basic side-chains. This effect is also found in the potent H_1-antihistaminic drug, triprolidine – where activity is restricted to the *cis* (H/pyrid-2-yl) isomer **(3.49)**.

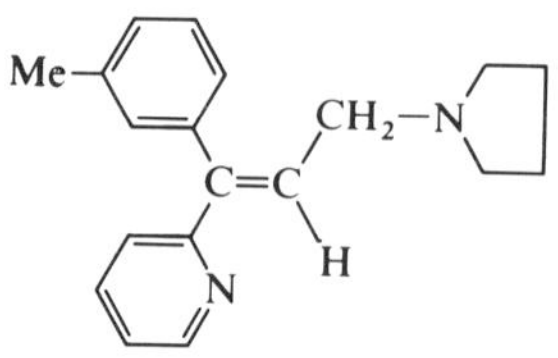

(3.49)

Another example is the synthetic analogue of oestrogen, stilboestrol, used for treating menopausal symptoms and cancer of the prostate gland in males (*see* p. 186). X-ray diffraction studies and ultra-violet absorption spectroscopy have revealed that not only is a *trans* structure associated with oestrogenic activity but that the two benzene rings are also twisted out of plane by the other alkene substituents **(3.50)**. The resultant degree of twisting imparts a thickness to the

(3.50)

molecule which compares with the dimensions of ring D and its angular methyl (C-18) group in the natural hormone, oestradiol. The distance between the two oxygen atoms (essential for activity) is also comparable in the two compounds.

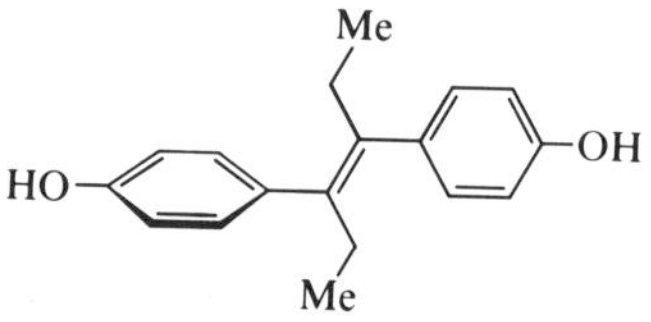

FURTHER READING

1. Albert A. (1979) *Selective Toxicity*, 6th ed. London, Chapman & Hall.
2. Stenlake J. B. (1979) *Foundations of Molecular Pharmacology*, Vol. 1, *Medicinal and Pharmaceutical Chemistry*, Vol. 2, *The Chemical Basis of Drug Action*, University of London, Athlone.
3. (*a*) Mautner H. G. (1980) Receptor theories and dose-response relationships. (*b*) Kuntz I. D. (1980) Drug–receptor geometry. (*c*) Kollman P. A. (1980) The nature of the drug–receptor bond. In Wolff M. E. (ed.) *Burger's Medicinal Chemistry*, 4th ed. Part 1. New York–London, Wiley, (*a*) pp. 271–84; (*b*) pp. 285–312; (*c*) pp. 313–30.
4. (*a*) Meienhofer J. (1980) Endogenous opioid agonists. (*b*) Hollstein U. (1980) Non-lactam antibiotics – anthracyclines and actinomycins. (*c*) Sweeney T. R. and Struke R. E. (1980) Antimalarials. (*d*) Montgomery J. A., Johnston T. P. and Fulmer Shealey Y. (1980) Drugs for neoplastic diseases – anthracyclines and actinomycins. In Wolff M. E. (ed.) *Burger's Medicinal Chemistry*, 4th ed. Part 2. New York–London, Wiley, (*a*) pp. 756–63; (*b*) pp. 181–6; 238–40; (*c*) pp. 333–414; (*d*) pp. 634–5.

5. (a) Johnson M. R. and Milne G. M. (1981) Analgetics. (b) Ganellin C. R. and Durant G. J. (1981) Histamine H-2 receptor agonists and antagonists. (c) Cannon J. G. (1981) Cholinergics. (d) Rama Sastry B. V. (1981) Anti-cholinergics: anti-spasmodic and anti-ulcer drugs. (e) Vernier V. G. (1981) Anti-Parkinsonism drugs. (f) Kaiser C. and Setler P. E. (1981) Antipsychotic drugs. (g) Kaiser C. and Setler P. E. (1981) Anti-depressant drugs. In Wolff M. E. (ed.) *Burger's Medicinal Chemistry*, 4th ed. Part 3. New York – London, Wiley, (a) pp. 699–754; (b) pp. 487–552; (c) pp. 339–60; (d) pp. 361–412; (e) pp. 413–30; (f) pp. 859–980; (g) pp. 997–1068.
6. Feinberg A. P., Creese I. and Snyder S. H. (1976) The opiate receptor: a model explaining structure–activity relationships of opiate agonists and antagonists. *Proc. Nat. Acad. Sci. U.S.A., Neurobiology*, **73**, 11, 4215–19.
7. Hughes J. (1981) Peripheral opiate receptor mechanisms. *Trends Pharmacol. Sci.* **2**, 21–4.
8. Simon E. J. (1981) Opiate receptors – some recent developments. *Trends Pharmacol. Sci.* **2**, 155–8.
9. Beddell C. R., Lowe L. A. and Wilkinson S. (1980) Endogenous opioid peptides – the enkaphalins and endorphins. In Ellis G. P. and West G. B. (ed.) *Prog. Med. Chem.*, Vol. 17. Amsterdam, Elsevier, pp. 1–39.
10. Adler M. W. (1980) Opioid peptides. *Life Sci.* **26**, 497–510.
11. Neidle S. (1979) The molecular basis for the action of some DNA-binding drugs. In Ellis G. P. and West G. B. (ed.) *Prog. Med. Chem.*, Vol. 16. Amsterdam, Elsevier, pp. 152–221.
12. Cheng C. C., Zee-Cheng R. K. Y., Narayanan V. L., Ing R. B. and Paull K. D. (1981) The collaborative development of a new family of antineoplastic drugs. *Trends Pharmacol. Sci.*, **2**, 223–4.
13. Mitchell R. C. (1980) An infra-red study of intramolecular hydrogen-bonding in histamine H_2-receptor antagonists. *J. Chem. Soc. Perkin Transact. II*, 915–18.
14. Bristol A. J. (1981) Agents for the treatment of peptic ulcer disease. In Hess H.-J. (ed.) *Annual Reports in Medicinal Chemistry*, Vol. 16. New York – London, Academic Press, pp. 83–91.
15. Wilhelm M. (1975) The chemistry of polycyclic psycho-active drugs-serendipity or systematic investigation. *Pharm. J.* **214**, 414–16.
16. Maj J. (1981) Antidepressant drugs – theories of action. *Trends Pharmacol. Sci.* **2**, 80–3.
17. (a) Antidepressants. (b) Antipsychotic agents. (c) Analgesics, endogenous opioids and opiate receptors. (d) Antineoplastic agents. (e) Antiparasitic agents. In Hess H.-J. (ed.) *Annual Reports in Medicinal Chemistry*. New York – London, Academic Press, Vol. 15, (a) pp. 1–11, (b) pp. 12–21, (c) pp. 32–40, (d) pp. 130–8, (e) pp. 120–9, and Vol. 16, (a) pp. 1–10, (b) pp. 11–20, (c) pp. 41–50, (d) pp. 137–48, (e) pp. 125–36.

Chapter 4

Design of enzyme inhibitors (antimetabolites) as drugs

Design of enzyme inhibitors (antimetabolites) as drugs

4.1 INTRODUCTION

Enzymes catalyse the reactions of their substrates by initial formation of a complex (ES) between the enzyme and substrate(s) at the active site of the enzyme. This complex then breaks down, either directly or through intermediary stages, to give the products (P) of the reaction with regeneration of the enzyme:

$$E + S \rightleftharpoons \underset{\substack{\text{enzyme–substrate} \\ \text{complex}}}{ES} \xrightarrow{k_{cat}} E + \text{products}, \qquad (4.1)$$

$$E + S \rightleftharpoons ES \xrightarrow{k_2} \underset{\substack{\text{intermediate} \\ + P_1}}{E'} \xrightarrow{k_3} E + P_2. \qquad (4.2)$$

k_{cat} is the overall rate constant for decomposition of ES into products, k_2 and k_3 are the respective rate constants for formation and breakdown of the intermediate E' (i.e. $k_{cat} = k_2\, k_3/(k_2 + k_3)$). Chemical agents, known as inhibitors, modify the ability of an enzyme to catalyse the reaction of its substrates. The term inhibitor is usually restricted to chemical agents, other modifiers of enzyme activity such as pH, ultra-violet light and heat being known as denaturizing agents.

4.1.1 Basic concept

The body contains several thousand different enzymes each catalysing a reaction of a single substrate or group of substrates. An array of enzymes is involved in a metabolic pathway, each catalysing a specific step in the pathway, i.e.

$$A \xrightarrow{E_1} B \xrightarrow{E_2} C \xrightarrow{E_3} \ \ldots \ \xrightarrow{E_n} \text{metabolite}.$$

These actions are integrated and controlled in various ways to produce a coherent pattern governed by the requirements of the cell.

There is evidence that a number of drugs in clinical use exert their action in the body by inhibiting a target-enzyme which is either normally present in mammalian tissue or has been introduced by a parasitic infection and is present in the parasite. The term, antimetabolite, is also widely used to describe an enzyme inhibitor to highlight the metabolite (substrate) whose metabolism is interrupted (antagonized) rather than the enzyme which is inhibited. Many of these drugs were not introduced into therapy on a rational basis as enzyme inhibitors/antimetabolites but were later found to exert their action in this manner.

In a clinical condition an inhibitor might be used to decrease the activity of an enzyme to decrease production of a metabolite. Inhibition of the enzyme in a pathway which governs the rate-controlling step in the series of reactions is most effective. Noradrenaline is synthesized at the nerve endings by a series of reactions from tyrosine. Many inhibitors of specific enzymes in the biosynthetic pathway have been designed with a view to decreasing the level of noradrenaline reaching the β-adrenergic receptors in the capillary vessels. This decreases the blood pressure of a hypertensive patient (*see* p. 108, 130).

In a parasitic infection, intense enzyme activity occurs with production of nuclear material for cell division followed by the spread of the infection. Inhibition of an enzyme in the bacterial biosynthetic pathway essential for purine or pyrimidine base synthesis prevents the spread of the infection so that it is contained and subsequently eliminated by the body's normal defence mechanisms. Inhibition of the enzyme dihydrofolate reductase, which produces the coenzyme tetrahydrofolate (essential for single carbon insertions in the intermediates of the base synthetic pathways), is sufficient to remove a wide spectrum of infections (*see* p. 102).

In addition to inhibiting the normal biotransformation effected by an enzyme it is also possible that a metabolite (or substrate) analogue may be transformed into a false building unit and subsequently incorporated into an essential macromolecule. Thus, 6-thioguanine owes its antileukaemic activity to incorporation into DNA in place of the normal nucleotide, guanylic acid (*see* p. 104). Further, certain antimetabolites may resemble the end product of an enzymic biosynthetic pathway and thus act as feedback inhibitors of an earlier *de novo* reaction. 6-Mercaptopurine probably owes its anticancer activity to inhibition of an early step in the synthesis of purine nucleotides (*see* p. 104).

4.1.2   Characteristics required of potential drugs

The basic concept of the use of enzyme inhibitors/antimetabolites as drugs requires in practice that the inhibitor has several acceptable features before it can be considered as a suitable candidate for clinical use.

Firstly, it must have a structural resemblance to the normal substrate/metabolite so that it may fit and bind to the enzyme in a similar manner. This structural similarity must not only be reflected in molecular dimensions but also in electron distribution since most enzymic active sites are highly polar. One effective method of obtaining a metabolite-antagonist is to substitute one electron-attracting (or repelling) group for another. Thus, the discovery of the metabolite–antimetabolite relationship of *p*-aminobenzoic acid (**4.1**) and sulphanilamide (**4.2**) in antibacterial therapy set the scene for the antimetabolite theory of drug action. Sometimes the substitution of atoms or groups with similar van der Waals' radii into the normal substrate have produced valuable antagonists, e.g. 5-fluorouracil inhibits the enzymic utilization of uracil in anticancer therapy (*see* p. 105).

$$H_2N\text{—}\langle\!\!=\!\!\rangle\text{—}R$$

(4.1)   R = COOH
(4.2)   R = SO_2NH_2

Secondly, the inhibitor must reach its site of action, the target-enzyme, and persist there; the factors involved here are the rates of excretion and metabolism as well as possession of the correct lipophilic/hydrophilic ratio for transport to the target.

Thirdly, its action must be restricted to the target-enzyme so that it shows specificity of action. Interference by the inhibitor with the action of other enzymes, or direct reaction with cellular constituents, essential to the well-being of the cell, could be followed by cellular imbalances which manifest themselves clinically as unwanted or perhaps dangerous side-effects.

Design of an inhibitor which had absolute specificity for a target-enzyme was at one time considered unobtainable and the aim was to limit the spectrum of the inhibitor's other targets and its relative potency towards them as much as possible. More recently, with the introduction of k_{cat} inhibitors (see p. 124) the development of more specific agents is promised. The problem of specificity is exacerbated when the target-enzyme is present in an invading parasite since the host and the parasite have enzymes which are common to both. However, nature herself occasionally helps in this situation by either providing the host with an isoenzyme which binds the inhibitor less firmly than the corresponding bacterial isoenzyme or, in rare cases, by absenting the target-enzyme from the host's tissues. Examples of a group of drugs which owe their relative non-toxic action to differences in isoenzyme patterns are the folate reductase inhibitors (see p. 102), whereas the sulphonamides are useful drugs due to a biochemical lesion (see p. 96).

4.2   TYPES OF INHIBITORS

Enzyme inhibitors are divided into two main classes depending on the manner in which they interact with the enzyme. Reversible inhibitors are bound to the enzyme by weak interatomic forces, such as van der Waals', hydrogen bonding, ionic, and hydrophobic forces, whereas irreversible inhibitors form a stable covalent bond with a functional group present on the enzyme:

$$\text{reversible}\quad E+I \underset{\longleftarrow}{\overset{K_i}{\longrightarrow}} EI,$$

(4.3)

$$\text{irreversible}\quad E+I \overset{k}{\longrightarrow} EI.$$

4.2.1   Reversible inhibitors

Reversible inhibitors may be competitive, non-competitive or uncompetitive depending upon their point of entry into the enzyme–substrate reaction scheme.

Competitive inhibitors, as their name suggests, compete with the substrate for the active site of the enzyme and by forming an inactive enzyme–inhibitor complex decrease the interaction between the enzyme and the substrate:

$$
\begin{array}{c}
E + S \underset{}{\overset{K_s}{\rightleftharpoons}} ES \xrightarrow{k_2} E + P \\[4pt]
I \updownarrow K_i \\[4pt]
EI
\end{array}
\qquad (4.4)
$$

inactive
enzyme–inhibitor
complex

The rate (v) of the enzyme-catalysed reaction in the presence of a competitive inhibitor is given by

$$
v = \frac{V_{max}}{1 + \dfrac{K_m}{[S]}\left(1 + \dfrac{[I]}{K_i}\right)}
\qquad (4.5)
$$

where K_m is the Michaelis constant which is a molar concentration of substrate at which $v = \frac{1}{2} V_{max}$. The extent to which the reaction is slowed in the presence of the inhibitor is dependent upon the inhibitor concentration [I], and the dissociation constant, K_i, for the enzyme–inhibitor complex. A small value for $K_i (\simeq 10^{-5}\text{–}10^{-8}\,\text{M})$ indicates strong binding of the inhibitor to the enzyme. With this type of inhibitor the inhibition may be overcome, for a fixed inhibitor concentration, by increasing the substrate concentration. This fact can be readily established by examination of Equation 4.5.

The value for K_i may be obtained by determining the initial rate of the enzyme-catalysed reaction using a fixed enzyme concentration over a suitable range of substrate concentrations in the presence and absence of a fixed concentration of the inhibitor. Rearrangement of Equation 4.5 gives

$$
\frac{1}{v} = \frac{1}{V_{max}} + \left(\frac{K_m}{V_{max}}\right)\left(\frac{1}{[S]}\right).
\qquad (4.6)
$$

A plot of $1/v$ against $1/[S]$, known as a Lineweaver–Burk plot (see Fig. 4.1), for the two series of experiments, gives two regression lines which cut at the same point on the $1/v$ axis (corresponding to $1/V_{max}$) but cut the $1/[S]$ axis at values corresponding to $-1/K_m$ and $-1/K_m(1 + [I]/K_i)$ in the absence and presence of the inhibitor respectively, from which K_m and K_i can be calculated.

Non-competitive inhibitors combine with the enzyme–substrate complex and prevent the breakdown of the complex to products (see Equation 4.7). These

$$
\begin{array}{c}
E + S \rightleftharpoons ES \longrightarrow E + P \\[4pt]
I \updownarrow K_i \qquad\qquad I \updownarrow K_i \\[4pt]
EI + S \rightleftharpoons EIS
\end{array}
\qquad (4.7)
$$

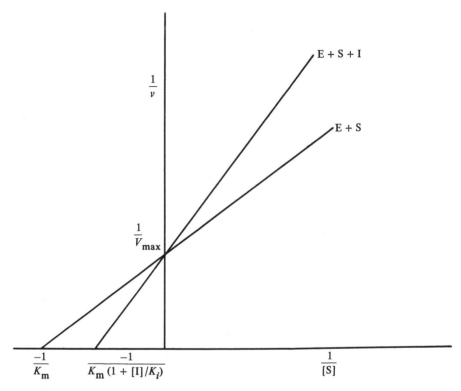

Fig. 4.1   Lineweaver–Burk plot for determining K_i for competitive inhibition of an enzyme-catalysed reaction.

inhibitors do not bind at the active site and only change the V_{max} parameter for the reaction. The kinetics for this type of inhibitor are given by

$$v = \frac{V_{max}/(1+[I]/K_i)}{(1+K_m/[S])} . \qquad (4.8)$$

The extent of the inhibition, by a fixed concentration of inhibitor, cannot be reversed by increasing the substrate concentration (contrast competitive inhibition) since substrate and inhibitor bind at different sites. A Lineweaver–Burk plot of $1/v$ against $1/[S]$ gives a straight line which cuts the $1/[S]$ axis at $-1/K_m$ and the $1/v$ axis at $(1+[I]/K_i)/V_{max}$. Other classes of reversible inhibitors are the uncompetitive and mixed inhibitors where K_m and V_{max} are both altered.

4.2.2   Reversible inhibitors as drugs

The majority of drugs, exerting their action as reversible inhibitors of an enzyme, are of the competitive type and a list of some of the more important reversible inhibitors which have been used clinically, together with the target enzyme, is given in Table 4.1. Much effort has been expended in the design and synthesis of

Table 4.1   Some reversible inhibitors used clinically

Drug	Enzyme inhibited	Clinical use
Allopurinol	Xanthine oxidase	Treatment of gout
Acetazolamide, Dichlorophenamide	Carbonic anhydrase	Diuretic
Trimethoprim, Pyrimethamine, Paludrine, Methotrexate	Dihydrofolate reductase	Antibacterial Antimalarial Anticancer agent
Aspirin	Prostaglandin synthetase	Anti-inflammatory
Cardiac glycosides	Na, K^+-ATPase	Heart ailments
Amphenone, Metyrapone	11β-Hydroxylase	Test for pituitary function
6-Mercaptopurine, Azathioprine	Riboxyl amidotransferase	Anticancer agent
5-Fluorouracil, Floxuridine	Thymidylate synthetase	Anticancer agent
Captopril	Angiotensin-converting enzyme	Hypotensive agent
Sulthiame	Carbonic anhydrase	Treatment of epilepsy
Sodium valproate	GABA transaminase (?)	Treatment of epilepsy
Idoxuridine	Thymidine kinase and thymidylate kinase	Antiviral agent
Cytosine arabinoside (Ara-C) 5-Fluoro-2,5′-anhydrocytosine arabinoside	DNA and RNA polymerases	Antiviral and anticancer agents

reversible competitive inhibitors of a wide range of mammalian enzymes but, frequently, potent *in vitro* inhibitors do not produce the required pharmacological effect when tested *in vivo*. The reason for apparent loss in potency on transference to the *in vivo* environment is not always clear. Possibly the inhibitor does not possess the correct lipophilic:lipophobic ratio to penetrate the many cellular membranes it encounters before reaching the target enzyme. Alternative and more likely explanations are: (*a*) the inhibitor reaches the target enzyme but can only exert a brief inhibitory effect on the enzyme before build-up of the substrate reverses the inhibition to a steady-state inhibition level which is below the threshold level necessary to produce the pharmacological response; (*b*) the target enzyme does not catalyse the rate-controlling step in a metabolic chain and operates well below its maximum efficiency so that inhibition has little effect on the overall pathway. The latter situation has been well established for the noradrenaline synthetic pathway where the enzyme dopa decarboxylase needs to be nearly completely inhibited before noradrenaline synthesis is affected since another enzyme, tyrosine hydroxylase, determines the overall turnover rate in the pathway (*see* p. 108).

Reversible inhibitors have a relatively short duration of action when used as drugs and administration of the drug at frequent intervals is required to maintain the clinical response. Frequent administration is required since, as the plasma level of the drug falls due to metabolism and excretion, the compartmental concentrations of the drug decrease and the enzyme is left to obey the requirements of the changing equilibrium.

4.2.3 Irreversible inhibitors

Irreversible inhibitors form a covalent bond with a functional group on the enzyme, usually at the active site or just outside depending on the molecular dimensions of the inhibitor.

There are two classes of irreversible inhibitors; the active site-directed inhibitors where the reactive function is already present and the k_{cat} inhibitors where this function is generated by the enzyme. Each class is discussed in detail elsewhere (*see* p. 115 and p. 124).

Irreversible inhibition renders the enzyme inactive to its substrate by blocking access to the active site and also, in certain instances, by removing the catalytic activity of the enzyme should reaction occur with a catalytic group within the active site.

This type of inhibitor either contains or develops a reactive functional group which may be either an alkylating or an acylating (phosphorylating) function. A list of functional groups usually used in active site-directed irreversible inhibitors is shown in Table 4.2. Also summarized in the table is the type of functional group present on the enzyme in the amino acid residue which subsequently is modified.

4.2.4 Kinetics of irreversible enzyme inhibition

In the previous discussion on reversible inhibitors, the potency of an inhibitor was shown to be reflected in the K_i value, which is characteristic of the inhibitor and independent of inhibitor concentration. However, the actual level of inhibition achieved in an enzyme system involves the use of equations into which inhibitor and substrate concentrations, as well as the K_m value for the substrate, need to be incorporated. Similarly, the potency of an irreversible inhibitor is given by binding and rate constants which are both independent of inhibitor concentration. This allows a precise comparison of the relative potency of inhibitors, which is necessary in the design and development of more effective inhibitors of an enzyme.

Irreversible inhibition of an enzyme by an active site-directed inhibitor can be represented by

$$E + I \xrightarrow{\ k\ } EI \tag{4.9}$$

Table 4.2   Reactive functional groups present in active site-directed irreversible inhibitors and enzymes

Functional groups on inhibitor
(1) Alkylating functions:

α-Halogenoketone

$$-\overset{\overset{\textstyle O}{\|}}{C}-CH_2Cl$$

Diazoketone — $-COCHN_2$

Maleamide

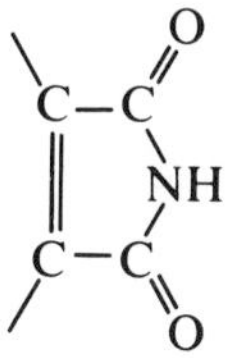

(2) Acylating function:

Phenylurethane

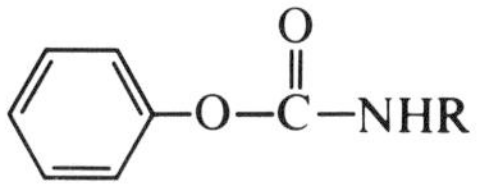

Sulphonyl halide — $-SO_2Cl$

Reactive ester

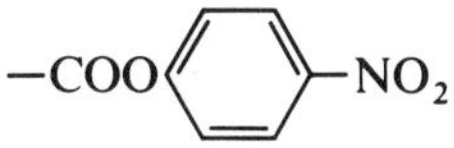

$$-COO-\!\!\!\!\bigcirc\!\!\!\!-NO_2$$

Functional groups on enzyme
Imidazole nitrogen (histidine residue)
Carboxylate (aspartate, glutamate) $-COOH$

Amino -α-amino (terminal)

$$-HN-\overset{\overset{\textstyle O}{\|}}{C}-\overset{\overset{\textstyle R}{|}}{CH}-NH_2$$

     -ε-amino (lysine) $-NH_2$
Methyl mercapto (methionine) $-S-CH_3$
Hydroxyl (serine) $-CH_2OH$

provided that complex formation between the inhibitor and the enzyme is ignored for the present time. The reaction is bimolecular, but, since the inhibitor is usually present in large excess of the enzyme concentration, the kinetics for inactivation of the enzyme follow a pseudo first-order reaction.

In the general case of a bimolecular reaction between two compounds A and B, the rate of reaction is given by

$$\frac{dx}{dt} = k_2(a-x)(b-x),\tag{4.10}$$

where k_2 is the second-order rate constant, a and b are the initial concentrations of A and B respectively and the concentration of product is x at time t. Integration and rearrangement of Equation 4.10 gives

$$k_2 = \frac{2 \cdot 303}{t(a-b)} \log \frac{b(a-x)}{a(b-x)}. \tag{4.11}$$

In the situation where $a \gg b$, this simplifies to

$$k_2 a = \frac{2 \cdot 303}{t} \log \frac{b}{(b-x)}. \tag{4.12}$$

Since $k_2 a = k_1$ where k_1 is the pseudo first-order reaction rate constant; then

$$k_1 = \frac{2 \cdot 303}{t} \log \frac{b}{(b-x)}. \tag{4.13}$$

A plot of $\log(b-x)$ versus t for the reaction as it proceeds, using a known concentration of the inhibitor, gives a regression line with slope $= -2 \cdot 303/k_1$, from which k_1 and k_2 may be obtained.

In practice in enzyme inhibition reactions it is sometimes found that k_1 is not directly proportional to a so that the value of k_2 is not constant with a change in the concentration of the inhibitor a. This is due to initial binding of the inhibitor to the active site of the enzyme before the irreversible inhibition reaction occurs:

$$\text{E}+\text{I} \underset{}{\overset{K_i}{\rightleftharpoons}} \underset{\text{complex}}{\text{(E)(I)}} \overset{k_{+2}}{\longrightarrow} \underset{\substack{\text{inhibited} \\ \text{enzyme}}}{\text{EI}} \tag{4.14}$$

The rate of the inactivation reaction is given by

$$\frac{dx}{dt} = \frac{k_{+2}[\text{E}]}{1 + K_i/[\text{I}]}, \tag{4.15}$$

where x represents the concentration of the inhibited enzyme (EI), K_i is the dissociation constant for the enzyme–inhibitor complex and k_{+2} is the first-order rate constant for the breakdown of the complex into products. Integration of Equation 4.15 gives

$$k_1 t = \ln \text{E} - \ln(\text{E}-x) \tag{4.16}$$

where k_1 is the observed first-order rate constant and

$$k_1 = \frac{k_{+2}}{1 + K_i/[\text{I}]}. \tag{4.17}$$

When Equation 4.17 is written in the reciprocal form

$$\frac{1}{k_1} = \frac{K_i}{k_{+2}[\text{I}]} + \frac{1}{k_{+2}}, \tag{4.18}$$

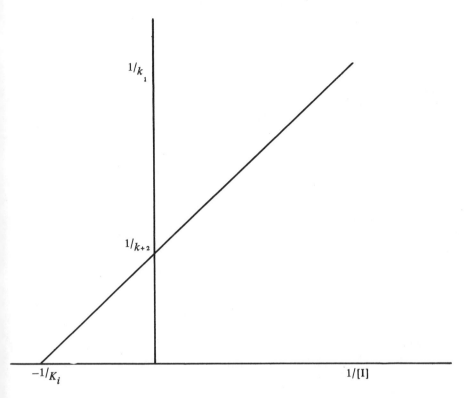

Fig. 4.2   Determination of K_i and k_{+2} for an irreversible inhibition reaction involving complex formation.

it can be seen that a plot of $1/k_1$ against $1/[I]$ gives a regression line from which k_{+2} and K_i may be evaluated (*see* Fig. 4.2).

4.2.5   Irreversible inhibitors as drugs

Irreversible inhibitors, by forming a firm bond to the enzyme, would be expected to produce a pharmacological effect of long duration so that infrequent administration of the drug would be required since the level of inhibition should be unaffected by clearance of excess drug from the body. In practice, more frequent administration is necessary to maintain the pharmacological effect due to resynthesis of fresh enzyme.

Irreversible inhibitors (except k_{cat} inhibitors, *see* p. 124) are reactive agents, and besides the target enzyme, will react with other constituents containing amino or thiol groups which are present in the cell or body tissues. Such reactions will produce toxic symptoms should constituents essential to the cell be appreciably depleted. Alternatively, reaction between the inhibitor and non-essential constituents at a rate comparable with the rate of inhibition of the target enzyme could deplete the levels of the inhibitor due to a mass-action effect before the inhibition reaction is complete. TLCK, a specific inhibitor for trypsin-like enzymes (*see* p. 117) reacts as rapidly with the thiol group of glutathione as with the enzyme. The glutathione concentration in the body's compartments varies from 0.62–5.7×10^{-3} M whereas the inhibitor concentration would be many orders lower; TLCK would not be a useful *in vivo* inhibitor.

A list of some irreversible enzyme inhibitors which have been used clinically is given in Table 4.3 together with their target-enzymes.

Table 4.3   Some irreversible inhibitors used clinically

Drug	Enzyme inhibited	Clinical use
Sulphonamides	Dihydropteroate synthetase	Antibacterials
Hydrazine derivatives	Monoamine oxidase	Antidepressants
Serazide, Carbidopa	Dopa decarboxylase	In conjunction with L-dopa in Parkinson's disease
Neostigmine, Eserine, Pyridostigmine, Benzpyrinium, Dyflos, Ecothiopate	Acetylcholinesterase	Glaucoma, myasthenia gravis
Penicillins, Cephalosporins	Transpeptidase	Antibiotics
Organoarsenicals	Pyruvate dehydrogenase	Antiprotozoal agents
O-Carbamyl-D-serine	Alanine racemase	Antibiotic
D-Cycloserine	Alanine racemase and other enzymes	Antibiotic
Azaserine	Formylglycinamide ribotide amido transferase	Anticancer agent
γ-Vinyl GABA	GABA transaminase	Anti-convulsant
Clavulanic acid	β-Lactamase	Adjuvant to penicillin antibiotics
α-Mono(di)fluoromethyldopa	Dopa decarboxylase (A.A.A.D.) (peripheral)	Hypotensive

4.3   EXAMPLES OF ENZYME INHIBITORS (ANTIMETABOLITES) USED AS DRUGS

4.3.1   Antibacterial sulphonamides

The discovery of this group of drugs had a dramatic impact on chemotherapy and also served to reawaken interest in enzyme inhibition as a mechanism of drug action.

Prior to the 1930–40 decade there was widespread scepticism regarding the possibility of successfully treating bacterial infections with synthetic organic substances introduced into the bloodstream. This outlook was shattered in 1935 when Domagk described the treatment of streptococcal infections with the drug prontosil (4.3) which had its origin in the German dyestuff industry and was, in fact, a red dye. Dyestuffs containing the sulphonamide ($-SO_2NH_2$) group had

$$H_2N-\text{⟨⟩}-N{=}N-\text{⟨⟩}-SO_2NH_2$$
$$\underset{NH_2}{}$$

(4.3)

long been known to become firmly attached to the proteins of wool, i.e. were 'fast to wool'. It was then conceived that this group might also become firmly 'attached' to the proteins of bacteria. Over one thousand azodyes were tested before the introduction of prontosil.

Later, at the Pasteur Institute in Paris, it was discovered that prontosil was reduced *in vivo* to liberate the active drug, sulphanilamide (4.4), which was detected in urine as its acetyl derivative. This discovery led to the search for other sulphonamide derivatives with improved therapeutic effect. However, due to the slow realization of the importance of these discoveries, it was not until 1937 that sulphapyridine (4.5), M and B 693, was marketed for treating pneumococcal

(4.4)   (4.5)

infections. Other heterocyclic derivatives were subsequently sought in order to reduce side-effects such as nausea and skin rashes so that by 1948 some 5000 sulphonamide derivatives had been prepared and biologically tested. Since the introduction of sulphonamides in 1935 some of the most lethal diseases, e.g. pneumonia, meningitis, cystitis, bacillary dysentery, gonorrhoea and trachoma, have become curable. Although many of these conditions are now controlled with antibiotics, the sulphonamides still retain an important role in treating systemic infections.

The sulphapyrimidines, sulphadiazine (4.6) and sulphadimidine (4.7), are absorbed slowly and completely from the intestine and acetylated (the acetyl derivative is not antibacterial) to a lesser extent than sulphanilamide, sulphapyridine and sulphathiazole (4.8). N^4-succinyl and phthalyl sulphathiazoles have low water solubilities but are highly ionized under the alkaline conditions of the intestines so that they are poorly absorbed and retained in the gut after oral administration. The carboxyamide group becomes hydrolysed by digestive and bacterial proteinases to release the parent sulphonamide enabling the treatment of intestinal infections such as bacillary dysentery. The increased acidity of sulphacetamide (4.9) explains why its water-soluble sodium salt is neutral in solution and consequently suitable for treating eye infections.

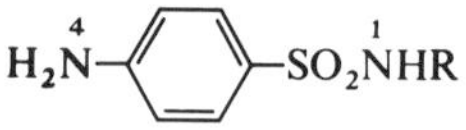

$$H_2\overset{4}{N}-\!\!\!\left\langle\bigcirc\right\rangle\!\!\!-SO_2\overset{1}{N}HR$$

(4.6)   R =

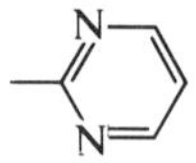

(4.7)   R =

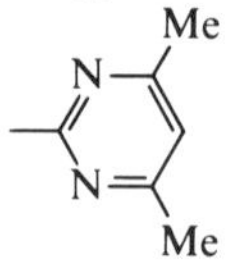

(4.8)   R =

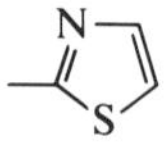

(4.9)   R = $-COCH_3$

(4.10)   R =

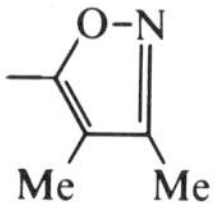

(4.11)   R =

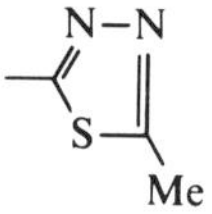

Other sulphonamides have been developed for their high aqueous solubility so that rapid elimination and high concentration in the urine is obtained. Thus, sulphafurazole (4.10) and sulphamethizole (4.11) are relatively strongly acidic (pK_a 4·9 and 5·5, respectively) and almost completely ionized at physiological pH. The additional high solubility of their acetyl derivatives avoids undesirable crystallization in the renal tubules. Such properties render these drugs eminently suitable for treating urinary tract infections.

Heterocyclic sulphonamides based on two ring nitrogen atoms and also substituted with methoxyl groups bind strongly to serum albumin due to their increased lipid solubility. These are eliminated very slowly and produce a sustained effect. Some doubt has, however, been expressed on their efficacy since adequate blood concentrations may not always be attained for antibacterial activity.

4.3.1.1   Mode of action

Theories related to the mode of action of the sulphonamides were developed from 1940 onwards. Initially, their antibacterial effect *in vitro* was found to be offset (antagonized) by the addition of extracts of pus and particularly, yeast. Since this activity resided in the alkali-soluble fraction of yeast and was lost on treatment with nitrous acid – the active antagonist was suggested to be an aromatic amino acid. By analogy with the few examples of enzyme competitive inhibition previously known it was suggested that the sulphonamide interfered with the utilization of a normal substrate (metabolite) by an enzyme present in the bacterial cell. This substrate was believed to be *p*-aminobenzoic acid because of the close resemblance to sulphanilamide. *p*-Aminobenzoic acid was subsequently isolated from yeast and also shown to be a necessary growth factor for bacteria.

Quantitative studies revealed that the *ratio* of the amount of *p*-aminobenzoic acid needed to antagonize the antibacterial effect of a given amount of sulphonamide was constant over a wide range of sulphonamide concentrations. Therefore, the sulphonamide was behaving as a typical competitive inhibitor. Later it was shown that the sulphonamide competed with *p*-aminobenzoic acid for an active site on the enzyme dihydrofolate synthetase which utilizes the natural metabolite to synthesize dihydrofolic acid (4.14). In this respect, the similarity in dimensions and electron distribution of the two molecules is of prime importance (4.12). Since the —NHR group protrudes away from the otherwise planar

(4.12)

molecule, the substitution of various groups R does not affect the ability of the molecule to fit the enzyme site. Unlike *p*-aminobenzoic acid, which is completely ionized as an acid (pK_a 4·9) at physiological pH, sulphanilamide is a weak acid (pK_a 10·3) although strong negative fractional charges reside on the sulphonyl oxygens.

The selective toxicity of the sulphonamides lies in the fact that mammals, unlike susceptible bacteria, do not need to synthesize dihydrofolic acid but absorb it from the diet.

The biosynthetic route to dihydrofolic acid has now been elucidated (Fig. 4.3). The pteridine alcohol, 2-amino-4-hydroxy-6-hydroxymethyl-7,8-dihydropteridine (4.13), is phosphorylated stepwise, by ATP, to give the 6-pyrophosphate which is then condensed with *p*-aminobenzoic acid or *p*-aminobenzoylglutamic acid to form dihydropteroic acid or dihydrofolic acid (4.14) respectively. The sulphonamides competitively inhibit the enzyme dihydrofolate synthetase which effects these condensations.

It has been proposed that there are two binding sites on the enzyme, located 0·67–0·70 nm apart, one being specific for binding the 4-NH_2 group and the other non-specific for binding the acidic group of *p*-aminobenzoic acid or a sulphonamide. X-ray crystallographic studies have revealed certain structural similarities between N_1-substituted sulphonamides and *p*-aminobenzoic acid glutamate which suggest that the N_1-substituent competes for a site normally reserved for the glutamate residue.

4.3.1.2 *Ionization of sulphonamides*

In 1942, Bell and Roblin found that the most active sulphonamides at physiological pH (7·3) were those possessing pK_a values for the sulphonamide (—SO_2NHR)

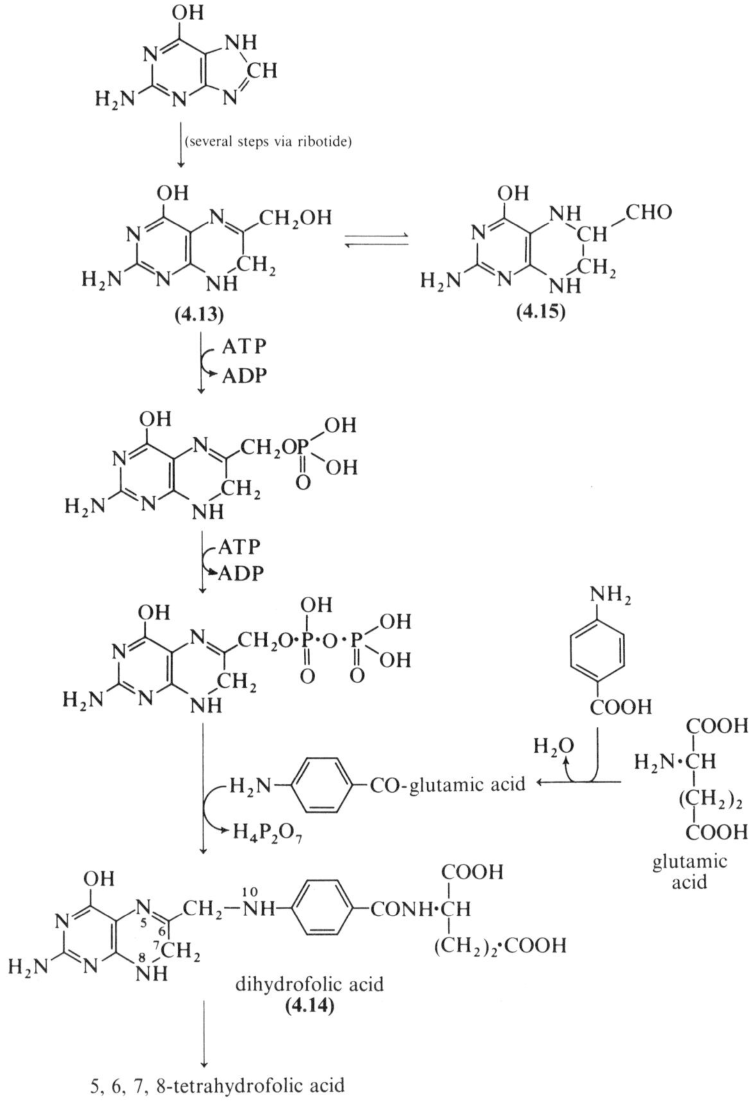

OH
NH
CH
H_2N N N

(several steps via ribotide)

OH
CH_2OH
CH_2
H_2N N NH
(4.13)

⇌

OH
NH CHO
CH
CH_2
H_2N N NH
(4.15)

ATP
ADP

OH
CH_2OP OH
OH
O
CH_2
H_2N N NH

ATP
ADP

OH
OH
$CH_2O·P·O·P$ OH
O O
CH_2
H_2N N NH

NH_2

COOH

H_2O

$-H_2N-$⟨⟩$-CO$-glutamic acid ←

$H_4P_2O_7$

COOH
$H_2N·CH$
$(CH_2)_2$
COOH
glutamic acid

OH
CH_2-NH-⟨⟩$-CONH·CH$
10
5 6
8 7CH_2
H_2N N NH
dihydrofolic acid
(4.14)

COOH
$(CH_2)_2·COOH$

5, 6, 7, 8-tetrahydrofolic acid

Fig. 4.3   Biosynthesis of tetrahydrofolic acid.

group, dissociating as an acid, in the range 6–8, i.e. about 50% ionized. These observations were interpreted by suggesting that the more negative the —SO_2 group became, the more closely it resembled the carboxylate anion of the *p*-aminobenzoic acid and the more effective would be the sulphonamide as an antagonist. Now, the —SO_2 group is enabled to become more negative in the anion of the sulphonamide **(4.16)**. However, although ionization is facilitated by electron-withdrawing R groups, e.g. π electron-deficient heterocyclic rings, these

$$Ph-\overset{\overset{O}{\parallel}}{\underset{\underset{O}{\parallel}}{S}}-\overset{}{N}-R \longleftrightarrow Ph-\overset{\overset{\overset{-}{O}}{\mid}}{\underset{\underset{O}{\parallel}}{S}}=N-R \longleftrightarrow Ph-\overset{\overset{O}{\parallel}}{\underset{\underset{O}{\mid}}{S}}=N-R$$

(4.16)

introduce an opposing factor (electron attraction) which offsets the ability of the sulphonyl oxygens to become more negative. At some point in these two opposing effects the antibacterial activity passes through a maximum corresponding to about 50% ionization. Another explanation for these observations is that since the bacterial cell wall is impermeable to the hydrophilic sulphonamide anion, maximum activity is obtained only by those compounds which possess ionized and un-ionized (lipophilic) forms in sufficient concentrations.

Other studies have revealed that the primary aromatic amino group of sulphonamides is important since alkyl substitution causes loss of bacteriostatic activity. Seydel, from infra-red studies, concluded that the negativity of the aromatic amino group was important for activity. The most active compounds were found to have pK_a values, for the basic group, lying within the range 1·91–2·34. This, and other accumulated evidence, suggests that sulphonamides interfere with the biosynthetic route to dihydrofolic acid by forming a Schiff's base (4.17) with pteridine aldehyde (4.15) (*see* Fig. 4.3) which exists in equilibrium with

$$R-\overset{}{\underset{\underset{H}{\mid}}{C}}=N-R'$$

R = pteridine
R' = *p*-sulphonamidophenyl

(4.17)

the corresponding alcohol (4.13). This reaction leads to depletion of pteridine alcohol and a slowing down of the production of dihydrofolic acid. Supporting this contention is the observation that *p*-aminobenzoic acid prevents the antibacterial action of the sulphonamides only when both are administered simultaneously. Delaying the addition of *p*-aminobenzoic acid for 1–2 hours does not reverse the action of the sulphonamide. The competitive inhibition and reversal effected by *p*-aminobenzoic acid when added simultaneously with sulphonamide is accounted for by the greater amount of *p*-aminobenzoic acid immediately available leading to a depletion of the pyrophosphate ester of the pteridine alcohol. In order to maintain the equilibrium between intermediates, this leads to depletion of pteridine alcohol and its aldehydic form so that less of the latter is available to react with the sulphonamide.

Experiments using folate-synthesizing enzymes in a cell-free system containing sulphamethoxazole and the pteridine alcohol (4.13) showed that the addition of *p*-aminobenzoic acid failed to reverse the enzymic inhibition. A condensation product of the sulphonamide (utilizing the *p*-amino group) and pteridine alcohol was subsequently isolated. This suggests the possibility of metabolic incorporation of the antimetabolite to give a sulphonamide analogue of dihydrofolic acid.

Other antimetabolites which may interfere with the biosynthetic route to dihydrofolic acid are 7,7-dialkyl-7,8-dihydropteridines. These compounds strongly inhibit the enzyme which phosphorylates the alcohol group. They may constitute potential chemotherapeutic agents.

The relevance of the mode of action of the sulphonamides is that it leads to the depletion not only of dihydrofolic acid but also 5,6,7,8-tetrahydrofolic acid formed by enzymic reduction of the former. Derivatives of tetrahydrofolic acid occupy a key role as coenzymes in the cellular production of purines and pyrimidines required for synthesis of nuclear DNA.

4.3.2 Role of tetrahydrofolic acid

Tetrahydrofolic acid is formed from dihydrofolic acid by means of the enzyme dihydrofolate reductase (hydrogenase). Subsequent modifications by various one-carbon substituents yield vital coenzymes such as N_{10}-formyl-5,6,7,8-tetrahydrofolic acid which effects the formylation of the intermediate ribotide (4.18) to give inosinic acid (4.19). This constitutes the insertion of C_2 into the

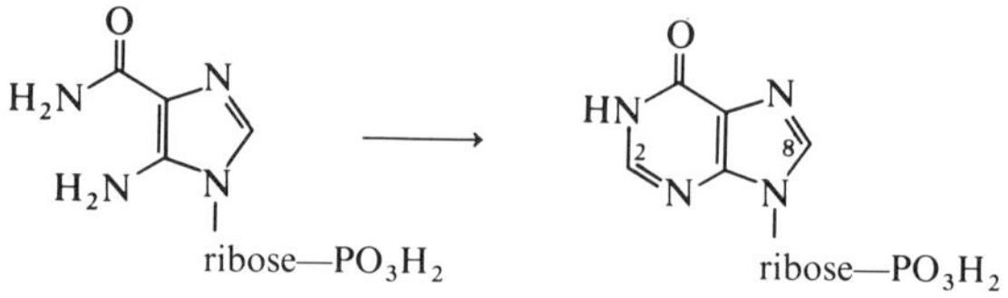

purine skeleton. Inosinic acid is further transformed to adenylic acid (4.20) and guanylic acid (4.21) required for DNA synthesis. An earlier stage in the biosynthetic route when C_8 is inserted involves the formylation of glycinamide ribotide to give (4.18). The coenzyme necessary for this is N_5,N_{10}-methenyl-tetrahydrofolic

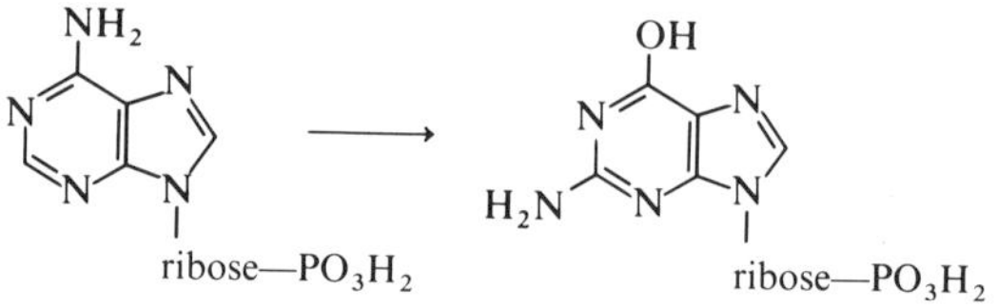

acid (4.22). Of all the reactions catalysed by tetrahydrofolic acid derivatives the synthesis of thymine (required for DNA) is the most sensitive to shortage of folic acid. (The addition of thymine has been shown to antagonize the action of sulphadiazine on streptococci.) The coenzyme participating in the methylation of

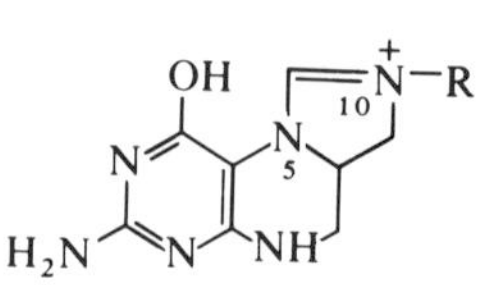

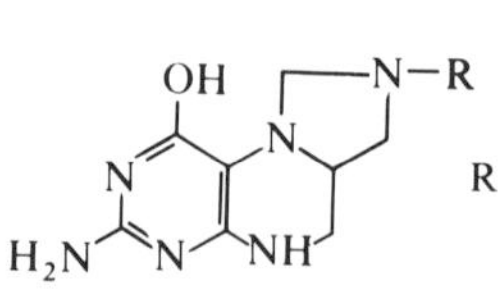

R = benzoylglutamic acid

uracil ribose-phosphate (uridylic acid (4.24a)) to give thymine ribose-phosphate (thymidylic acid (4.24b)) is N_5,N_{10}-methylene-tetrahydrofolic acid (4.23). (The enzyme thymidylate synthetase is involved in the transference of the methyl group

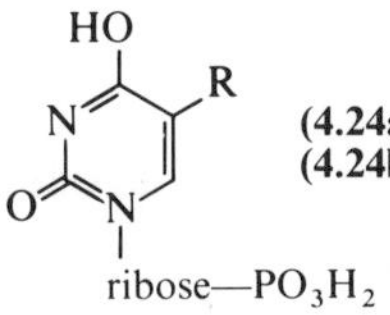

(4.24a) R = H
(4.24b) R = Me

from the coenzyme.) Another coenzyme, N_5-methyl-tetrahydrofolic acid, participates in the synthesis of methionine. DNA polymerases are subsequently involved in the elaboration of DNA from purine and pyrimidine nucleotides.

4.3.2.1 Folic acid analogues in cancer chemotherapy

Because of the high turnover of DNA in rapidly dividing cancer cells, it was thought that inhibition of the biosynthesis of tetrahydrofolic acid could produce beneficial results in the treatment of malignant tumours. Consequently, analogues of folic acid (4.25) were prepared to compete with the normal substrate (metabolite), dihydrofolic acid, for the active site of the enzyme dihydrofolate reductase. This, in turn, would inhibit the coenzymic mediated production of purine and pyrimidine nucleotides necessary for DNA. Slight modification of folic acid produced the first antimetabolite, aminopterin (4.26), to be used in the treatment of cancer. Clinical trials conducted from 1958 onwards revealed amethopterin (methotrexate (4.27)) to be more selective. Amethopterin has been shown to bind more strongly, by a factor of 10^4, than the natural substrate to dihydrofolate

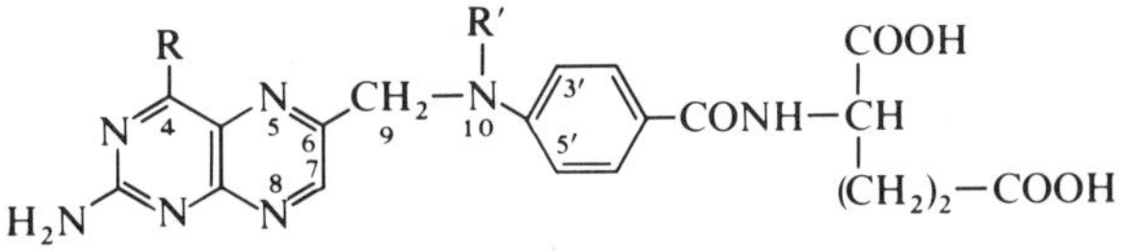

(4.25) R = OH, R′ = H   folic acid
(4.26) R = NH$_2$, R′ = H   aminopterin
(4.27) R = NH$_2$, R′ = Me   methotrexate

reductase. This has been related to the higher basic strength resulting from the replacement of —OH on C-4 by an amino group. Examination of the dihydro-folate reductase–methotrexate complex by X-ray diffraction reveals the pyrimidine ring to be situated in a lipophilic cavity where the protonated N-1 group is ionically bound to a juxtapositioned carboxylic acid group. Methotrexate produces a remarkable remission of symptoms for about a year in lymphoblastic leukaemia but the cells eventually develop resistance by increasing the production of dihydrofolate reductase. Choriocarcinoma – a fast growing tumour of pregnancy previously with a high death rate – is rapidly and completely cured with methotrexate. Dramatic cures have also been obtained in Burkitt's lymphoma which is a highly malignant carcinoma of the lymph glands.

Disadvantages in the use of methotrexate stem from its adverse effect on the production of red blood cells leading to macrocytic anaemia. Gastrointestinal ulceration, kidney and liver damage are other side-effects requiring careful monitoring. Although one of the earliest cytotoxic drugs, more effective ways of using it are being discovered. In high dose intermittent schedules the adverse effect on the bone-marrow is relieved by the periodic administration of N_5- formyltetrahydrofolic acid (folinic acid), which, being a precursor of the coenzymic N_{10}-formyl derivative, enables blockade of tetrahydrofolic acid production to be by-passed (folinic acid 'rescue' procedure).

A number of derivatives of methotrexate have been prepared with a view to reducing its toxicity. The phenyl substituted 3′,5′-dichloro derivative is significantly less toxic, probably due to its ease of metabolism to 3′,5′-dichloro-7-hydroxymethotrexate which is equally effective in inhibiting dihydrofolate reductase.

4.3.2.2 *Folic acid analogues in bacterial (and protozoal) chemotherapy*

A search for inhibitors of dihydrofolate reductase as potential antimalarials revealed that aminopterin and methotrexate were not toxic to protozoa since, like folic acid, they are not readily absorbed by the micro-organisms. In order to facilitate absorption, a substantial slice of the molecule of aminopterin was dispensed with, leaving a diaminopteridine nucleus which was then substituted with lipophilic phenyl or alkyl groups. Thus, 2,4-diamino-6,7-diphenylpteridine produced antimalarial activity comparable with quinine. Further modification of the pteridine nucleus, omitting nitrogen at position 5 and retaining lipophilic alkyl groups, gave analogues of greater penetrating power. (4.28) was found to inhibit dihydrofolate reductase isolated from various bacterial species in proportion to its effect on intact bacteria. More recently, some powerful antifolates have been obtained by also omitting N-8 to give a series of 2,4-diaminoquinazolines.

(4.28)   (4.29)

The continuing simplification of such molecules revealed that simple 2,4-diaminopyrimidines possessed considerable antifolate activity in micro-organisms. These investigations led to the development of the highly potent antimalarial, pyrimethamine (4.29). Selectivity for the malarial dihydrofolate reductase is aided by the high lipid solubility conferred by chlorophenyl and ethyl substituents. This facilitates penetration of the lipid membrane of red cells infected with erythrocytic forms of the parasite. Selectivity of action is also a result of a much greater sensitivity towards the drug shown by the parasitic enzyme compared to that of the host. The plasmodial enzyme has a molecular weight 10 times greater than the mammalian enzyme and is probably an isoenzyme. Cycloguanil (4.31), the active form produced *in vivo* on administering proguanil (4.30), also owes its antimalarial activity to inhibition of dihydrofolate reductase.

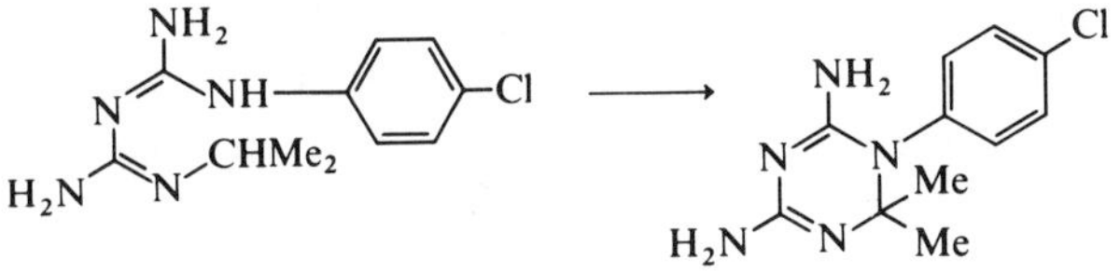

(4.30)   (4.31)

In a search for antibacterial 2,4-diaminopyrimidines, a group of 5-benzyl substituted derivatives were synthesized. When the lipophilicity was slightly reduced by substitution of methoxy groups in the phenyl nucleus optimal activity was obtained. Thus, trimethoprim (4.32) represents a simple analogue of folic acid with a relatively small lipophilic group which is absorbable by bacteria.

Some ten or so years ago it was observed that when trimethoprim was administered in conjunction with a sulphonamide (sulphamethoxazole (4.33))

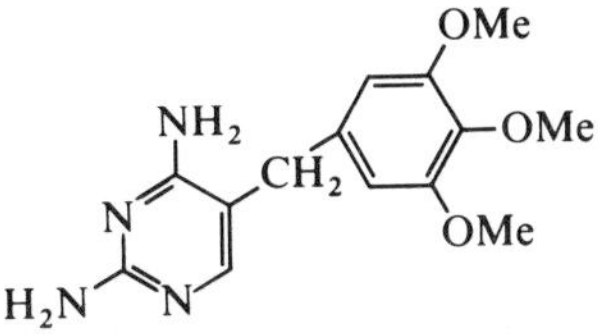

(4.32) 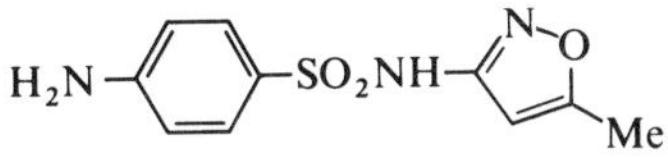   (4.33)

possessing similar pharmacokinetic properties, a considerably increased antibacterial action resulted. This is due to a synergistic effect arising from the 'sequential inhibition' of both dihydrofolate synthetase and dihydrofolate reductase in the metabolic pathway leading to tetrahydrofolic acid (*see* Fig. 4.3) (*see also* Section 9.6.5).

The same synergistic principle has been used in the treatment of malaria. Here, pyrimethamine is combined with a long-acting sulphonamide which acts in phase with the relatively long-lasting dihydrofolate reductase inhibitor. Such combinations have been found to be active in cases resistant to quinine and chloroquine. This is important since in South America and South East Asia resistance of parasites to synthetic antimalarials is widespread. Since both drugs are long-acting a single intramuscularly injected dose ensures effective concentrations in the body for 1 week.

4.3.3   Purine analogues in cancer chemotherapy

Purine (and pyrimidine) analogues inhibit a later stage in the synthesis of DNA than dihydrofolate reductase inhibitors.

6-Mercaptopurine (4.35) is well established in the treatment of acute childhood leukaemias, especially chronic myelocytic leukaemia where the remission rate is about 50%. The free base is converted *in vivo* by sensitive neoplasms to the ribonucleotide (MPRP (**4.37**)). This results from the reaction of the base with 5-phosphoribosylpyrophosphate (**4.38**) catalysed by the enzyme hypoxanthine-guanine phosphoribosyl-transferase. Resistance to 6-mercaptopurine arises due to loss of this enzyme within the neoplasm. Although MPRP inhibits several enzymic pathways in the biosynthesis of purine nucleotides, including the conversion of inosine-5'-phosphate (**4.19**) to adenosine-5'-phosphate (**4.20**), the main inhibition appears to be at an early stage when 5-phosphoribosylpyrophosphate is converted to phosphoribosylamine (**4.39**) by phosphoribosylpyrophosphate amido-transferase. Allopurinol is sometimes also administered to inhibit xanthine oxidase degradation of 6-mercaptopurine to thiouric acid which may cause renal damage.

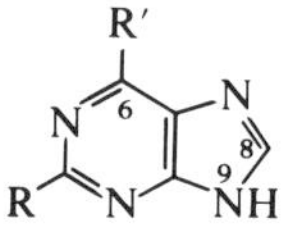

(**4.34**)   R = H, R' = NH$_2$
(**4.35**)   R = H, R' = SH
(**4.36**)   R = NH$_2$, R' = SH

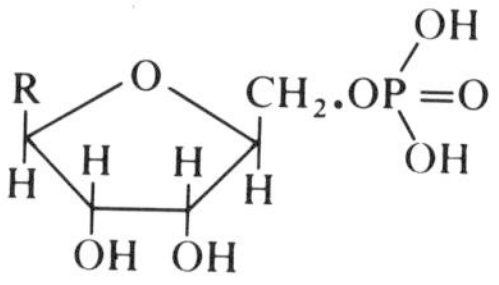

(**4.37**)   R = 6-mercaptopurin-9-yl
(**4.38**)   R = pyrophosphate
(**4.39**)   R = NH$_2$

Another cytotoxic drug, 6-thioguanine (**4.36**), used for treating myeloblastic leukaemia, is also metabolized to the 9-(1'-ribosyl-5'-phosphate) in the neoplasm. However, in contrast to MPRP, this does not inhibit an enzyme but is further phosphorylated to the triphosphate and incorporated by an unknown biosynthetic pathway into DNA as a false nucleotide. Lack of selectivity towards tumour cells is due to rapid incorporation of thioguanine into DNA of bone-marrow cells. 8-Azaguanine exerts its anticancer action in a similar manner.

Immunosuppression is a major side-effect which may complicate cancer chemotherapy. This has led to the design of drugs to prevent rejection following organ transplant surgery. The unsuitability of 6-mercaptopurine for this purpose, due to a high rate of elimination, has led to its conversion to the S-(1-methyl-4-nitroimidazol-5-yl) derivative, azathioprine (imuran), which has a more sustained effect. The electron-attracting properties of the nitro group renders the C—S bond amenable to progressive *in vivo* enzymic cleavage.

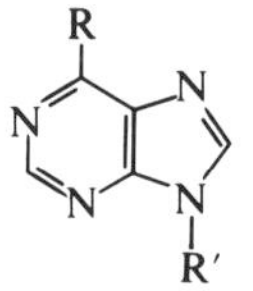

(**4.40**)   R = NH$_2$, R' =

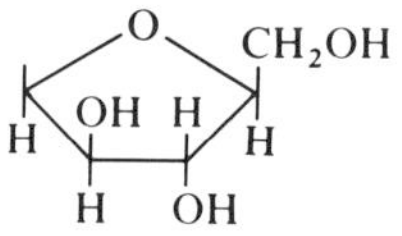

(**4.41**)   R = NH$_2$, R' =

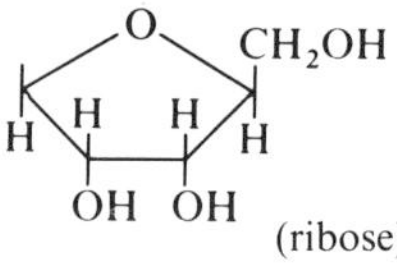

(**4.42**)   R = OH, R' = arabinose

Adenine arabinoside, 9-β-D-arabinofuranosyladenine, **(4.40)** is an analogue of the natural adenosine riboside **(4.41)** and is one of several adenine nucleosides tested for anti-tumour activity. Cytotoxic activity in leukaemias follows conversion to the triphosphate, and non-competitive inhibition of DNA polymerase acting on its normal ribotidal metabolite. Extensive deamination to the inactive inosine analogue **(4.42)** has been inhibited by co-administration of further analogues containing modified pyrimidine nuclei.

4.3.4   Pyrimidine analogues in cancer (and viral) chemotherapy

Of the several halogeno-pyrimidines investigated only fluoro derivatives have appreciable anticancer activity. 5-Fluorouracil **(4.43)** is highly selective, as a 5% cream, in treating skin cancer. It is also used in the palliative treatment of certain solid tumours, e.g gastrointestinal tract, breast, pancreas, for which surgery or irradiation is not always possible. Solutions for injection may be prepared with the aid of sodium hydroxide.

5-Fluorouracil (FU, **(4.43)**) has been shown to be initially bioconverted to the 2'-deoxyribonucleotide, 5-fluoro-2'-deoxyuridylic acid (FUdRP **(4.44)**) which is a potent competitive inhibitor of thymidylate synthetase. This is the enzyme which effects transference of a methyl group from the coenzyme, methylenetetrahydrofolic acid, to deoxyuridylic acid **(4.45)** yielding thymidylic acid **(4.46)** which is

(4.43)   R = F, R' = H(FU)

(4.44)   R = F, R' = (dRP)

(4.45)   R = H, R' = dRP
(4.46)   R = Me, R' = dRP

subsequently incorporated into DNA. The inhibitor has been shown to have an affinity for the enzyme which is several thousand times greater than that of the natural substrate. This remarkable inhibitory effect is associated with the unique properties of the fluorine atom whose van der Waals' radius compares with that of hydrogen. The electronegativity of fluorine also has an effect on electron distribution conferring an acid strength 30 times that of uracil. These features enable FUdRP to fit the active site of the enzyme particularly well. Further studies have suggested that FUdRP forms a covalent bond with the active site via a nucleophilic sulphydryl group. The increased size and decreased electronegativity of other halogens confer much less activity on analogous molecules. The high selectivity of FU, especially in skin treatments, may be related to the fact that enzymes which readily metabolize uracil also readily degrade FU in normal cells but not in cancer cells.

6-Azauridine **(4.47)** – another antagonist of pyrimidine synthesis – is poorly absorbed after oral administration, remaining largely in the intestines. Conversion to

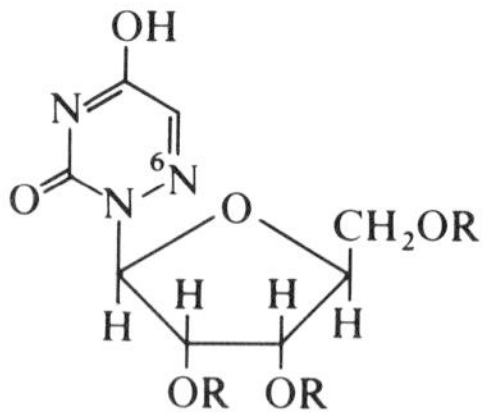

(4.47) R = H
(4.48) R = —COCH$_3$

the triacetate **(4.48)** increases lipophilic properties so that effective absorption, proceeded by deacetylation in the bloodstream, occurs.

Other halogenated 2′-deoxypyrimidine nucleosides have found use as antiviral agents. Thus, 5-iodo-2′-deoxyuridine, idoxuridine (IdU **(4.49)**), becomes converted in cells to the mono-, di- and triphosphate forms which are thought to compete with thymidine phosphates for enzymes such as thymidine kinase and thymidylate kinase involved in the further utilization of thymidine. However, antiviral activity is mediated principally by incorporation into viral DNA in place of thymidine **(4.50)**. Since the drug is also incorporated into the DNA of normal cells it must not be administered systemically. The biochemical similarity between IdU and thymidine is related to comparable van der Waals' radii of the 5-substituted methyl and iodo groups.

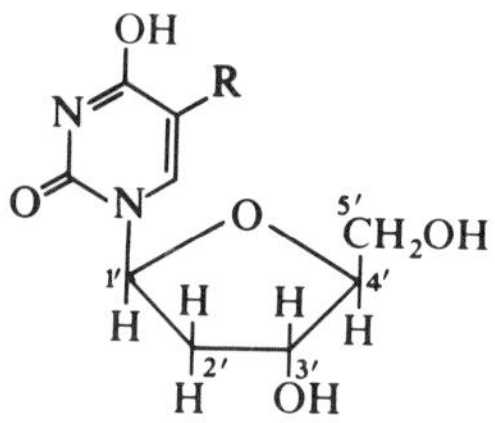

(4.49) R = I
(4.50) R = Me
(4.51) R = —CF$_3$

Clinically, IdU has been successful in curing a virus infection of the eye, herpetic keratitis, due to herpes simplex. This was hitherto a serious disease which was painful and long lasting and had no effective remedy. Selectivity depends upon the barrier imposed by the conjunctiva which prevents diffusion to other parts of the eye. IdU is also used in the treatment of herpes zoster (shingles) when it is applied as a solution in dimethylsulphoxide to the lesions.

Markedly less toxic is the analogous 5-iodo-5′-amino-2′,5′-dideoxyuridine whose 5′-N-phosphate is incorporated only into viral DNA.

The substitution of groups of comparable van der Waals' radii has led to the preparation of the trifluoromethyl analogue **(4.51)** of thymidine. Antiviral activity here proceeds via phosphorylation by thymidine kinase to the 5′-phosphate which is a potent inhibitor of thymidylate synthetase.

A more selective pyrimidine antimetabolite is cytosine arabinoside (1,β-D-arabinofuranosylcytosine, cytarabine, Ara-C **(4.52)**) used for treating generalized herpes infection by continuous intravenous infusion without seriously affecting the bone-marrow. The nucleoside is converted to the 5′-phosphate by deoxycytidine

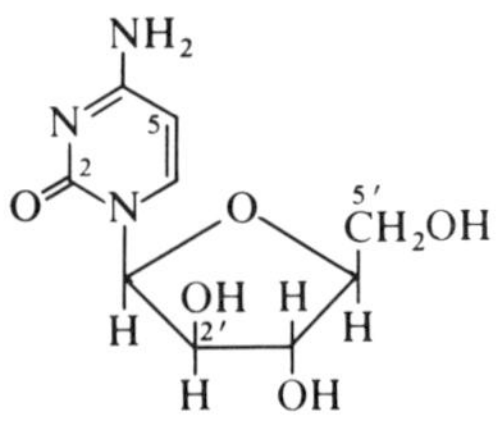

(4.52) 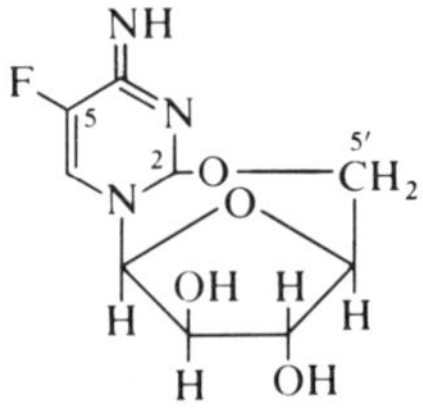   (4.52a)

kinase. This is followed by conversion to the triphosphate which has been shown to inhibit both DNA and RNA polymerases. Cytosine arabinoside further inhibits a nucleotide reductase enzyme which converts cytidine diphosphate to $2'$-deoxy cytidine diphosphate required for DNA synthesis.

Cytosine arabinoside is also one of the most effective single agents available for treating acute myeloblastic leukaemia, achieving remission rates of about 25% when used as a single agent. When combined with thioguanine or the cytotoxic antibiotic, daunorubicin, remission rates are increased to 50%. Newer combinations including vincristine have led to claims of 70% remission. Some long term survivals of myeloblastic leukaemia are being reported.

A disadvantage of cytosine arabinoside arises from rapid hepatic deamination by cytosine deaminase to the inactive uracil derivative. This short activity in the plasma is counteracted by continuous infusion methods of administration. Rapid deamination has led to a search for pyrimidine nucleoside deaminase inhibitors which could be given simultaneously. Lack of success here has led to the formulation of O-acyl derivatives which may be slowly cleaved by esterases to sustain low blood levels. 5-Fluoro-2,5'-anhydrocytosine arabinoside (4.52a) – a novel cyclonucleoside – is slowly non-enzymically hydrolysed in vivo to Ara-C. It has significant anti-tumour activity in adenocarcinoma of the stomach and pancreas.

A relatively new entry to the antiviral scene is the azole nucleoside, ribavirin, virazole, 1-β-D-ribofuranosyl-1,2,4-triazole-3-carboxamide (4.53). It is active against type A hepatitis, influenza A and B, measles and cutaneous infections caused by herpes viruses. There is some evidence to indicate that ribavirin inhibits the conversion of inosine-5'-phosphate to xanthosine-5'-phosphate in the biosynthetic route to nucleic acid. It may also selectively inhibit the synthesis of virus induced polypeptides without affecting normal cellular polypeptide synthesis.

It is widely held that many cancers may be virally induced. This has suggested

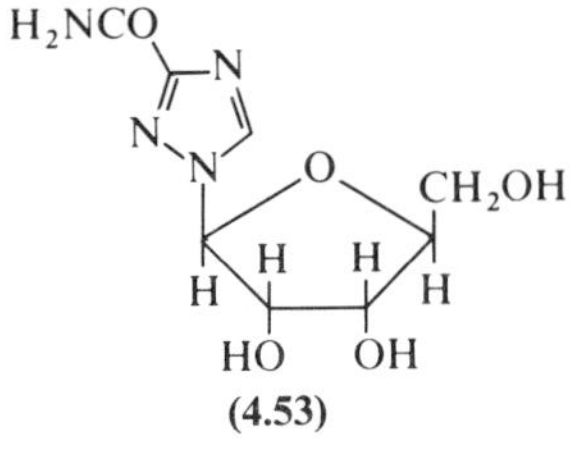

(4.53)

that a suitable antiviral agent may prevent reinduction of a cancer previously controlled by other chemical means. Attempts have been made to cure animal tumours by inhibiting reverse transcriptase from RNA viruses using cytosine arabinoside and virazole in addition to other anticancer drugs.

4.3.5 Peripheral aromatic amino acid decarboxylase (A.A.A.D.) inhibitors

Noradrenaline is synthesized at the nerve endings of the postganglionic fibre by a series of reactions from tyrosine (see Equation 4.19), the rate-determining step for the sequence being the hydroxylation of tyrosine by tyrosine hydroxylase.

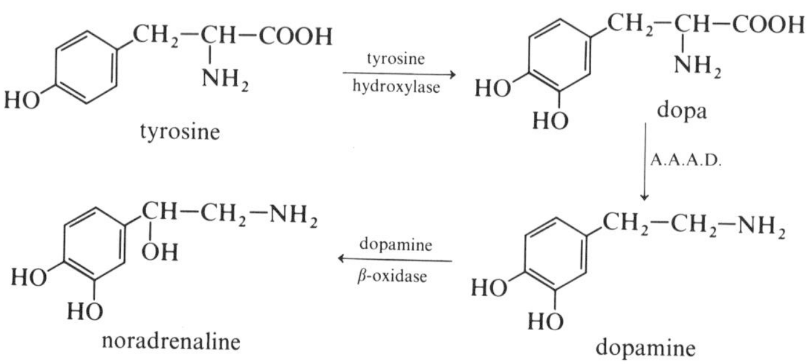

$$(4.19)$$

Inhibitors of A.A.A.D. have been synthesized as potential antihypertensive drugs on the basis that a decrease in the biosynthesis of noradrenaline would deplete noradrenaline stores at the nerve endings and lead to a decrease in blood pressure. Although many inhibitors of the enzyme are known from *in vitro* studies (e.g. methyldopa (4.55a)) only a few exert an antihypertensive action *in vivo* and probably by an alternative mechanism since the rate-determining step for the sequence is governed by tyrosine hydroxylase (see p. 130). However, this work led to the discovery of the inhibitors serazide (4.54) and carbidopa (4.55b) which have

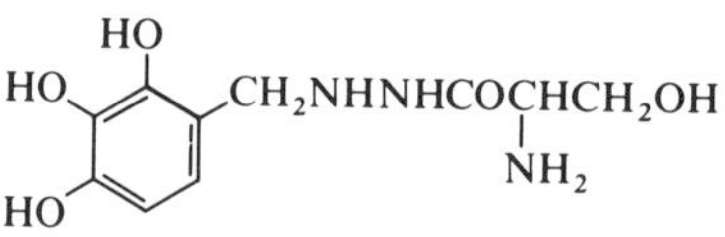

serazide
(4.54)

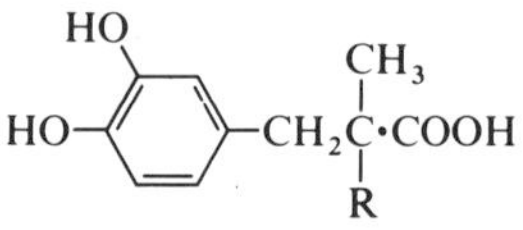

(4.55a) R = NH$_2$ methyldopa
(4.55b) R = NHNH$_2$ carbidopa

proved useful as adjuvants in the treatment of Parkinson's disease with L-dopa, L-dopa penetrates into the basal ganglia of the brain where it is decarboxylated to the active agent, dopamine. Large doses of L-dopa are required in therapy since it is depleted in the plasma by peripheral A.A.A.D. to dopamine which is readily removed by monoamine oxidase. Combination of L-dopa with serazide or carbidopa leads to decreased metabolism of L-dopa so that smaller effective doses can be used in therapy which have fewer side-effects than large doses. Necessary features of these inhibitors are that they do not penetrate the blood–brain barrier and interfere with the decarboxylation of L-dopa to dopamine in the brain and neither do they reduce the synthesis of endogenous amines in the peripheral tissues.

4.3.6 Carbonic anhydrase inhibitors

The enzyme carbonic anhydrase is well distributed in the body but that situated in the cells lining the renal tubule is responsible for regulating acid–base balance. This is achieved by catalytic hydration of carbon dioxide to carbonic acid which then enables the exchange of hydrogen ions for sodium ions in the tubular urine, the latter being reabsorbed. Inhibitors of the enzyme exert a diuretic effect since the excreted sodium ions carry a shell of water molecules with them.

One of the early noted side-effects of sulphanilamide therapy was the production of an alkaline urine and this was eventually associated with inhibition of kidney carbonic anhydrase. Since then, many less toxic molecules containing the sulphonamide group have been synthesized as potential diuretics. One of the first drugs used clinically was acetazolamide (4.56) which was not useful for the treatment of chronic conditions since the acidosis produced in the body by excretion of sodium bicarbonate decreased its activity. Related developments led to the discovery of the chlorthiazide (4.57) group of diuretics in current use, where

$$CH_3CONH \overset{N-N}{\underset{S}{\bigtriangleup}} SO_2NH_2$$

acetazolamide
(4.56)

chlorthiazide
(4.57)

diuresis is associated with loss of sodium and chloride ions so that long-term treatment does not cause acidosis. The chlorothiazide group of drugs, although inhibitors of carbonic anhydrase, are not considered at the dose-levels used in therapy to primarily exert their action in this manner, but act by reducing the reabsorption of electrolytes from the renal tubules thereby increasing the excretion of sodium and chloride ions. Sulthiame, tetrahydro-2-p-sulphamoylphenyl-2H-1,2-thiazine-1,1-dioxide, is a carbonic anhydrase inhibitor which is used in epilepsy associated with behaviour disorders. Sulthiame inhibits brain carbonic anhydrase which results in an increased carbon dioxide level in the brain. Excess carbon dioxide decreases nerve conduction and consequently electrical activity in the brain.

4.3.7 Acetylcholinesterase inhibitors

Acetylcholine is the chemical transmitter released at the nerve endings in the parasympathetic and motor nervous systems following a nervous impulse. After a response from the tissue the acetylcholine is removed by hydrolysis to inert

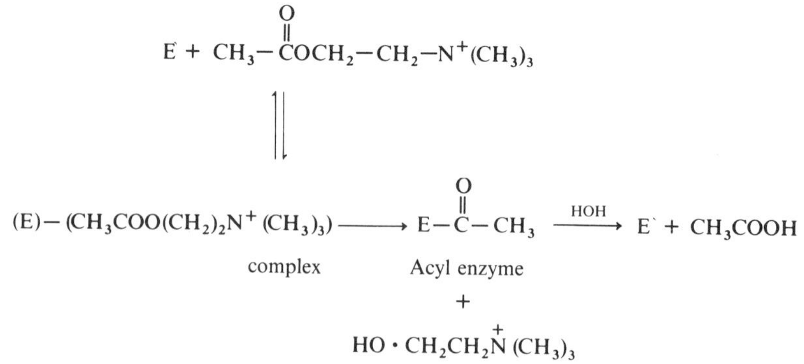

$$E + CH_3 - \overset{\overset{\displaystyle O}{\|}}{C}OCH_2 - CH_2 - N^+(CH_3)_3$$

$$(E) - (CH_3COO(CH_2)_2N^+(CH_3)_3) \longrightarrow E - \overset{\overset{\displaystyle O}{\|}}{C} - CH_3 \overset{HOH}{\longrightarrow} E + CH_3COOH$$

complex   Acyl enzyme

+

$$HO \cdot CH_2CH_2\overset{+}{N}(CH_3)_3 \qquad\qquad (4.20)$$

products by acetylcholinesterase (see Equation 4.20) in the proximity. Inhibitors of acetylcholinesterase allow a build-up of acetylcholine at the nerve endings so that a more prolonged effect is produced which is useful in the treatment of myasthenia gravis, a disease associated with the rapid fatigue of muscles, as well as in the treatment of glaucoma where stimulation of the ciliary body improves drainage from the eye and decreases intra-ocular pressure.

Inhibitors of acetylcholinesterase fall into two groups: the 'reversible' carbamate inhibitors such as eserine (physostigmine (4.63)), neostigmine (4.58) and benzyl-pyrinium (4.59) and the irreversible organophosphorus inhibitors, dyflos (4.60a) and ecothiopate (4.60b). The carbamates carry a positive charge and are bound at the anionic site (carboxylate ion) of the enzyme and correctly positioned to form a carbamyl enzyme with the serine hydroxyl group at the esteratic site (see Equation 4.21). The carbamyl enzyme is only slowly decomposed ($t_{\frac{1}{2}} = \simeq 20$ min) and in the presence of excess inhibitor the enzyme is partially locked up in this form so that its activity towards the substrate acetylcholine is decreased. Dilution or removal of excess inhibitor leads to a shift in the steady-state inhibition level with an increase

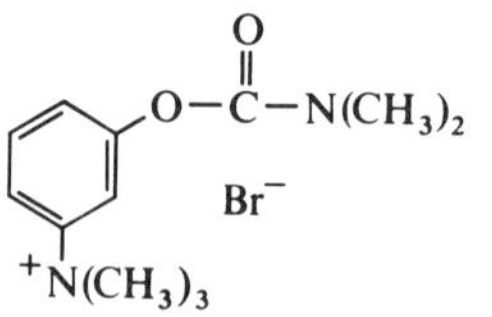

neostigmine
(4.58)

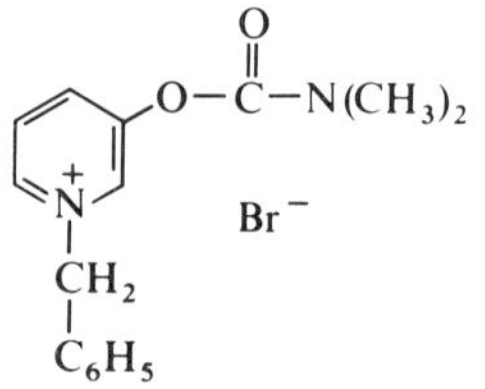

benzylpyrinium
(4.59)

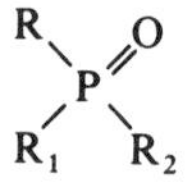

(4.60a) $R = R_1 = -OCH(CH_3)_2$, $R_2 = F$ dyflos
(4.60b) $R = R_1 = -OCH_2CH_3$, $R_2 = -S \cdot CH_2 \cdot CH_2 \cdot NMe_3$ ecothiopate
(4.60c) $R = -CH_3$, $R_1 = -O \cdot CH(CH_3)_2$, $R_2 = F$ sarin
(4.60d) $R = -O \cdot CH_2 \cdot CH_3$, $R_1 = N(CH_3)_2$, $R_2 = -CN$ tabun

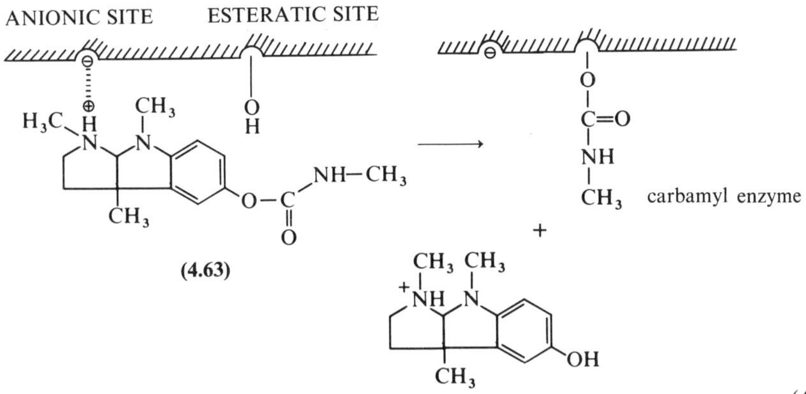

(4.21)

in activity of the enzyme. This observation originally gave the impression that the carbamates were reversible competitive inhibitors of the enzyme.

The organophosphorus compounds rapidly react with the enzyme to form a stable phosphoryl enzyme and the enzyme is irreversibly inhibited (*see* Equation 4.22).

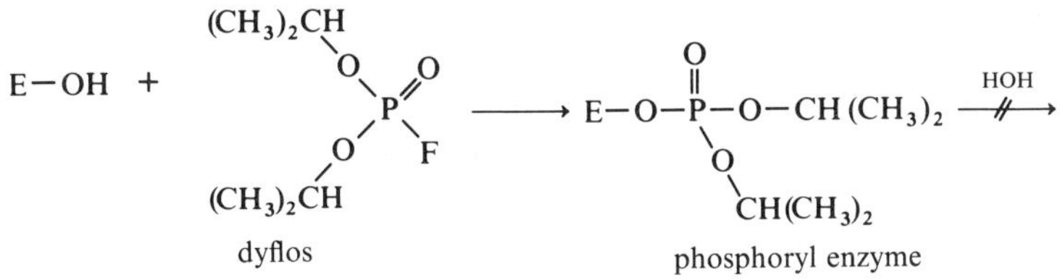

(4.22)

The organophosphorus compounds have a long duration of action in the body after a single dose of the drug and enzyme activity only returns after synthesis of fresh enzyme. Due to dangers of overdosage, as well as handling, they are little used except for treatment of glaucoma where the other less toxic carbamate drugs have not proved satisfactory in a particular therapy,

Volatile organophosphorus compounds such as sarin (**4.60c**) and tabun (**4.60d**) have been prepared for use as nerve gases in war and other less volatile compounds have been used as insecticides for the spraying of crops. Inhibition of the mammalian or insect enzyme leads to a build-up of acetylcholine and death from accumulated acetylcholine poisoning.

Much research has been carried out to find antidotes, for nerve gas poisoning, which could be distributed to the population in the event of war. One of these discoveries, pyridine-2-aldoxime mesylate (pralidoxime (**4.61**) has been successfully used, in conjunction with atropine to block the action of acetylcholine on receptors, in the treatment of accidental poisoning during crop spraying. Pralidoxime is considered to complex at the anionic site where it is firmly held by electrostatic attraction in the correct spacial configuration for attack by the oxime anion on the phosphorus atom with displacement of the inhibitor residue from the

pralidoxime
(4.61)

TMB-4
(4.62)

enzyme. A more recent development was the compound TMB-4 **(4.62)** which is a more powerful reactivator of the inhibited enzyme than pralidoxime but its use has been restricted to animal experiments.

4.3.8 Angiotensin-converting enzyme inhibitors

Angiotensin-converting enzyme (peptidyldipeptide carboxy hydrolase) converts the inactive decapeptide angiotensin I (AI) to the vasoconstrictor octapeptide angiotensin II (AII) (*see* Equation 4.23) and is a key enzymic component of the

$$\text{Asp-Arg-Val-Tyr-Ile-His-Pro-Phe}|\text{His-Leu} \xrightarrow[\text{enzyme}]{\substack{\text{angiotensin}\\\text{converting}}} \text{Asp-Arg-Val-Tyr-Ile-His-Pro-Phe}$$

angiotensin I   angiotensin II   (4.23)

renin–angiotensin system which helps to maintain blood pressure following events such as haemorrhage, which lower the blood volume. Studies on peptides isolated from snake venoms showed that the pentapeptide, Glu-Lys-Trp-Ala-Pro was an inhibitor of the enzyme and had a short-acting antihypertensive action. Many analogues were subsequently synthesized and the nonapeptide, Glu-Trp-Pro-Arg-Pro-Gln-Ile-Pro-Pro (SQ, 20 881, teprotide) was studied clinically and shown, on parenteral administration, to be a safe and effective antihypertensive drug for treatment of many forms of hypertension, although it had the disadvantage of not being orally active and less useful for long term therapy. Little was known at that time concerning the structure of the active site of the enzyme and the manner in which the natural substrate was bound, so insufficient information was available from this source for the design of more stable and efficient inhibitors. The observation that the enzyme was a zinc metalloprotein and the fact that its substrate specificity resembled that of the zinc-containing carboxypeptidase A about which much was known (*see also* p. 147) led to the premise that the active sites of the two enzymes bore some similarity although there were obvious differences. Cleavage of carboxyl-terminal dipeptides occurred with angiotensin-converting enzyme whereas only single carboxyl-terminal amino acids were released by carboxypeptidase A. Guesses were made as to the structural features present in angiotensin-converting enzyme which could account for these differences and these guesses provided a basis for the design of potential inhibitors of the enzyme. This work eventually led to the discovery of captopril **(4.64)** which is a non-toxic orally active antihypertensive agent which exerts its action by specifically inhibiting angiotensin-converting enzyme. However, whether its clinical effect is due to either inhibiting the formation of angiotensin II or by inhibiting destruction of the vasodilator peptide, bradykinin, (another action of the enzyme) is not clear.

4.3.9 β-Lactamase inhibitors

β-Lactamases are enzymes produced by certain bacteria (*see* p. 253) which catalyse the hydrolysis of the β-lactam ring of certain penicillins (4.65) and cephalosporins

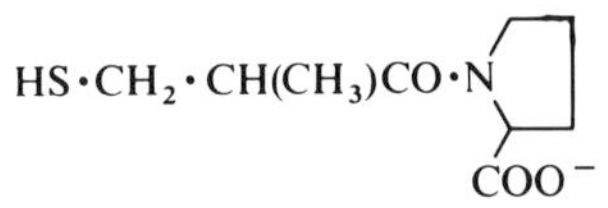

captopril
(4.64)

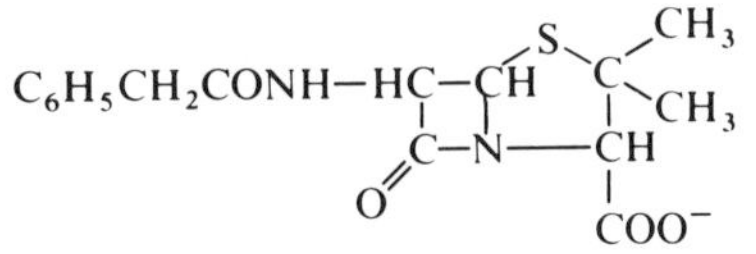

benzyl penicillin
(4.65)

(4.66) to give inert products so that the organism is resistant to these types of antibiotics. This resistance to β-lactam antibiotics can be overcome by the use of β-lactamase inhibitors as adjuvants in therapy.

Clavulanic acid (4.67), isolated from *Streptomyces clavigerus*, although a poor antibiotic, is an irreversible inhibitor of β-lactamases and lowers the effective β-lactam antibiotic concentration towards a large number of resistant bacteria. The sulphone, CP-45 899 (4.68) has a similar spectrum of synergistic action.

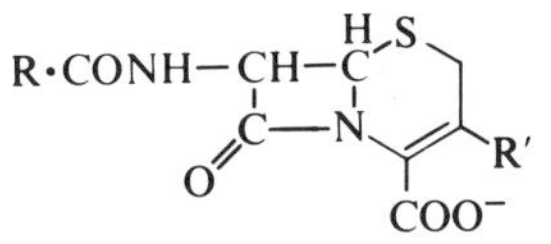

cephalosporin
(4.66)

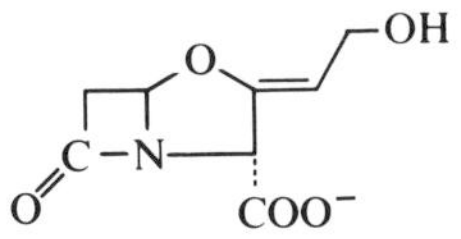

clavulanic acid
(4.67)

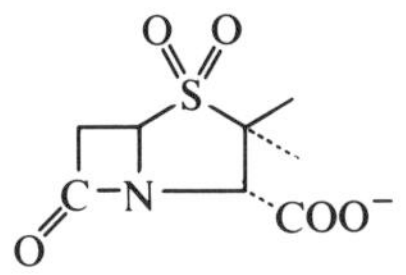

CP-45 899
(4.68)

β-Lactam antibiotics probably form an acyl-enzyme with the β-lactamase, as shown in (4.69), which is hydrolysed to the products of the reaction, the 6-substituent determining the rate of hydrolysis. Reaction with clavulanic acid or CP-45 899 is considered to proceed in a similar manner. However, clavulanic acid is a poor substrate of the enzyme so that the lifetime of the acyl-enzyme is extended and this permits the lactam residue of the acyl-enzyme to undergo other reactions

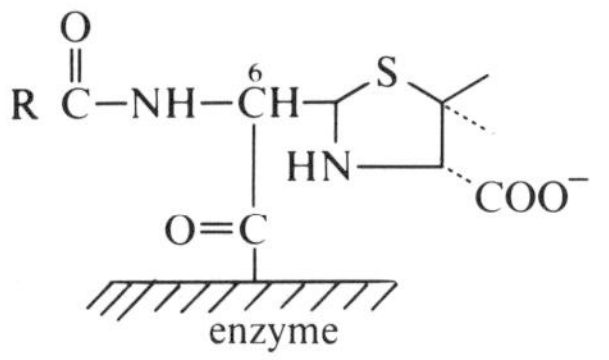

enzyme
(4.69)

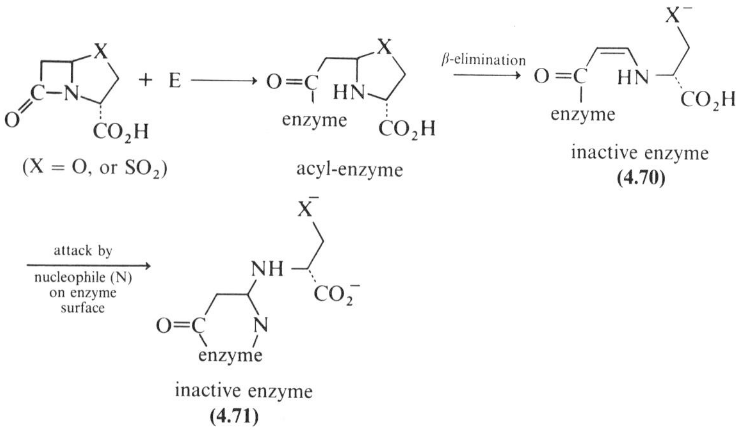

$$(4.24)$$

whilst still attached to the protein. A proposed reaction (*see* Equation 4.24) is a β-elimination to give the inactive enzyme (**4.70**). Further reaction occurs within (**4.70**) whereby a nucleophile on the protein surface reacts with the inhibitor residue to give another form (**4.71**) of the inactive enzyme. Although the main pathway for the reaction is deacylation of the acyl-enzyme, clavulanic acid inhibits the enzyme after 150 turnovers due to progressive conversion of the acyl enzyme to (**4.70**) and (**4.71**), whereas CP-45 899 (**4.68**) inhibits after 4500 turnovers. These inhibitors could be termed k_{cat} inhibitors (*see* p. 124).

A mixture of amoxycillin and clavulanic acid in the ratio 2:1 for oral administration has recently been marketed. The two components have identical rates of absorption, which is a necessary requirement for this type of preparation, otherwise the antibiotic would be depleted in the tissues by the β-lactamase before the inhibitor becomes available.

4.4 CURRENT RATIONAL APPROACHES TO THE DESIGN OF ENZYME INHIBITORS

4.4.1 Introduction

The majority of drugs exert their action in the body by interacting with a collection of atoms or groups of atoms constituting a drug receptor. The receptor for enzyme inhibitors is a specific enzyme which, fortunately for design purposes, can usually be isolated and studied *in vitro*. These studies provide relevant information concerning its substrate specificity, coenzyme activators, the functional groupings present at the active site and even the precise arrangement and composition of the active site when crystallographic studies are possible. From this knowledge, predictions can be made regarding the structural features required in inhibitors of the enzyme.

Current research on the rational design of inhibitors falls mainly into three areas: active site-directed irreversible inhibitors, transition state analogues as reversible inhibitors and k_{cat} inhibitors (suicide inactivators). There has been interest, recently, in classical reversible inhibitors but the most profitable work has been restricted to the angiotensin-converting enzyme inhibitors (*see* p. 112) and anticancer drugs (*see* p. 106) considered previously.

4.4.2   Active site-directed irreversible inhibitors

These inhibitors resemble the substrate sufficiently to form a reversible enzyme–inhibitor complex, analogous to the enzyme–substrate complex, within which reaction occurs between functional groups on the inhibitor and enzyme. A stable covalent bond is formed with irreversible inhibition of the enzyme. Active site-directed irreversible inhibitors are designed to exhibit specificity towards their target-enzymes since they are structurally modelled on the specific substrate of the enzyme concerned. This approach has also been referred to as affinity-labelling.

4.4.2.1   *α-Chymotrypsin inhibitors*

One of the first inhibitors to be designed using this concept was toluenesulphonyl-L-phenylalanyl chloromethylketone (TPCK **(4.72)**) which is an inhibitor of α-chymotrypsin. Substrates of α-chymotrypsin bind in a hydrophobic cavity, at the

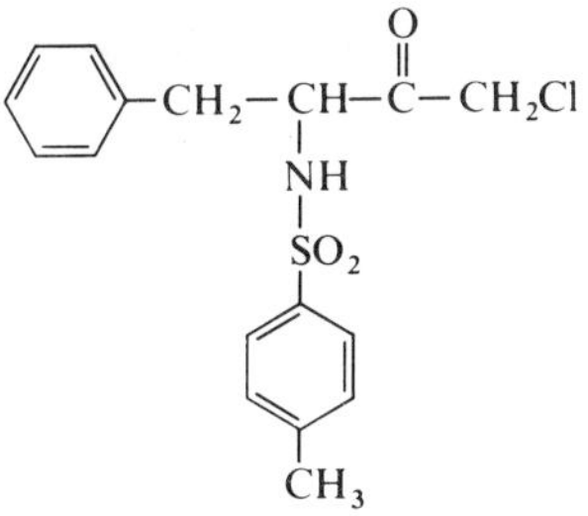

(4.72)

active site, by means of the flat aromatic or hetero-aromatic rings of their phenylalanyl, tyrosinyl or tryptophanyl residues. Additional hydrogen bonding between the Ser-214 hydroxyl group and the α-NH group of the substrate correctly positions the labile ester, amide or peptide linkage for reaction with the Ser-195 hydroxyl group with formation of an acyl-enzyme. The hydroxyl function is activated by the electron relay system, Asp-102 – His-57 – Ser-195, which forms the catalytic part of the active site. Deacylation to give the product of the reaction, with regeneration of the enzyme, is catalysed by the same relay system where the nucleophile is water.

TPCK is based on a substrate of the enzyme, ethyl toluenesulphonyl-L-phenylalanine, where the labile ester group has been replaced by an alkylating chloromethylketone group. When the inhibitor is bound at the active site, the alkylating function is positioned in a similar manner to the ester group of the substrate and is able to alkylate His-57 (*see* Fig. 4.4 and Equation 4.25). This

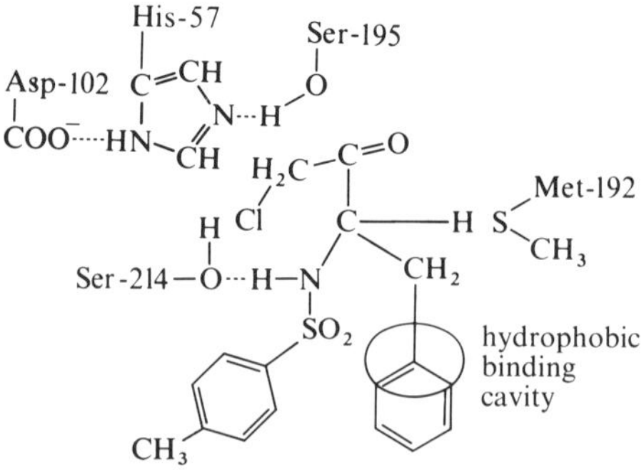

Fig. 4.4 Schematic representation of binding of TPCK at active site of α-chymotrypsin.

reaction removes the catalytic properties of the enzyme as well as blocking access of substrate molecules to the site.

Other active site-directed inhibitors of α-chymotrypsin, without the α-NH group, are not bound in the same stereochemical disposition as TPCK so that the alkylating function has a greater choice of nucleophilic group with which to react. Phenacyl chloride (4.73) reacts with the thiomethyl group of Met-192, which forms a lid to the hydrophobic cavity, to give the sulphonium salt (see Equation 4.26).

Other proteases which have similar substrate specificities and so are clearly

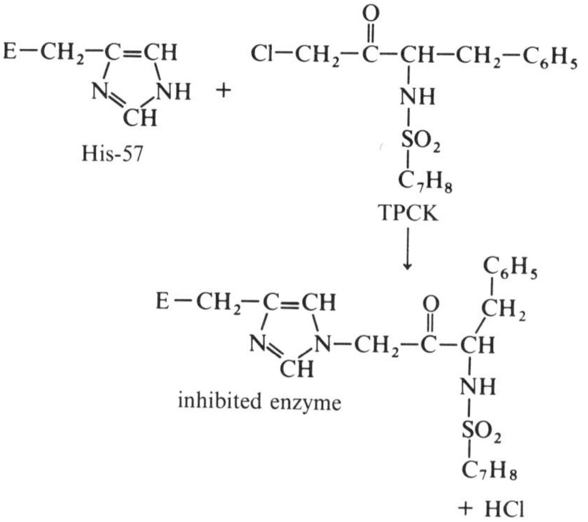

(4.25)

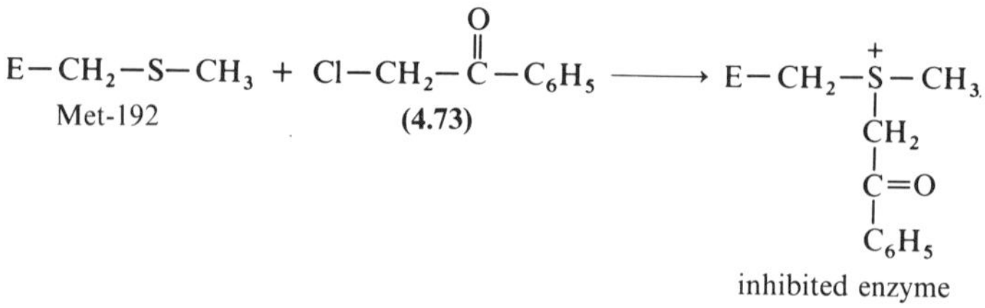

(4.26)

related to α-chymotrypsin are also inhibited by TPCK, but proteases with widely different substrate specificites such as trypsin and elastase are not inhibited.

4.4.2.2   *Trypsin and trypsin-like enzyme inhibitors*

The active site of trypsin is similar to that of α-chymotrypsin except that a carboxyl ion (from Asp-177) occurs at the bottom of the binding cavity. Trypsin shows specificity to suitably substituted derivatives of lysine and arginine where the protonated basic side-chains are bound in the cavity. TLCK, the lysine analogue of TPCK, is a good inhibitor of trypsin. The inhibitor is bound at the active site of trypsin, in a similar manner to that described for the binding of TPCK to α-chymotrypsin, and alkylates the catalytic His-46 residue (equivalent to His-57 in α-chymotrypsin). TLCK does not inhibit α-chymotrypsin since the protonated side-chain of the lysine residue cannot be accommodated, on thermodynamic grounds, in the hydrophobic cavity of α-chymotrypsin.

There are many enzymes with trypsin-like activity in the body which exert different functions in the processes of blood coagulation, fibrinolysis, kinin production, complement action and fertilization. TLCK is an inhibitor of trypsin-like enzymes and this lack of specificity precludes its possible use as a drug for potentially thrombolytic patients where inhibition of the enzyme thrombin, as it is released in the blood-clotting process, would prevent clot formation.

Polypeptide inhibitors based on a terminal chloromethyl ketone derivative of arginine have been recently designed which are capable of differentiating between the enzymes of this group. One of the inhibitors, D-Phe-Pro-Arg-CH$_2$Cl, inhibits thrombin very fast, at concentrations as low as 10^{-9} M, with a second-order rate constant (k_2, *see* p. 92) which is about 2500 times greater than that for the reaction with kallikrein. The reactions with the closely related enzymes, Factor Xc and plasmin, are even slower. The selectivity of this type of *flexible* active site-directed polypeptide inhibitor, within this group of enzymes, is due to the affinity (K_i) of the inhibitor for the active site. This is made possible by differences in binding at sub-sites associated with amino acid residues on the enzyme surface outside the primary hydrophobic binding site. Effectiveness for thrombin inhibition depends particularly upon binding by the second from terminal amino acid residue of the inhibitor where enhanced binding occurs with a D-amino acid residue.

4.4.2.3   *Elastase inhibitors*

It is a general belief that pulmonary emphysema results from the uninhibited proteolysis of lung tissue (elastin) by elastase and related neutral proteases derived from lysosomes released from degraded leukocytes and macrophages. Under normal circumstances, where infection or inflammation of the lung leads to increased lysosome release, proteolytic digestion of lung tissue is warded off by the circulating macromolecular protease inhibitor, α-antitrypsin. Individuals with an α$_1$-antitrypsin deficiency are not protected in this manner and develop emphysema.

Synthetic elastase inhibitors could be useful agents for the treatment of this disease.

Elastase possesses an active site similar in structure to that for α-chymotrypsin, trypsin and subtilisin but with only a small cup for the hydrophobic binding site due to protrusion of Val-209 and Thr-221 residues into the cavity. These two amino acids replace the smaller glycine residues in α-chymotrypsin. Since the natural substrate (elastin) has a high content of alanine, proline and glycine residues, synthetic polypeptide inhibitors have been designed containing alanine and proline residues together with a terminal alanyl chloromethyl ketone residue, e.g. Ac-Ala-Ala-Pro-Ala-CH$_2$Cl.

Studies with peptide substrates have shown that elastase possesses an extended substrate binding site consisting of a main hydrophobic binding 'cavity' (P_1) together with, at least, four binding sub-sites (P_2–P_5). The reactivity of the alanine peptide chloromethyl ketones towards elastase is related to the number of amino acid residues present in the inhibitor. The tetrapeptide inhibitors, which possess a residue for binding to the sub-site P_4, are usually 10–50 times more reactive than the tripeptides.

Simple analogues of peptide chloromethyl ketones, e.g. Tos-Ala-CH$_2$Cl (c.f. TPCK and TLCK), do not inhibit elastase. This difference shows the importance in elastase of cumulative binding of its substrates and inhibitors at several points on the enzyme surface. This is due to relative weak binding at the hydrophobic 'cavity' (P_1) in contrast to the stronger binding which occurs in the deeper cavity of α-chymotrypsin and trypsin.

4.4.3   Transition state analogues as reversible enzyme inhibitors

4.4.3.1   *Introduction*

An organic reaction between two types of molecules is considered to proceed through a high energy activated complex known as the transition state which is formed by collision of molecules with greater kinetic energy than the majority present in the reaction. The energy required for formation of the transition state is the activation energy for the reaction and is the barrier to the reaction occurring spontaneously. The transition state may break down to give either the components from which it was formed or the products of the reaction. The transition state for the reaction between hydroxyl ion and methyl iodide is shown in Equation 4.27

$$
\text{OH}^- + \underset{\substack{\\ \text{H} \quad \text{H}}}{\overset{\text{H}}{\text{C}}}\!\!-\!\!\text{I} \;\longrightarrow\; \left[\text{HO}\cdots\underset{\substack{\\ \text{H} \quad \text{H}}}{\overset{\text{H}}{\text{C}}}\cdots\text{I}\right]^- \;\longrightarrow\; \text{HO}-\underset{\substack{\\ \text{H} \quad \overset{}{\text{H}}}}{\overset{\text{H}}{\text{C}}} \; + \text{I}^- \qquad (4.27)
$$

and the energy diagram for the reaction in Fig. 4.5. The transition state shown depicts both commencement of formation of a C—OH bond and the breaking of the C—I bond. Enzymes catalyse organic reactions by lowering the activation

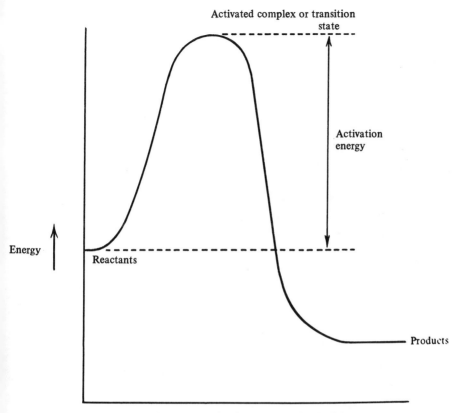

Fig. 4.5   Energy changes for the reaction between methyl iodide and hydroxyl ion.

energy for the reaction and one view is that they accomplish this by straining or distorting the bound substrate towards the transition state. Equation 4.28 shows a single substrate–enzymatic reaction and the corresponding non-enzymatic reaction where $ES^{\ddagger}$ and $S^{\ddagger\prime}$ represent the transition states for the enzymatic and non-enzymatic reaction, respectively, and $K_N^{\ddagger}$ and $K_E^{\ddagger}$ are equilibrium constants, respectively, for their formation. K_S is the association constant for formation of ES from E and S, and K_T is the association constant for the hypothetical reaction involving the binding of $S^{\ddagger\prime}$ to E. Analysis of the relationships between these equilibrium constants shows that $K_T K_N^{\ddagger} = K_S K_E^{\ddagger}$. Since the equilibrium constant for a reaction is equal to the rate constant multiplied by h/kT, where h is Planck's constant and k is Boltzmann's constant, then $K_T = K_S(k_E/k_N)$, where k_E and k_N

$$
\begin{array}{ccccc}
E + S & \xrightarrow{K_N^{\ddagger}} & E + S^{\ddagger\prime} & \longrightarrow & E + P \\
K_s \updownarrow & & K_T \updownarrow & & \updownarrow \\
ES & \underset{K_E^{\ddagger}}{\rightleftharpoons} & ES^{\ddagger} & \longrightarrow & EP
\end{array}
\qquad (4.28)
$$

are the first-order rate constants for breakdown of the ES complex and the non-enzymatic reaction, respectively. Since the ratio k_E/k_N is usually of the order 10^{10} or greater, it follows that $K_T \gg K_S$. This means that the transition state $S^{\ddagger\prime}$ is considered to bind to the enzyme at least 10^{10} times more tightly than the substrate.

4.4.3.2   *Transition state analogues*

A transition state analogue is a stable compound that structurally resembles the substrate portion of the unstable transition state of an enzymic reaction. Since the bond-breaking and bond-making mechanism of the enzyme-catalysed and non-enzymatic reaction are similar, then the analogue will resemble $S^{\ddagger\prime}$ and have an enormous affinity for the enzyme compared to the substrate and consequently will be bound more tightly. It would not be possible to design a *stable* compound which mimics the transition state closely since the transition state itself is unstable by possessing partially broken and/or made covalent bonds. Even crude transition state analogues of substrate reactions would be expected to be sufficiently tightly bound to the enzyme to be excellent reversible inhibitors. This expectation has been borne out in practice.

4.4.3.3   *Design of transition state analogues*

Design of a transition state analogue for a specific enzyme requires a knowledge of the mechanism of the enzymatic reaction. Fortunately the main structural features of the transition states for the majority of enzymatic reactions are either known or can be predicted with some confidence. Examples are now considered of transition state analogues which are inhibitors of enzymes catalysing reactions with a wide variety of transition state structures.

(a) Analogues of carbanion-like transition states   Several enzyme-catalysed reactions pass through a transition state resembling an enolate ion **(4.74)** and these systems are inhibited by a carboxylate ion **(4.75)** due to the resemblance in charge distribution between the two ions. Phosphoglycolic acid **(4.76)** resembles the metastable enediolate intermediate **(4.77)** that occurs in the interconversion of

dihydroxyacetone phosphate and glyceraldehyde-3-phosphate, catalysed by triosephosphate isomerase (*see* Equation 4.29), and is a reversible inhibitor of the enzyme. The potency (P) of the inhibitor is given by the ratio, association constant for binding of inhibitor : association constant for binding of substrate and equals 75.

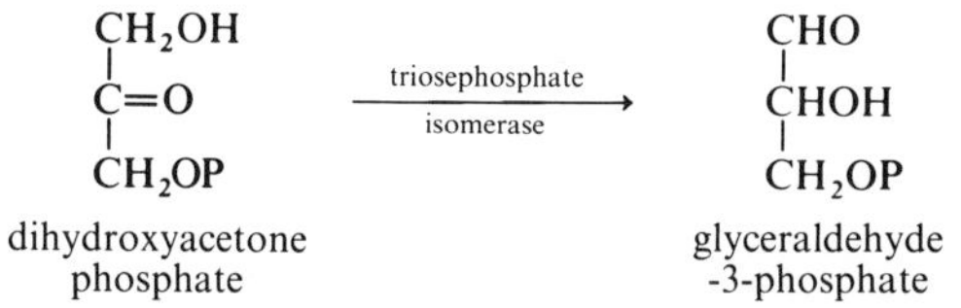

$$
\begin{array}{ccc}
\begin{array}{c} CH_2OH \\ | \\ C=O \\ | \\ CH_2OP \end{array}
& \xrightarrow[\text{isomerase}]{\text{triosephosphate}} &
\begin{array}{c} CHO \\ | \\ CHOH \\ | \\ CH_2OP \end{array}
\end{array}
\qquad (4.29)
$$

dihydroxyacetone
phosphate   glyceraldehyde
-3-phosphate

(b) Carbonium ion-like transition state   Glycosyl-transferring enzymes catalyse reactions which pass through a transition state, comprising an alkoxy carbonium ion **(4.78)**, where a positive charge is distributed over the sugar ring oxygen and the C-1 carbon atom. D-Glucono-δ-lactone **(4.79)**, which has a similar charge distribution on the ring oxygen and C-1 carbon atoms and a similar half chair conformation as the transition state **(4.78)**, is an inhibitor of these reactions ($P = 10\,000$). The antibiotic norjirimycin **(4.80)** is an even better transition state analogue inhibitor of the enzyme for the same reason.

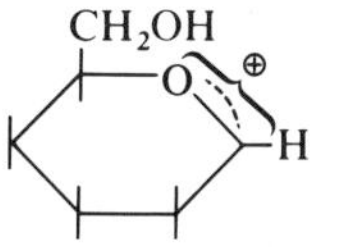

(4.78) 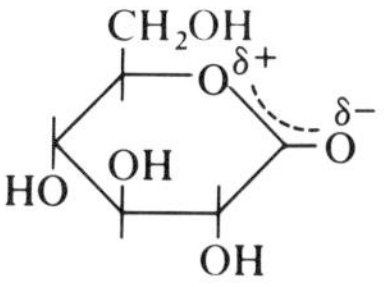   **(4.79)** 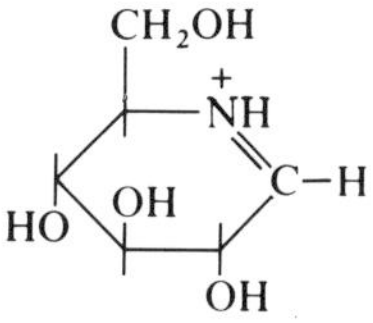   **(4.80)**

(c) Phosphoryl transfer   The transition state for most phosphoryl transfer reactions is probably a trigonal bipyramid of pentacovalent phosphorus, with entering and leaving groups (X and Y) as shown in **(4.81)**.

Ribonuclease catalyses the hydrolysis of uridine-2′,3′-cyclic phosphate **(4.83)** to uridine-3′-phosphate **(4.85)** through the transition state **(4.84)** (*see* Equation 4.30).

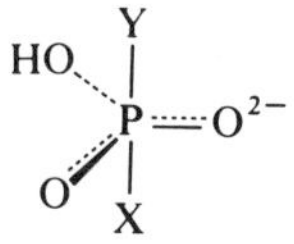

(4.81)

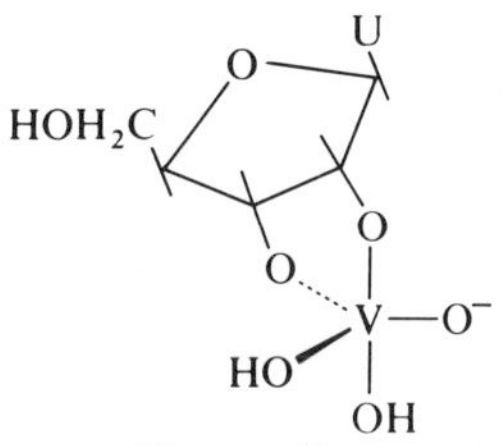

U = uracil
(4.82)

The oxovanadium ion–uridine complex **(4.82)** is an inhibitor of this reaction ($P = 1700$) due to its close resemblance to the transition state **(4.84)**.

(d) Tetrahedral transition states   It has been established that many proteases and esterases catalyse the reactions of their substrates through an acyl-enzyme intermediate which is subsequently hydrolysed to the products of the reaction. (*see*

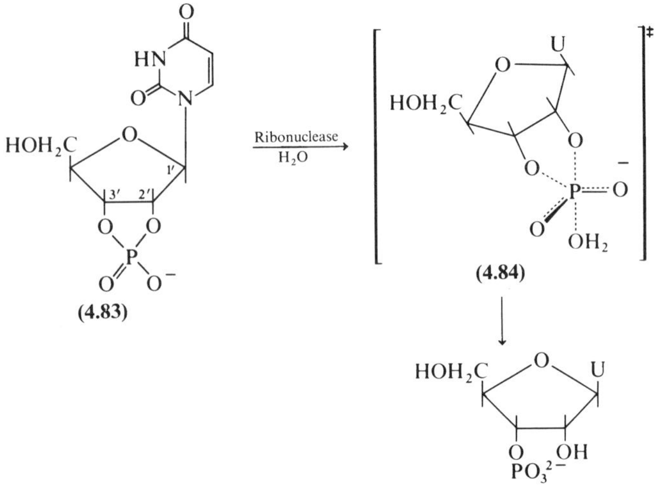

(4.83)

(4.84)

(4.85)

$$(4.30)$$

$$E + S \rightleftharpoons \underset{\text{complex}}{ES} \xrightarrow{k_2} \underset{\substack{\text{acyl-enzyme} \\ + P_1}}{ES'} \xrightarrow[\text{HOH}]{k_3} E + P_2$$

$$(4.31)$$

Equation 4.31). The ES-complex breaks down through a tetrahedral transition state which is probably very similar to the tetrahedral intermediate **(4.86)** as illustrated for α-chymotrypsin-catalysis in Equation 4.32.

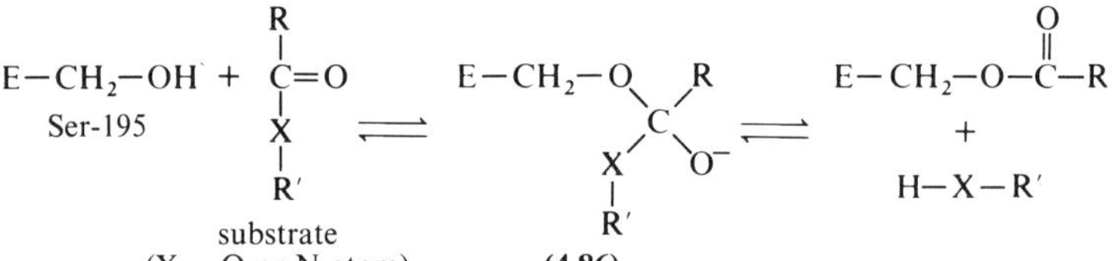

$$(4.32)$$

2-Phenylethane boronic acid **(4.87)** is an inhibitor of α-chymotrypsin. Its specificity is derived from the aryl residue which can bind in the hydrophobic cavity at the active site (*see* p. 115) and its resemblance to the transition state **(4.86)** is due to its ability to form an anionic tetrahedral adduct **(4.88)** in dilute basic solution. The adduct **(4.89)** formed here is not considered to be derived from hydroxyl ion in the media but from the activated hydroxyl group of Ser-195 normally involved in catalysis of the substrate.

Other boron derivatives are specific inhibitors of other enzymes, their specificity being derived from the structure of the side-chain, e.g. subtilisin ($C_6H_5 \cdot B(OH)_2$, $P = 2 \times 10^2$), acetylcholinesterase (($CH_3)_3\overset{+}{N}(CH_2)_3 \cdot B(OH)_2$, $P = 10^4$), glutamyl transpeptidase ($-OOC-CH(\overset{+}{N}H_3)CH_2OB(OH)_2$, $P = 10^6$) and lipase ($CH_3(CH_2)_{16}B(OH)_2$, $P = 2 \cdot 5 \times 10^3$).

Elastase is a serine protease and hydrolyses suitable substrates containing proline or alanine residues on the carboxyl side of these residues. The reaction

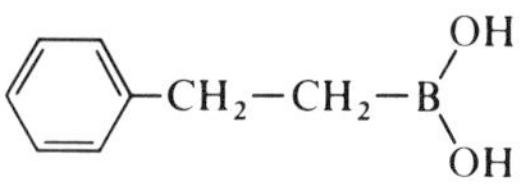

(4.87)

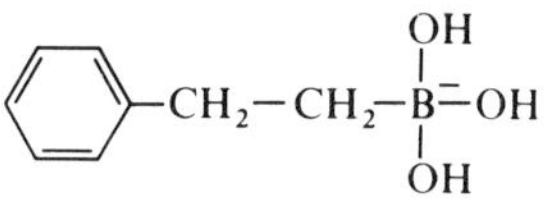

(4.88)

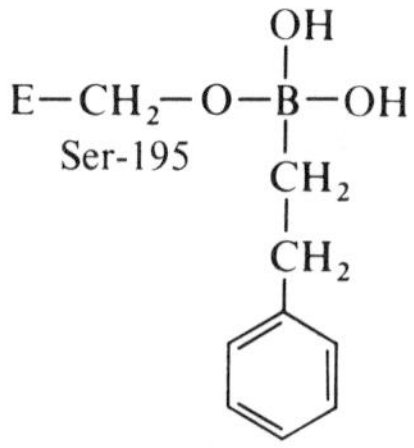

(4.89)

sequence is similar to that for α-chymotrypsin and passes through a tetrahedral intermediate and acyl-enzyme.

A number of polypeptides, where the terminal carboxyl group has been replaced by an aldehyde group, are potent competitive inhibitors of elastase. Aldehydes form stable tetrahedral addition complexes such as the hydrate and hemiacetal which are sometimes more stable in solution, e.g. glucose. It has been suggested that aldehyde inhibitors form a stable hemiacetal structure (4.90) with the

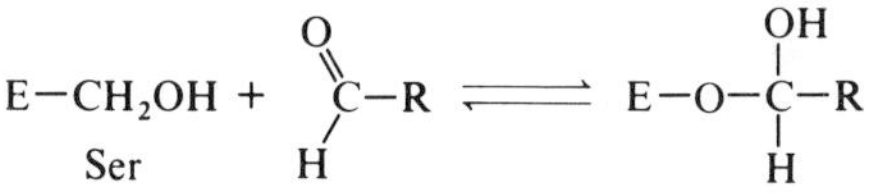

(4.33)

(4.90)

hydroxyl function of serine at the active site and this resembles the tetrahedral transition state for the enzyme-catalysed reaction. The aldehyde inhibitor, Ac-Pro-Ala-Pro-Alaninal, binds 5000 times more strongly to the enzyme than the corresponding amide (substrate) and 750 times more strongly than the corresponding alcohol.

Another type of enzyme, adenosine deaminase, converts adenosine (4.91) to inosine (4.93) and is also capable of displacing other groups and atoms from the 6-position of purine ribonucleotides. The tetrahedral intermediate (4.92) is considered to have a similar structure to the transition state for the reaction. One of

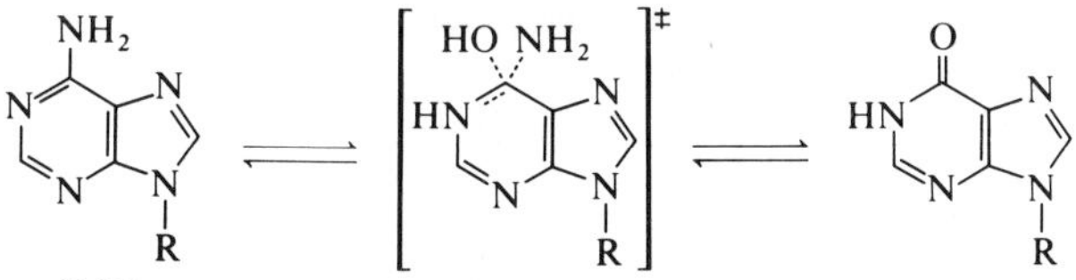

(4.91)   (4.92)   (4.93)

(4.34)

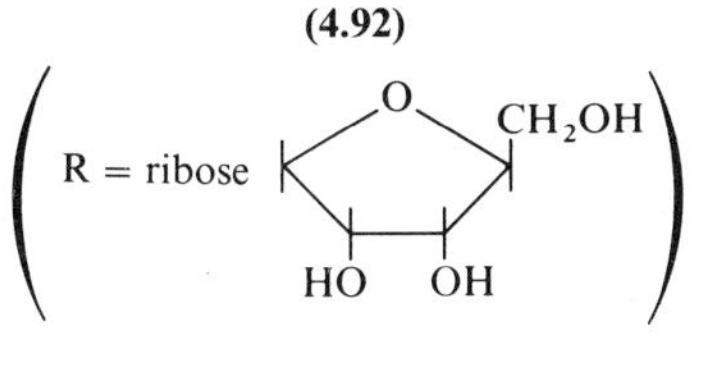

R = ribose

the diastereoisomers of 1,6-dihydro-6-hydroxymethylpurine (4.94) is a potent inhibitor of the enzyme due to its resemblance to the transition state.

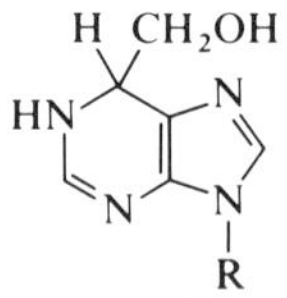

(4.94)

4.4.3.4   *Summary*

The transition state analogue concept has been used to explain the high potency of many competitive reversible inhibitors in terms of their ability to bind more strongly to the enzyme than to the normal substrate. Present day design of a transition state analogue inhibitor, for a specific enzyme catalysing a reaction of its substrate by a predictable reaction mechanism pathway, is a realistic proposition and has been successfully accomplished in many instances.

By binding so much more strongly to the enzyme than does the substrate, it is more likely that this type of competitive reversible inhibitor would be more useful in therapy than the classical type of inhibitor which only resembles the structure of the substrate. This is because the action of the transition state analogue is less likely to be reversed by build-up of substrate (*see* p. 88). This point can readily be demonstrated by rearranging Equation 4.5 which gives the rate of the enzyme-catalysed reaction in the presence of a competitive inhibitor, to

$$v = \frac{V_{max}}{1 + \dfrac{K_m}{[S]} + \dfrac{K_m [I]}{[S] K_i}} \qquad (4.35)$$

This shows that, as the substrate concentration builds up, the second and third terms in the denominator decrease and v approaches V_{max}. However, if K_m/K_i is large (i.e. 10^3), for example when transition state analogues are used, the third term becomes less sensitive to an appreciable increase in the substrate concentration and the inhibition is, therefore, more persistent.

4.4.4 k_{cat} Inhibitors as irreversible enzyme inhibitors

Many irreversible inhibitors of certain enzymes have previously been recognized in which the range of electrophilic centres normally associated with active site-directed irreversible inhibitors were absent (*see* Table 4.2), so that the means by which they inhibited the enzyme was not understood. More recently the action of these inhibitors has become explicable since they have become characterized as k_{cat} inhibitors. k_{cat} Inhibitors bind to the enzyme through the K_S parameter and are modified by the enzyme in such a way as to generate a reactive group which irreversibly inhibits the enzyme by forming a covalent bond with a functional group present at the enzyme active site. These inhibitors are substrates of the enzyme as suggested by the term k_{cat} which is the overall rate constant for the decomposition of the enzyme–substrate complex in an enzyme-catalysed reaction. k_{cat} Inhibitors have also been referred to as 'suicide enzyme inactivators' or 'suicide substrates' especially in connection with the inhibition of pyridoxal phosphate-dependent enzymes.

   k_{cat} Inhibitors do not generate a reactive electrophilic centre until acted upon by the target-enzyme. Reaction may then occur with a nucleophile on the enzyme surface or alternatively the species may be degraded to innocuous products. Consequently the reactive electrophilic species, by not being free to react with other molecules in the biological media, has a high degree of specificity for its target-enzyme.

4.4.4.1 k_{cat} Inhibitors of flavin-linked monoamine oxidase

Monoamine oxidases (MAO), some of which contain flavin as a prosthetic group, catalyse the oxidative deamination of aliphatic amines to aldehydes (Equation 4.36) and control the levels of biogenic amines such as noradrenaline in the body. The proposed mechanism for the reaction

$$R \cdot CH_2 \cdot NH_2 \xrightarrow{\text{MAO}} R \cdot CHO \qquad (4.36)$$

with the flavin-linked enzyme involves nucleophilic attack on the flavin by the amino group of the substrate to form a covalently bound intermediate. The intermediate subsequently breaks down by electron rearrangements due to the labilization of the α-C—H bond with formation of an intermediate aldimine which, on hydrolysis, gives the aldehyde (see Equation 4.37).

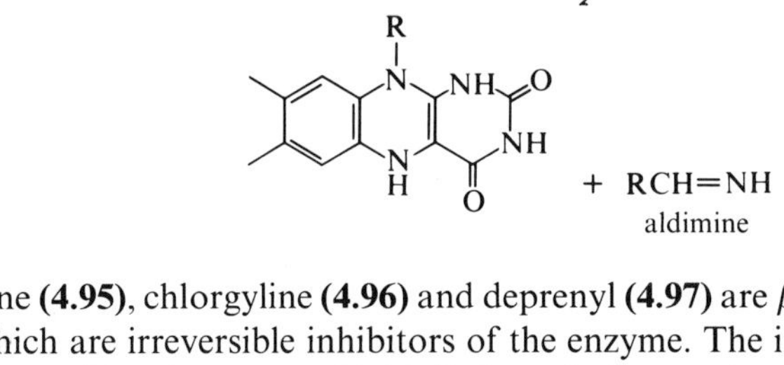

$$(4.37)$$

Pargyline (4.95), chlorgyline (4.96) and deprenyl (4.97) are β,γ-acetylenic tertiary amines which are irreversible inhibitors of the enzyme. The irreversible inhibition reaction is considered to proceed initially by a similar mechanism to that operating with the normal substrate except that the electrons flow from the labile α-C—H

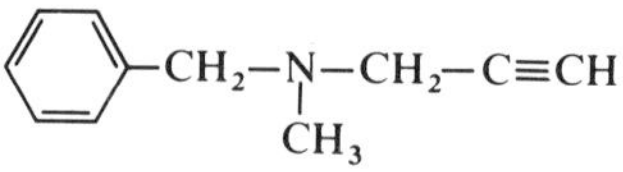

$$\text{Ph}-\text{CH}_2-\underset{\underset{\text{CH}_3}{|}}{\text{N}}-\text{CH}_2-\text{C}\equiv\text{CH}$$

(4.95)

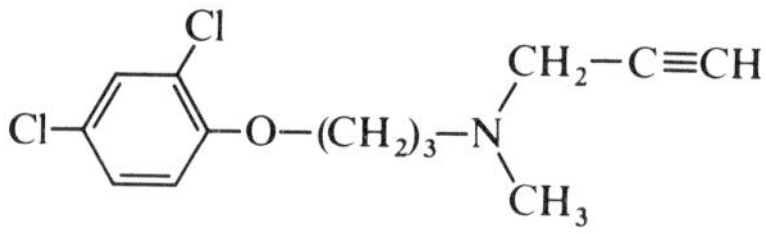

(4.96)

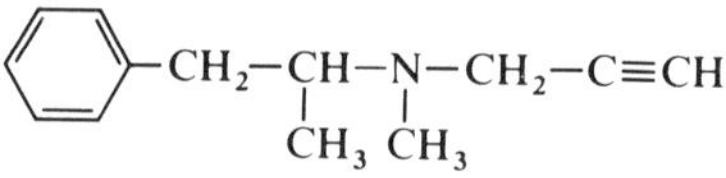

$$\text{Ph}-\text{CH}_2-\underset{\underset{\text{CH}_3}{|}}{\text{CH}}-\underset{\underset{\text{CH}_3}{|}}{\text{N}}-\text{CH}_2-\text{C}\equiv\text{CH}$$

(4.97)

bond towards the acetylenic group with production of a reactive allene. The reaction sequence for propargylamine **(4.98)** is illustrated in Equation 4.38. The firmly bound modified flavin molecule reacts with a functional group on the enzyme surface through its highly reactive alkylating arm. This reaction renders

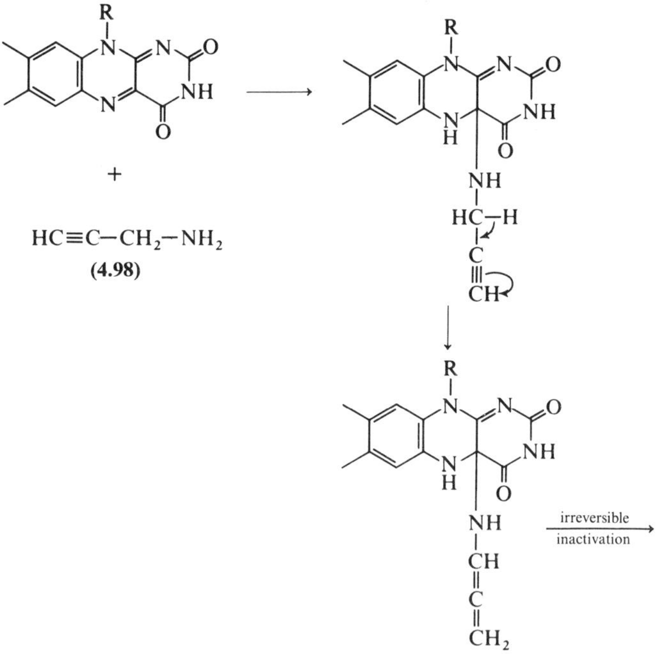

$$\text{HC}\equiv\text{C}-\text{CH}_2-\text{NH}_2$$

(4.98)

(4.38)

the enzyme inactive to the normal substrate. *cis*-Bromoallylamine is also an inhibitor of the enzyme. Here the unreactive vinyl bromide is converted to a reactive alkylating alkyl bromide by the action of the enzyme (*see* Equation 4.39). The two types of inhibitors described here are substrates of the enzyme but the nature and position of additional functions, present in their structures and absent in normal substrates of the enzyme, dictates that a different pathway is followed in decomposition of the residue attached to the flavin. A reacting alkylating arm is generated followed by inhibition of the enzyme.

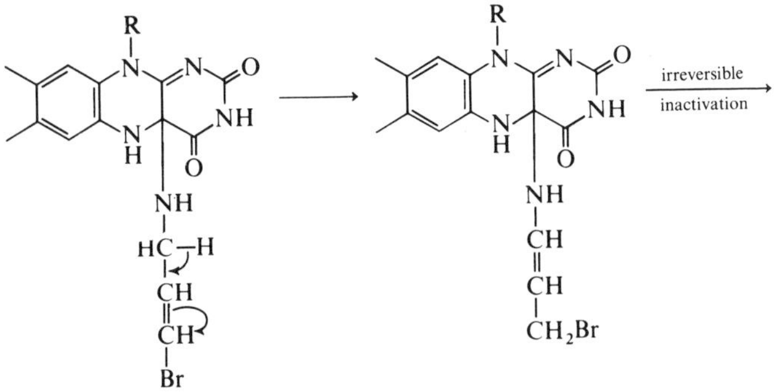

$$(4.39)$$

4.4.4.2 *Pyridoxal phosphate-dependent enzymes*

Many enzymes, using pyridoxal phosphate as a coenzyme to catalyse several different types of reactions of amino acid substrates, are inhibited by k_{cat} inhibitors. Here, the spectrum of activity shown by the inhibitors is restricted to amino acid-metabolizing enzymes.

The coenzyme pyridoxal phosphate is bound to the enzyme by formation of an aldimine with the ω-amino group of a lysine residue. The first step in the reaction with the amino acid substrate is an exchange reaction to form an aldimine with the α-amino group of the amino acid (*see* Equation 4.40). The aldimine then breaks

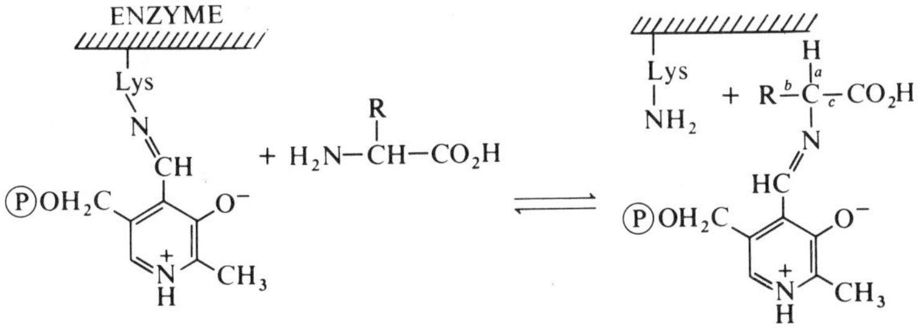

$$(4.40)$$

down by fission of bond *a*, *b* or *c* with a flow of the electron pair towards the nitrogen to give a ketimine which subsequently degrades to the product of the reaction. Fission of bond *a* occurs in racemization, α,β-elimination, β-substitution and transamination reactions, whereas fission of *b* gives glycine and fission of *c* leads to decarboxylation. The direction of the fission which occurs is dictated by the nature of the protein at the active site so that a specific enzyme catalyses a particular type of reaction.

Inactivators of pyridoxal phosphate-dependent enzymes fall into two groups: (*a*) β-haloalanines and other agents which lose the elements HX (e.g. HCl, H_2O) with the formation of an unsaturated aldimine; (*b*) olefinic (all ⸗nylic) and acetylenic (alkynylic) amino acids.

An example of inhibition by an inactivator belonging to the first group of reagents is the inhibition of bacterial threonine dehydrase by serine. This enzyme

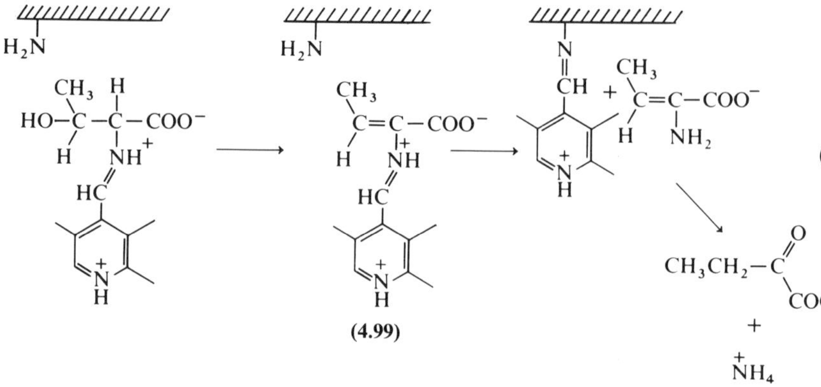

(4.41)

(4.99)

converts its natural substrate threonine to ketobutyrate by the pathway shown in Equation 4.41. The α-C—H bond in the aldimine is cleaved in a carbanion-forming step with elimination of hydroxyl ion to give the unsaturated aldimine (4.99) which breaks down to the products of the reaction. L-Serine is an inhibitor of this enzyme since the α,β-unsaturated aldimine produced with serine as substrate forms a covalent bond, at the β-carbon atom, with a nucleophilic group (probably —SH of a cysteine residue) on the enzyme surface. This results in irreversible inhibition of the enzyme. The β-carbon atom is an electrophilic centre and carries a partial positive charge due to the electron-withdrawing properties of the coenzyme imine residue which may be represented by the canonical forms (4.100). Serine is metabolized to pyruvate by the enzyme through the intermediate alkylating species and, although only about 1 in 10 000 turnovers of the enzyme leads to an

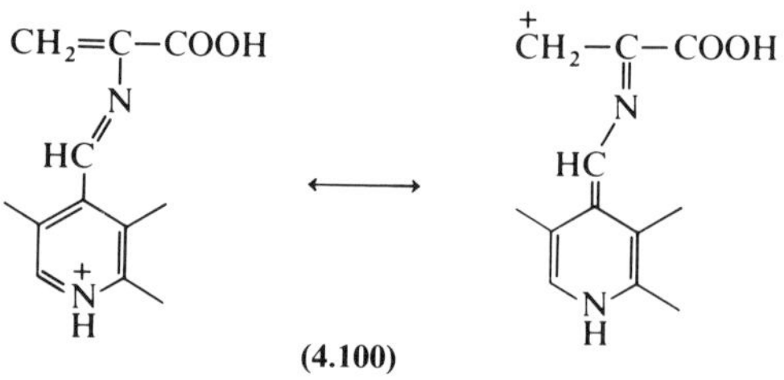

(4.100)

alkylation reaction, the enzyme is progressively inhibited. L-β-Chloroalanine inhibits the enzyme in a similar manner but is less specific than L-serine since it also inhibits enzymes catalysing other types of reactions. The second group of inhibitors contain α,β-unsaturated linkages. L-2-Amino-4-methoxy-*trans*-3-butenoic acid (AMB) is an inhibitor of aspartate aminotransferase. The α-C—H bond of the aldimine formed with AMB is cleaved and an unsaturated aldimine (4.101) is formed by movement of a pair of electrons to the α,β-position with acceptance of a proton by the γ-carbon (*see* Equation 4.42). (4.101) can inhibit the enzyme by reaction of the electrophilic β-carbon atom with a nucleophile on the enzyme.

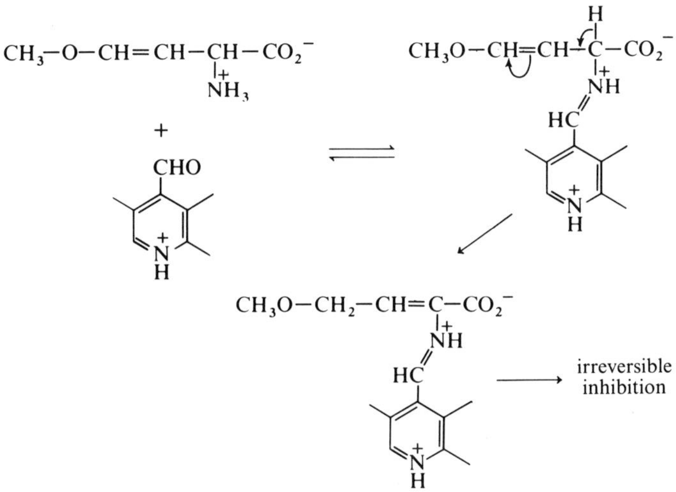

$$CH_3-O-CH=CH-CH-CO_2^-$$
$$\overset{|+}{NH_3}$$

$$CH_3O-CH=CH-\overset{H}{\underset{\underset{HC}{\overset{|+}{NH}}}{C}}-CO_2^-$$

$+$

CHO

$\rightleftharpoons$

(4.42)

$$CH_3O-CH_2-CH=C-CO_2^-$$
$$\overset{|+}{NH}$$

HC

$\longrightarrow$ irreversible inhibition

(4.101)

L-Chloroalanine, L-vinylglycine and L-propargyl glycine are also inhibitors of this enzyme, the ratio of catalytic turnovers : inactivation being unity for L-vinylglycine and 1700 for β-chloroalanine. L-Propargylglycine **(4.102)** probably gives the reactive allene intermediate **(4.103)** by a similar mechanism to that described for AMB.

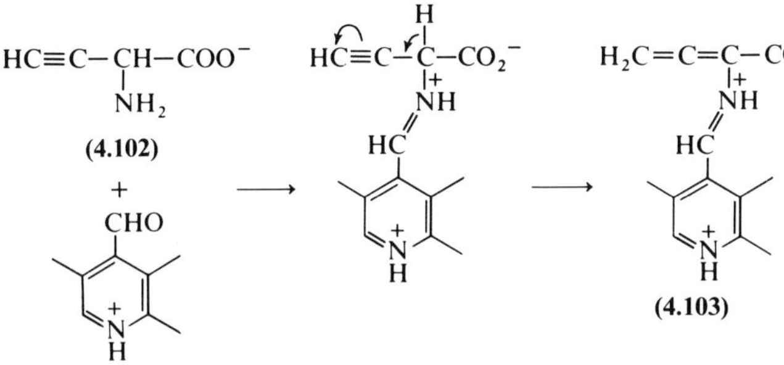

$$HC\equiv C-CH-COO^-$$
$$\overset{|}{NH_2}$$

(4.102)

$$HC\equiv C-\overset{H}{\underset{\underset{HC}{\overset{|+}{NH}}}{C}}-CO_2^-$$

$$H_2C=C=C-CO_2^-$$
$$\overset{|+}{NH}$$

HC

$+$

CHO

$\longrightarrow$ $\longrightarrow$ (4.43)

(4.103)

There has been much interest recently in the design of inhibitors of the pyridoxal phosphate-dependent enzyme, α-ketoglutarate-GABA transaminase. This enzyme governs the levels of the inhibitory neurotransmitter γ-amino butyric acid (GABA) in the brain (see Equation 4.44). Inhibitors of the enzyme would allow a build-up of GABA and could be used as anticonvulsant drugs for the treatment of epilepsy.

$$H_2N-CH_2-CH_2-CH_2-CO_2H \xrightarrow[\text{transamine}]{\text{GABA}} \overset{O}{\overset{\|}{C}}-CH_2-CH_2COOH \quad (4.44)$$

GABA

succinic semialdehyde

$$HC\equiv C-\underset{\underset{NH_2}{|}}{CH}-CH_2-CH_2-CO_2H \qquad H_2C=CH-\underset{\underset{NH_2}{|}}{CH}-CH_2-CH_2-CO_2H$$

$$\textbf{(4.104)} \qquad\qquad\qquad\qquad \textbf{(4.105)}$$

Two irreversible k_{cat} inhibitors of the enzyme, γ-ethynyl GABA **(4.104)** and γ-vinyl GABA **(4.105)**, have been developed and **(4.105)** has reached the clinical trial stage. These inhibitors are considered to act by inhibiting the enzyme by the general mechanism shown in Equations 4.43 and 4.42 respectively.

Another potent irreversible inhibitor of GABA transaminase is gabaculine **(4.106)**, which is a naturally occurring neurotoxin isolated from *Streptomyces toyocaenis*. Although not of clinical application this inhibitor is interesting since it is considered to inhibit the enzyme by a different mechanism to that previously described for suicide inactivators. Gabaculine acts as a substrate and is converted in the normal manner to the ketimine **(4.107)**. This then aromatizes under the influence of a basic group to form a stable enzyme-bound pyridoxamine derivative and the enzyme is inactivated.

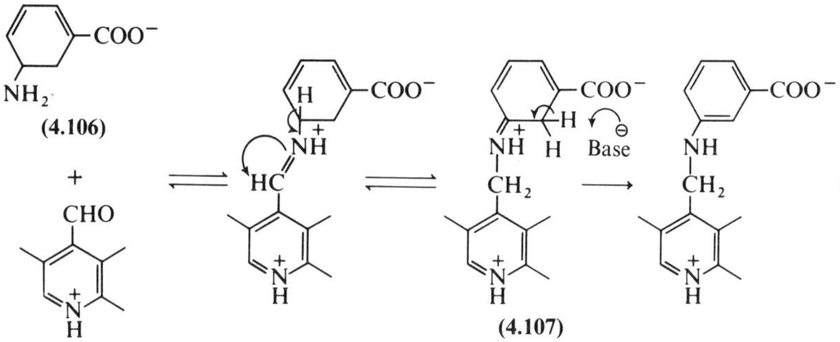

$$(4.45)$$

As previously described (*see* p. 108) the A.A.A.D. inhibitors carbidopa and serazide are useful adjuvants in the treatment of Parkinson's disease using L-dopa. Neither penetrates into the brain to inhibit the normal action of A.A.A.D. in converting L-dopa to dopamine, the active form of the drug. Difluoromethyl dopa **(4.108)** behaves in a similar manner but whereas monofluoromethyl dopa acts peripherally in small doses, in large doses it acts centrally to reduce the level of biosynthesis of biogenic amines (*see* p. 108).

Difluoromethyl, and monofluoromethyl dopa are k_{cat} inhibitors of the enzyme and are considered to effect inhibition by the mechanism shown in Equation 4.46 for difluoromethyl dopa.

α-Monofluoromethyldopa has a more intense action on A.A.A.D. than the difluoro-compound. Thus, it is able to reduce the level of A.A.A.D. activity in the brain by over 99% which affects catecholamine synthesis in spite of lack of involvement of the enzyme in the rate-determining step of hormonal biosynthesis.

Although at present these two inhibitors are only valuable tools used in research on brain catecholamines they may find therapeutic applications in the future.

(4.108)

(4.46)

(4.109)

FURTHER READING

1. Powers J. C., Carroll D. L. and Tuhy P. M. (1975) Synthetic active site-directed inhibitors of elastolytic proteases. *Ann. N.Y. Acad. Sci.* **256**, 420–5.

2. Lindquist R. N. (1975) The design of enzyme inhibitors. In Ariens E. J. (ed.) *Drug Design*, Vol. V. New York, Academic Press, pp. 24–80.

3. Smith H. J. and Spencer P. S. J. (1975) Enzyme inhibitors – active in therapy. *Manufacturing Chemist and Aerosol News.* Sept., pp. 57–61; Oct., pp. 43–8.

4. Shaw E. (1980) Design of irreversible inhibitors. In Sandler M. (ed.) *Enzyme Inhibitors as Drugs.* London, MacMillan, pp. 25–42.

5. Albert A. (1979) Metabolites, enzymes and metabolite analogues. In: *Selective Toxicity,* 6th ed. London, Chapman & Hall. pp. 289–329.

6. Stenlake J. B. (1979) Characteristics of drug–receptor interaction. In *Foundations of Molecular Pharmacology:* Vol. 2, *The Chemical Basis of Drug Action.* University of London, Athlone. pp. 1–39.

7. Santi D. V. and Kenyon G. L. (1980) Approaches to the rational design of enzyme inhibitors. In Wolff M. E. (ed.) *Burger's Medicinal Chemistry,* 4th ed., Part I. New York, Wiley, pp. 349–91.

8. (*a*) Anand N. (1980) Sulphonamides and sulphones. (*b*) Montgomery J. A., Johnston T. P. and Fulmer Sheally Y. (1980) Drugs for neoplastic diseases – antimetabolites. (*c*) Sweeney T. R. and Strube R. E. (1980) Anti-malarials. (*d*) Hess F. K. and Freter K. R. (1980) Agents affecting the immune response. (*e*) Sidwell R. W. and Witkowski J. T. (1980) Anti-viral agents. In Wolff M. E. (ed.) *Burger's Medicinal Chemistry,* 4th ed. Part 2. New York, Wiley, (*a*) pp. 1–40, (*b*) pp. 598–618, (*c*) pp. 333–414, (*d*) pp. 617–704, (*e*) pp. 543–94.

9. Drach J. C. (1980 and 1981) Anti-viral agents. In Hess H.-J. (ed.) *Annual Reports in Medicinal Chemistry,* Vols. 15 and 16. New York, Academic Press, pp. 149–61 (1980), pp. 149–59 (1981).

10. Rando R. R. (1974) Chemistry and enzymology of k_{cat} inhibitors. *Science* **185**, 320–4.

11. (*a*) John R. A. (1980) Enzyme-induced inactivation of pyridoxal phosphate-dependent enzymes: approaches to the design of specific inhibitors. (*b*) Knoll J. (1980) Monoamine oxidase inhibitors: chemistry and pharmacology. In Sandler M. (ed.) *Enzyme Inhibitors as Drugs.* London, Macmillan, (*a*) pp. 73–93, (*b*) pp. 151–71.

12. Metcalf B. W. (1981) Recent progress in the design of suicide enzyme inhibitors. In Hess H.-J. (ed.) *Annual Reports in Medicinal Chemistry,* Vol. 16. New York, Academic Press, pp. 289–97.

13. Baker B. R. (1967) *Design of Active Site-Directed Irreversible Enzyme Inhibitors.* New York, John Wiley & Sons.

Chapter 5

Metal complexation, isosteric modification and salt formation in drug design

Metal complexation, isosteric modification and salt formation in drug design

5.1 METAL COMPLEXES IN DRUG ACTION AND BIOLOGICAL SYSTEMS

5.1.1 Introduction

Traces of certain metals, functioning as cations in the living cell, are essential for all forms of life. The heavy metals copper, iron, manganese, molybdenum, cobalt, zinc and the lighter metals calcium, magnesium, potassium and sodium are amongst those which play an important role in numerous essential life processes. Thus, copper, iron, molybdenum and cobalt are necessary for establishing certain oxidation–reduction equilibria and are cofactors for some enzymes. Zinc and magnesium are required for the normal functioning of certain enzymes concerned with hydrolysis or the transfer of groups.

Copper is also an essential constituent of many enzymes. Cytochrome oxidase, present in the respiratory chain, contains two iron and two copper ions per molecule. The action of dopamine hydroxylase, a key enzyme in the biosynthesis of catecholamine hormones, requires copper. This element is also known to be concentrated in sympathetic nerve-endings and synaptic vessels of the brain where it probably assists in storing noradrenaline and 5-hydroxytryptamine respectively, complexed with adenosine triphosphate.

Iron occurs as a vital component of the porphyrin enzymes; catalase, peroxidases and cytochromes which are concerned with decomposition of hydrogen peroxide (H_2O_2), substrate oxidation with H_2O_2 and cellular oxidations respectively. The respiratory pigment haemoglobin also contains iron.

Cobalt is needed for several biochemical processes. It is a cofactor for carboxypeptidase breakdown of various kinins which are inflammation-inducing peptides. Cobalt is also found in the centre of a tetrapyrrole (corrin) structure which forms the nucleus of the cobamide group of coenzymes. Hydroxocobalamine and cyanocobalamine (vitamin B_{12}) are formed by the cleavage of these coenzymes during isolation from the liver. These coenzymes also catalyse the reduction of ribonucleotides to deoxyribonucleotides.

Calcium is needed for creating structures such as bones and teeth and to confer rigidity to tendons. It also has a role in association with phosphate anions, in controlling the permeability of semipermeable membranes. Calcium plays a part in the release of acetylcholine, both at synapses and the neuromuscular junction, during the passage of a nerve impulse.

Chromium, vanadium, nickel and tin are other heavy metals which are believed to be essential, although required in smaller amounts.

Apart from sodium and potassium, the role of the above metals in living cells (and in some drug actions) depends on the formation of metal ion complexes with organic molecular species or ions and it is pertinent to consider some fundamental aspects of the formation of such complexes.

5.1.2 Coordination complexes

A metal ion complexing agent is any electron-donating molecule or ion, referred to as a ligand. Examples of neutral molecules which function as ligands are amines, imines and sulphides whilst typical anions which function as ligands include carboxylate, cyanide, phenolate and thiophenolate. Complexes involving simple ligands (such as CN^-, COO^- and NH_3, each of which is capable of forming only one bond with the metal ion) are called coordination compounds. The metal in such complexes will have different properties from those of the free metal ion. Thus, the metal ion may not be precipitated from the complex by the usual precipitating agent, e.g. (a) ferric iron complexed as potassium ferricyanide, $K_3Fe(CN)_6$, does not precipitate as ferric hydroxide with alkali, (b) copper is not precipitated as the sulphide from potassium cuprocyanide, $K_3Cu(CN)_4$, by hydrogen sulphide. Further the higher valency state of an ion is stabilized by complex formation, e.g. the addition of potassium iodide to acidified sodium cupritartrate, rather than cupric sulphate, does not yield cuprous iodide.

The electrovalency of a complex ion is equal to the positive charge on the metal ion only when this is coordinated with neutral molecules, e.g. $Cu(NH_3)_4^{2+}$. If anions such as Cl^-, CN^-, COO^- are complexed with the metal ion the positive charge is reduced by one unit for each univalent negative ion. When the negative valency of the ions exceeds the positive valency of the central metal ion, the

Table 5.1   Electronic structure of ferrocyanide ion

	1 s	2 s p	3 s p d	4 s p d f
Fe	2	2 6	2 6 2 1 1 1 1	2
Fe^{2+}	2	2 6	2 6 2 2 2 —	
$Fe(II)(CN)_6^{4-}$	2	2 6	2 6 2 2 2 2 2	2 2 2 2 2 2

complex as a whole becomes negatively charged and associated with a corresponding number of 'external' positive ions, e.g. $[Fe(III)(CN)_6]^{3-}$ $3K^+$, $[Fe(II)(CN)_6]^{4-}$ $4K^+$.

The nature of the bonds binding one ferrous, Fe^{2+}, and six cyanide, $^-C{\equiv}N$, ions in the ferrocyanide complex can be elucidated by examination of the electronic configurations involved in complex ion formation (*see* Table 5.1). When Fe^{2+} is formed, two 4s electrons are lost and four unpaired 3d electrons pair up, leaving two 3d orbitals unoccupied. When six ^-CN anions become coordinated to Fe^{2+}, six electron pairs are donated. Four electrons fill up the vacant 3d orbitals, two electrons fill the vacant 4s orbital and six electrons fill the vacant 4p orbital. Thus, electrons forming the six Fe—CN bonds consists of two pairs of 3d, one pair of 4s and three pairs of 4p, making six hybrid d^2sp^3 bonds. Such hybridization, using electrons from different shells, only becomes possible when their energy levels are approximately equal, e.g. 3d and 4s. The six hybrid bonds are directed at right angles to one another in an octahedral configuration (5.1) as revealed by molecular orbital considerations. The shapes of complexes are important in the biological role of metals.

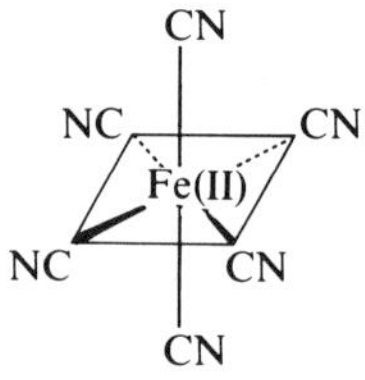

(5.1)

5.1.3 Coordination number

Werner (1891) first noticed that for each metal atom there is a limit to the number of small groups which can be accommodated around it. This is referred to as Werner's coordination number, which depends entirely on steric considerations and is in no way related to the valency of the ion. Thus, although the valency shell of the third period elements can expand to 18 electrons, the number of small groups capable of binding is restricted by the space available around the metal ion. In the second period of the periodic table, the maximum coordination number is 4 whilst in the third period the number is 6. Thus, in AlF_6^{3-} the outer shell contains 12 electrons and cannot expand to 18 since the maximum coordination number of 6 has been reached.

Within the limits imposed by Werner's coordination number there is a tendency, when forming a complex, for a metal to attain, or approach, a stable inert gas electronic structure (*see* Table 5.2).

5.1.4 Chelating agents and chelation

Whereas coordination compounds are formed from simple ligands, each forming one bond with a metal ion, ligands having more than one electron-donating group

Table 5.2   Electronic configuration of complex ions

Metal ion	Electronic configuration	Complex ion	Electronic configuration
Co^{3+}	2, 8, 14	$[Co(NH_3)_6]^{3+}$	2, 8, 18, 8
Cu^{2+}	2, 8, 17	$[Cu(NH_3)_4]^{2+}$	2, 8, 18, 7
Hg^{2+}	2, 8, 18, 32, 18	$[Hg(CNS)_4]^{2-}$	2, 8, 18, 32, 18, 8
Fe^{2+}	2, 8, 14	$[Fe(CN)_6]^{4-}$	2, 8, 18, 8
Fe^{3+}	2, 8, 13	$[Fe(CN)_6]^{3-}$	2, 8, 17, 8

are called chelating agents and are able to grip the metal with two or more bonds to give a cyclic structure or chelate. In this way, ethylenediamine, 1,2-diaminoethane, and glycine, aminoacetic acid, chelate cupric and cobaltous ions to give 1 : 1 or 1 : 2 complexes (5.2). Examination of electronic configurations involved in the (1 : 2)

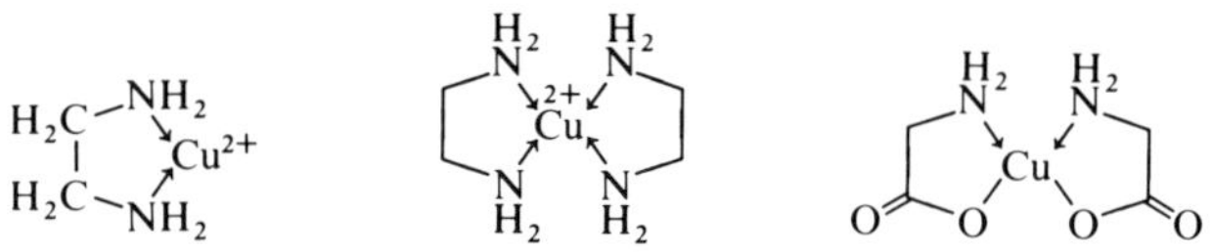

(5.2)

Table 5.3   Electronic configuration of Cu(II) $(-NH_2)_4^{2+}$

	1	2	3	4
	s	s p	s p d	s p d f
Cu	2	2 6	2 6 10	1
Cu^{2+}	2	2 6	2 6 9	
Cu(II) $(-NH_2)_4^{2+}$	2	2 6	2 6 10	2 5

ethylenediamine complex (*see* Table 5.3) reveals that four amine, $-NH_2$, groups donate eight electrons to the cupric ion whereby one electron fills the vacant 3d orbital, two electrons fill the vacant 4s orbital and 5 electrons occupy the vacant 4p orbital. Thus, the electrons forming the four $Cu^{2+}-NH_2$ bonds consist of one 3d, two 4s and five 4p electrons, giving rise to four dsp^2 hybrid bonds which are revealed, by orbital considerations, to be directed equidistantly apart in a planar configuration (5.3).

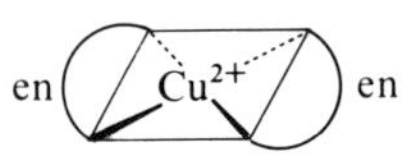

en = $H_2N\cdot CH_2\cdot CH_2\cdot NH_2$

(5.3)

Other bivalent cations, such as Ca^{2+} and Mg^{2+}, also form (with suitable chelating agents) complexes of coordination number 4 utilizing bonds which are

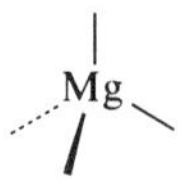

$$\overset{\displaystyle |}{\underset{\displaystyle /}{\cdots Mg}}\diagdown$$

(5.4)

sp^3 hybridized and consequently tetrahedrally directed (5.4). Table 5.4 shows that when electron-donating groups, :X or X^-, supply 8 electrons to a magnesium ion, Mg^{2+}, two electrons fill the vacant 3s orbital and six electrons fill the 3p orbital so that the four Mg—X bonds are sp^3 hybridized (5.4).

Table 5.4   Electronic configuration of magnesium complex

	1	2		3		
	s	s	p	s	p	d
Mg	2	2	6	2		
Mg^{2+}	2	2	6			
$Mg(X)_4$	2	2	6	2	6	

Divalent ferrous, zinc and cobaltous ions have sufficient vacant orbitals to exhibit a coordination number of 6 towards ligands of the ethylenediamine type. The ligands are gathered around the metal in a configuration determined by octahedral disposition of the d^2sp^3 hybridized bonds so that the metal ion will be common to three 5-membered rings (5.5). Since the structure has no plane of symmetry it can exist in two optically active, $(+)$ and $(-)$, forms illustrating that stereoisomerism is not confined to carbon compounds but arises whenever molecular asymmetry occurs.

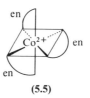

(5.5)

Ethylenediamine is an example of a bidentate ligand, forming a single ring in a 1:1 metal complex. Tri-, tetra- and polydentate ligands are also known. The significance of their chelating action in biological media is that bonds formed with metal ions are stronger than ordinary ionic bonds since they are partially covalent in character. The structures of the ligands must be such as to permit the formation of rings and the greater the number of rings formed the more stable will be the chelate.

5.1.5   Ligand selectivity

Metal and organic ligands show a definite order of affinity for one another. One method of quantifying this degree of tightness in binding is to employ stability constants which are related to mass-action equilibria between metal ion and ligand or ligands. Thus for the $1:1$ glycine—Cu^{2+} complex the equilibrium is

$$K_1 = \frac{[H_2N \cdot CH_2 \cdot \overset{\frown}{COOCu^+}]}{[Cu^{2+}][H_2N \cdot CH_2 \cdot COO^-]},$$

where K_1 is the stability constant. A second constant K_2 describes the stability of the $2:1$ complex, so that cumulative stability constants β are needed. These may be determined by potentiometric titration methods where two other variables: $\bar{n}$, the average number of complex-forming ligands bound by one metal ion and L, the concentration of the free chelating species, must be considered. Since these are also dependent on the pK_a of the ligand and pH of the medium, calculations will require computer programming. Such methods do not, however, offer a sure way of predicting stability constants of chelates in advance. This has led to the elaboration of ligand field theory, which in turn has been developed from a study of crystal field phenomena. Here the influences of ligand donor electrons on d electron energy levels of the metal, when they become combined, is evaluated. The energy liberated by this effect varies with the ligand and the number of d electrons associated with different metals and thus gives a measure of bond stability.

Another method of evaluating bond strength in chelation is based on the concept of hard and soft bases and acids. The atom donating electrons is considered as a base whilst that accepting the electrons is referred to as an acid. This treatment requires the strength of acids and bases to be expressed in terms of intrinsic strength, S, and softness, σ: the latter reflecting the mobility of the electrons. The relationship between two atoms A and B may be expressed as: $\log K = S_A S_B + \sigma_A + \sigma_B$. If both atoms A and B show similar electron mobility (high or low) then the bonding electrons are more evenly distributed, giving rise to a stable bond. However, if one of the atoms shows high electron mobility, the bond is less stable. Atoms showing high electron mobility are referred to as soft acids or bases whilst those showing low electron mobility are hard acids or bases. Stable bonds arise from hard–hard or soft–soft combinations of atoms, whilst hard–soft combinations yield less stable bonds.

Electron mobility or softness is determined by such considerations as size, charge, electronegativity or electropositivity, the number of outer shell electrons, accessibility of unoccupied orbitals and type of bond involved when complexing. Examples of hard and soft acids and bases are given in Table 5.5.

5.1.6   Medicinal applications

In a living system, the concentrations of metal ions are controlled within narrow limits. If the natural balance of these concentrations is disturbed by internal or external causes then the organism can no longer behave normally and disorder

Table 5.5   Hard and soft acids and bases

	Acids			Bases	
Hard	Ca^{2+} Mg^{2+} Be^{2+} Fe^{3+}	H_2O HO^- F^- Cl^-	ROH RO^- ROR $R \cdot COR$	$R \cdot COO^-$ CO_3^{2-}	NH_3 $R \cdot NH_2$ $NH_2 \cdot NH_2$
	Fe^{2+} Co^{2+} Zn^{2+} Ni^{2+} Cu^{2+} Pb^{2+}	Br^- NO_2^- SO_3^{2-}	$Ph \cdot NH_2$ Pyridine $-N{=}N-$		
Soft	Pd^{2+} Cd^{2+} Pt^{2+} Hg^{2+}	I^- CN^- CO NO	RSR' RSH RS^-	$R \cdot CH{=}CH \cdot R'$ Benzene	

results. Thus, a number of diseases are associated directly with changes in the concentration of trace metal ions in certain tissues and body fluids. Several medicinal compounds have been employed for their metal chelating properties, in order to correct these imbalances. Chelating agents have also proved valuable in arresting toxicity due to ingestion of certain metals, whilst the established biological actions of some other drugs have been associated with metal complexation. For chelating agents to be active in a biological environment their stability constants must be of the same order as those of tissue amino acids. Too high values would result in saturation of ligands before reaching their site of action. Drug design should also enable the attainment of hard–hard or soft–soft acid–base metal–ligand bonds. If penetration of cells is desirable then lipophilic groups such as carbon, halogens and sulphur should be built into the structure of the chelating agent.

The disodium salt of ethylenediamine-N,N,N',N'-tetraacetic acid, EDTA, utilizes hydrophilic groups to chelate metal ions yielding water-soluble complexes. Such chelating agents are termed sequestering agents. Disodium edetate injection (the tetrasodium salt is too alkaline) is used to diminish blood calcium levels in hypercalcaemia. The hard basic groups, $-COO^-$ and $-NH_2$ of the tetradentate ligand form a stable water-soluble complex with hard Ca^{2+} ions (5.6) which is excreted via the kidney. Disodium edetate has also been used for treating lime-burns of the cornea, decalcifying stenosed valves in the heart and for restoring the

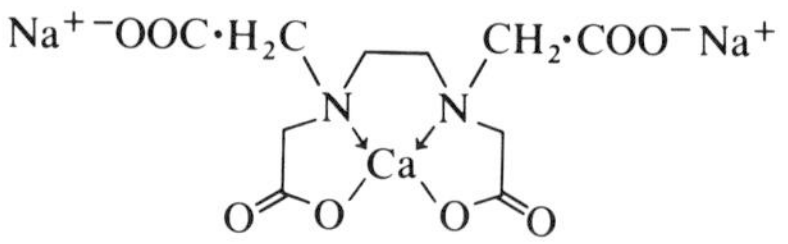

$Na^+ {}^-OOC \cdot H_2C$ $CH_2 \cdot COO^- Na^+$

(5.6)

K^+/Ca^{2+} balance in cardiac arrhythmias accidentally brought on by digitalis. Disodium edetate has been used in pharmaceutical analysis for assaying hardness of water, calcium gluconate injections and bismuth preparations. It has also been employed as an antioxidant for the stabilization of preparations containing adrenaline, ascorbic acid and chloroxylenol, which rapidly deteriorate in the presence of trace metals. The calcium chelate of disodium edetate is preferred for treating lead or mercury poisoning. Toxicity arises because soft heavy metal ions such as Pb^{2+} and Hg^{2+} combine with soft basic groups such as sulphydryl (of cysteine residues) to form strongly bonded complexes at enzymic active sites. The calcium disodium edetate antidote exchanges Ca^{2+} for uncomplexed Pb^{2+} ions and thus disturbs the equilibrium between unbound and enzyme-bound lead in favour of the former. Using calcium disodium edetate avoids the depletion of blood Ca^{2+} which would otherwise occur with disodium edetate.

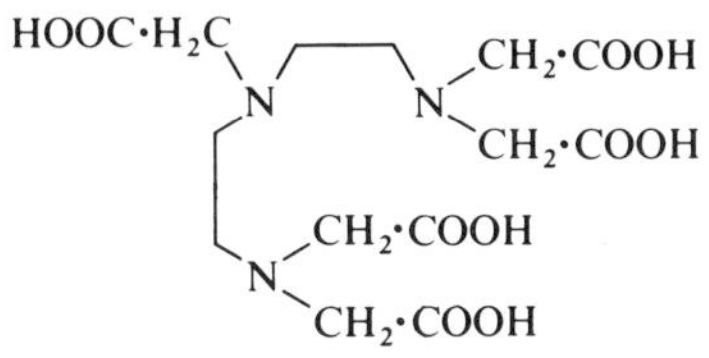

$$HOOC \cdot H_2C$$

$$CH_2 \cdot COOH$$
$$CH_2 \cdot COOH$$
$$CH_2 \cdot COOH$$
$$CH_2 \cdot COOH$$

(5.7)

Injections of diethylenetriaminepentacetic acid (5.7) are employed for treating contamination by plutonium in personnel working at nuclear energy establishments. In the treatment of cyanide poisoning the bi-(tridentate)dicobaltous chelate of ethylenediaminetetraacetic acid (5.8) is used since the soft Co(II) has a strong

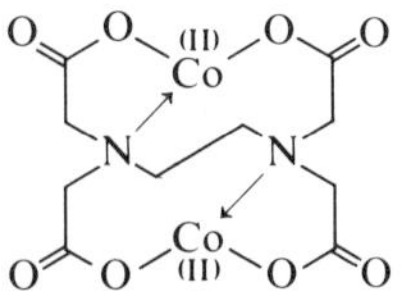

(5.8)

affinity for the soft CN^- anion. The action of the antidote depends on the metal ion increasing its coordination number from three to four or six by coordinating with CN^- ions. Cyanide poisoning arises due to the effect of CN^- on the cytochromes, of the respiratory chain, which are involved in electron transfer reactions pertinent to cellular oxidations. During this process the iron–porphyrin complex experiences an interchanging valency state of the metal. CN^- interferes with this by stabilizing the cation in the lower oxidation state – an effect which is characteristic of soft bases. Iron-containing catalase and peroxidase enzymes are affected by CN^- in a similar manner.

   D-(−)-Penicillamine, a hydrolysis product of various penicillins, is an effective antidote for copper poisoning. It is also used for treating Wilson's disease which is an inherited metabolic disorder associated with decreased excretion of copper. Dietary copper becomes stored in the liver, kidney and brain in excess causing fatalities in early life. Oral adminstration of penicillamine removes protein-bound copper as a soluble complex (5.9) which is excreted in the urine. Penicillamine-treated patients need careful monitoring because of its serious side-effects on the bone-marrow. These have been overcome by the use of triethylenetetramine which is a tetradentate ligand (5.10). Mercury poisoning has also been combated with penicillamine although the N-acetyl derivative with its softer basic group is considered to be more effective.

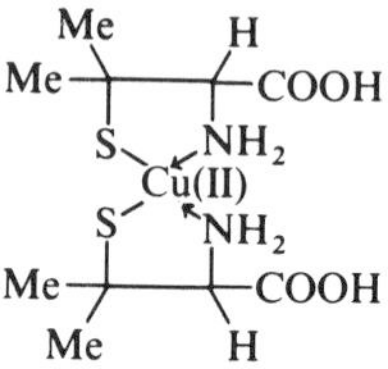

Me   H
Me─┬───┬─COOH
   S＼ ＿NH₂
    ＼Cu(II)
   S＿ ＼NH₂
Me─┬───┬─COOH
   Me   H
      (5.9)

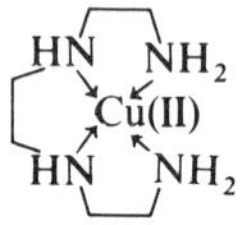

HN   NH₂
  ＼ ／
   Cu(II)
  ／ ＼
HN   NH₂
    (5.10)

Poisoning by mercury, arsenic, gold or antimony may be treated with dimercaprol, one of the first complexing agents to be used medicinally. Dimercaprol provides soft basic sulphydryl groups which bind these (soft) metals to produce water-soluble complexes (5.11). An intramuscular injection of the ligand in arachis oil is administered.

Another chelating agent, utilizing the soft sulphydryl group, is cysteamine (5.12) which removes excess copper and iron deposited in the bone-marrow, adrenals,

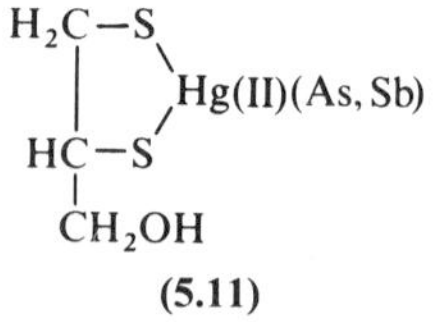

H_2C-S
| ＼
| Hg(II)(As, Sb)
$HC-S$ ／
|
CH_2OH
     (5.11)

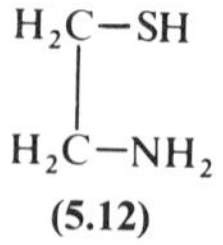

H_2C-SH
|
H_2C-NH_2
     (5.12)

liver, lungs and other organs as a result of radiation injury. Other similar compounds to cysteamine have been designed for this purpose.

Several chelating agents, including EDTA, have been examined for the possible treatment of chronic iron poisoning. One form of iron toxicity arises from the need to treat thalassaemia (the anaemia arising from the genetically determined disease) with repeated blood transfusions. This treatment results in excessive accumulation of iron in the kidneys, liver and heart. The most effective antidote for this at present is a polymer, hexapeptide, formed by condensing the amino and hydroxy-amino groups of N-hydroxyornithine with succinic acid. Desferrioxamine (5.13) is

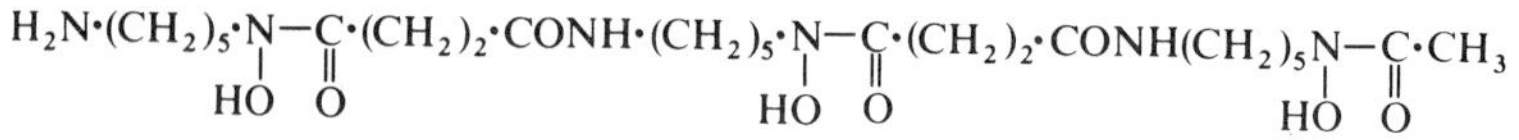

$H_2N\cdot(CH_2)_5\cdot N-C\cdot(CH_2)_2\cdot CONH\cdot(CH_2)_5\cdot N-C\cdot(CH_2)_2\cdot CONH(CH_2)_5 N-C\cdot CH_3$
$\quad\quad\quad\quad HO\ \ O \quad\quad\quad\quad\quad\quad\quad HO\ \ O \quad\quad\quad\quad\quad\quad HO\ \ O$
(5.13)

a powerful chelating agent with a specific affinity for iron as a result of the formation of a stable hard acid–hard base complex. Stability constant measurements show that the iron is bound more strongly than in the Fe–EDTA complex. Examination of the complex by X-ray diffraction has revealed the ferric iron(III) to be octahedrally bound to the three—N(OH)CO— groups. Desferrioxamine is given intramuscularly or by continuous intravenous infusion as its soluble methanesulphonate, mesylate, salt.

The antirheumatic effect of aspirin may be due to hydrolysis to salicylic acid which chelates copper associated with prostaglandin synthetase and so reduces prostaglandin synthesis. Salicylic acid or its sodium salt may also be used for treating beryllium poisoning when the formation of a soluble hard acid–hard base complex facilitates removal of the element.

Hydroxyurea exerts its anticancer effect by inhibiting the enzyme, ribonucleoside diphosphate reductase, which reduces ribonucleotides to 2'-deoxyribonucleotides required for DNA synthesis. This inhibition is thought to occur by chelation of iron, required for normal enzymic activity.

Numerous drugs form complexes with metals. Although formation of a chelate may have no relationship to the main pharmacological activity of the drug, it may cause some of the side-effects. Thus, hydrallazine (5.14) in producing its antihypertensive action may induce anaemia due to its ability to complex iron. The antitubercular drug, isonicotinic acid hydrazide, isoniazid (5.15), may induce histamine-like actions due to complexing of the metal from a copper-catalysed enzyme responsible for the destruction of histamine.

HN·NH₂

CONH·NH₂

(5.14)   (5.15)

5.1.7 Metal chelation in antibacterial activity

8-Hydroxyquinoline, oxine, has the advantage over many antibacterials of acting rapidly and possessing fungicidal properties. In ointments, it is valuable for treating skin rashes due to resistant staphylococci and for treating infected forms of eczema.

The lack of antibacterial action with O-methyl, N-methyl and isomeric hydroxy derivatives suggested that the activity of oxine involved chelation. In this respect, traces of ferric iron were shown to be required for activity, which depended on the formation of oxine–iron complexes involving hard acid–base bonding. Although 1:1, 2:1 and 3:1 complexes may be formed, the toxic effect is believed to be associated specifically with the 1:1 complex (5.16). Evidence suggests that the site of action is inside the bacterial cell or at least within the cytoplasmic membrane, since derivatives of oxine having increased hydrophilic properties and also able to chelate iron, e.g. 8-hydroxyquinoline-5-sulphonic acid, are not antibacterial. The oxine–iron complex, as a result of rearrangement of the orbitals of the ferric ion, is

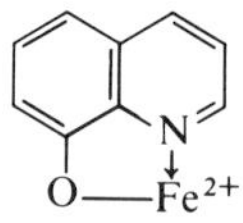

(5.16)

able to catalyse the oxidation of thiol groups in lipoic acid, thiocytic acid (5.17), which is an essential coenzyme required by the bacterium for oxidative decarboxylation of pyruvic acid. The importance of lipophilic properties is illustrated by the activity of halogenated derivatives such as 5,7-diiodo-8-hydroxyquinoline and 5-chloro-8-hydroxy-7-iodoquinoline used for treating bacterial dysentery.

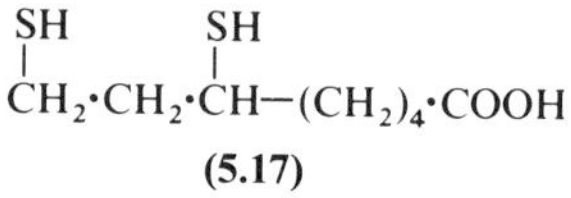

(5.17)

Isonicotinic acid hydrazide, isoniazid (5.15) probably owes its anti-tubercular properties to conversion of therapeutic quantities of the drug to a lipid-soluble chelate by interaction with serum Cu^{2+}. This facilitates uptake of the drug by the bacterial cell. Other anti-tubercular drugs whose absorption is assisted by copper(II) chelation are thiacetazone (5.18) and ethambutol (5.19). The antiviral activity of methisazone (5.52) also appears to be related to its ability to complex copper by utilization of the ring carbonyl oxygen and second nitrogen atom of the thiosemicarbazide side chain. Such chelates have been shown to interact with nucleic acids.

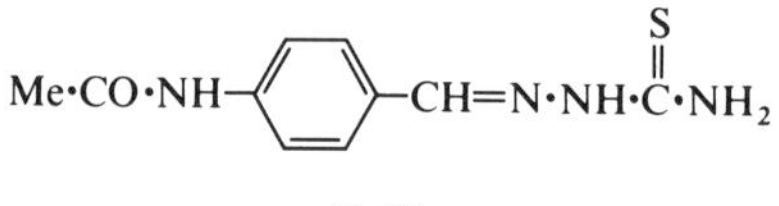

(5.18) 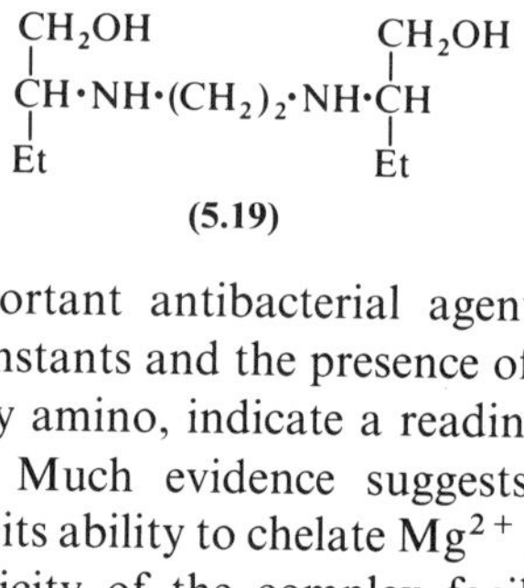   (5.19)

The tetracyclines constitute a group of important antibacterial agents for treating systemic bacterial infections. Stability constants and the presence of hard basic groups, such as acidic hydroxyl and tertiary amino, indicate a readiness to chelate hard ions such as Ca^{2+} and Mg^{2+}. Much evidence suggests that tetracycline (5.20) owes its antibacterial activity to its ability to chelate Mg^{2+} in the bacterial cell membrane. The increased lipophilicity of the complex facilitates concentration in the bacterial cell, where the eventual action is to impair their ability to synthesize proteins on the ribosomes.

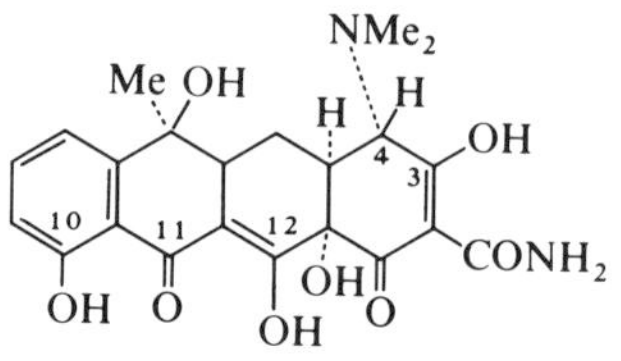

(5.20)

There has been much speculation regarding the precise location of groups on the molecule which are involved in metal ion binding. Phenolic, ketonic and hydroxyl groups at positions 10, 11 and 12, respectively, may be involved but the acidic 3-hydroxyl and basic 4-dimethylamino groups are also strong contenders. 2:1 complexes involving the latter two groups are known.

The chelating properties of tetracyclines render them less effective therapeutically when administered simultaneously with milk (Ca^{2+}), antacids (Ca^{2+}, Mg^{2+} and Al^{3+}) or iron preparations, due to delayed gastric absorption. Tetracyclines may also discolour growing teeth by accumulation of the yellow calcium chelate.

5.1.8   Chelation in anticancer activity

An important discovery of the past decade revealed that coordination compounds of platinum possessed anticancer activity. This evolved from the observation, in 1964, that when an alternating electrical field was applied using platinum electrodes across an electrical cell, containing *Eschericha coli*, all cell division was arrested. The effective agents were identified as platinum complexes, produced electrolytically, at concentrations of about 10 parts per million. Several such complexes were shown to possess anticancer activity but only one, *cis*-diamminedichloroplatinum, cisplatin **(5.21)**, has been extensively investigated

$$H_3N \diagdown \nearrow Cl$$
$$Pt(II)$$
$$H_3N \diagup \diagdown Cl$$

(5.21)

clinically. Molecular orbital considerations establish that the structure is planar so that *cis–trans* isomerism becomes possible. This stereochemical property is critical to activity since *trans* isomers are inactive. Such observations have suggested that anticancer activity is due to chelation, since replacement of two chlorine atoms in the *trans* isomer is unlikely. It has been proposed that bidentate bonding of DNA occurs, both on one strand and between two strands, involving interaction with all the bases except thymine.

Cisplatin was introduced clinically in the U.K. early in 1979, when it was claimed to be the first heavy metal compound marketed for use in oncology. It is given intravenously, the dose being limited by nephrotoxicity and damage to the eighth cranial nerve. Combined with vinblastine (*see* section 6.3), in clinical trials it produced complete remission for 59% of patients with cancer of the testis and 30% remission for cancer of the ovary. It is also active in squamous cell carcinoma of the head and neck, carcinoma of the bladder and drug-resistant choriocarcinoma.

5.1.9   Iron preparations

Iron is an essential constituent of the body, where it is required for haemoglobin formation and the oxidative processes of living tissues. The body contains about 3·5 g of iron, two-thirds of which is present in haemoglobin whilst most of the remainder occurs as the storage form, ferritin. Only a small proportion ($\simeq 10\%$) of iron ingested in food is absorbed and 15–20 mg daily in the diet is sufficient. Much of the iron in food is in the insoluble ferric state but reducing agents also present in the diet, e.g. ascorbic acid and glutathione, reduce ferric to ferrous iron which is more water-soluble. Medicinal iron preparations should, therefore, be taken at meal times. When needed, iron passes through the intestinal mucosa as the ferrous, Fe^{2+}, form. In the mucosal cell Fe^{2+} is oxidized to Fe^{3+}, with the formation of colloidal particles of ferric hydroxide. These particles occupy interstitial spaces in the protein apoferritin, to yield ferritin. When the iron content of blood falls below its normal level, ferritin gives up its Fe^{3+} which is reduced by mucosal cell enzymes to the ferrous state. On passing into the bloodstream it is immediately reoxidized to Fe^{3+}. Two Fe^{3+} ions combine with the protein siderophilin to give transferrin which is a circulating form of iron. Transferrin is a glycopeptide in which Fe^{3+} is chelated between imidazole and tyrosine residues.

Medicinally, iron is required as a dietary supplement in conditions of iron deficiency associated with secondary anaemias. Generally, large doses of ferrous salts are therapeutically most effective since only a small proportion of iron administered orally will be absorbed. Although ferrous sulphate is a convenient means of administration it can be accompanied by astringency and gastric irritation. In order to reduce these side-effects other ferrous preparations which combine iron in a chelated form are used. One of the most successful is ferrous gluconate whilst ferrous fumarate, ferrous succinate and ferrous glycine sulphate are also available.

Although ferric compounds have poor absorption properties they continue to be used for treating anaemia. Ferric iron is formulated in complexes which have reduced gastric irritation and whose solubility enables administration in aqueous solution. In ferric ammonium citrate, iron is present as a citrate complex of unknown composition whereas ferrocholinate is a chelate formed by reacting freshly precipitated ferric hydroxide with choline dihydrogen citrate (5.22). Iron is thought to be bound by two carboxyl groups in a 5-membered ring. Although this complex is much more soluble than ferrous sulphate and ferrous gluconate, and its use is accompanied by much reduced toxicity, there is no evidence for improved oral effectiveness.

$$Me_3\overset{+}{N}\cdot CH_2\cdot CH_2\cdot O\cdot CO\cdot CH_2$$
$$\underset{\overset{|}{C}H_2\cdot COOH}{\overset{|}{C}(OH)COOH}$$

(5.22)

Other iron preparations have been sought when oral medication is not practicable due to adverse gastrointestinal conditions, or when rapid attainment of high serum-iron is required (as in emergency surgery). Iron–dextran is a sterile colloidal solution containing a complex of ferric hydroxide with partially hydrolysed dextran, possessing a lower molecular weight than that used as a blood volume expander. The dextran consists of a polymer of anhydroglucose units consisting mainly of 1,6-linked glucopyranose structures (5.23) although 1,4- and

$$\left[\begin{array}{c} -O-CH_2 \\ \end{array} \right]_n$$

(5.23)

1,3-linkages also occur, giving branched chains. The iron–dextran complex is relatively non-irritating when injected intramuscularly and absorption is virtually complete. Iron–sorbitol injection is a sterile colloidal solution of a complex of ferric iron, sorbitol (a reduction product of glucose) and citric acid, stabilized with dextrin. This is absorbed even more rapidly than iron–dextran.

5.1.10   Metal-binding in enzyme action

Several enzymes require a metal cofactor which, as a result of coordination linkages 'bridges' the substrate and the active site so as to facilitate their interaction. Metal-binding may also enable a polypeptide chain to assume a correct tertiary folding so that relevant isolated regions of the structure might be assembled in relatively close proximity to consitute an active site.

Polypeptide structures in living cells are well-endowed with metal-binding groups, such as the imidazole ring of histidine, the thiol group of cysteine and ionized carboxyl groups of numerous other amino acid residues. The haem–iron proteins found in cytochromes and peroxidases are all derivatives of porphyrin in which the pyrrole hydrogens are replaced by side-chains. In the structure of haem, ferrous iron is essentially square-planar coordinated between four pyrrole nitrogen atoms. A coordination number of 6 for iron permits an extra one or two ligands of the peptide chains to be bound axially to the porphyrin ring. The required oxidation of ferrous to ferric iron readily occurs in such complexes.

Zinc is a necessary cofactor for several enzymes including carboxypeptidases, which hydrolyse peptides and carbonic anhydrase, which accelerates the otherwise slow conversion of carbonic acid to carbon dioxide. Zn^{2+} may also be coordinated to purine bases during the winding and unwinding of DNA.

The structure of the active site of carboxypeptidase A was the first to be determined for an enzyme associated with a metal. It has a molecular weight of about 35 000, contains 307 amino acid units and one zinc atom. Carboxypeptidase A is an important enzyme secreted by the pancreas and which hydrolyses peptides with hydrophobic side-chains at the terminal carboxyl end. This enzyme was also the first to provide evidence that substrates, with the help of metal coordination, can distort the active site of enzymes, i.e. induce conformational changes. Figure 5.1 illustrates the hydrolysis of glycyl-L-tyrosine by carboxypeptidase A. Zn^{2+} lies in a shallow depression, adjacent to a deep lipophilic cavity, where it is coordinated via the imidazole nitrogen atoms of histidine-69 and histidine-196 and the carboxylate anion of glutamic acid-72. The coordination number of 4 is completed with a water molecule (not shown). This water molecule is subsequently displaced

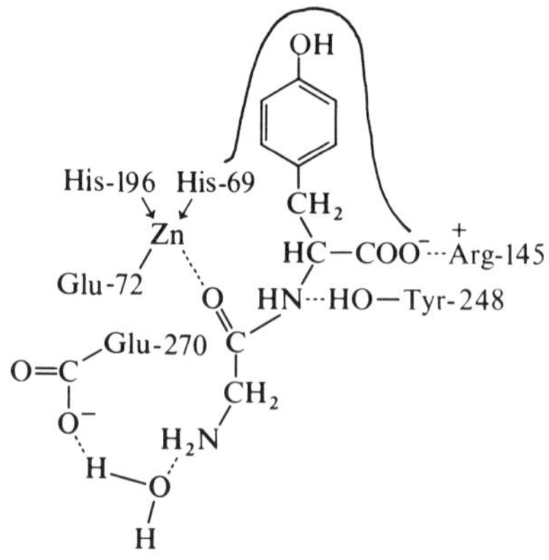

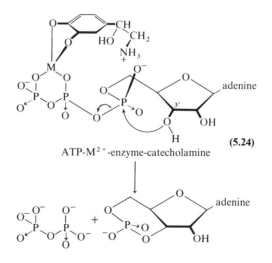

Fig. 5.1   Carboxypeptidase-Zn-glycyl-L-tyrosine.

by a carbonyl oxygen of the peptide link of the substrate which is forced towards the zinc as a result of consolidation of the benzyl group of the substrate within the cavity by van der Waals' binding and hydrophobic forces. The substrate is also ionically bound by its terminal —COO^- to the ionized guanidinium group of arginine-145 which consequently moves through 0.2 nm with the disruption of hydrogen bonds. The resultant disturbance causes a free —OH group of tyrosine-248 to rotate through $120°$ to a position close enough for hydrogen bonding to the —NH of the peptide. The zinc ion facilitates hydrolysis by increasing the polarization of the amide C=O bond for nucleophilic attack, on the electron-deficient carbon, by a carboxylate anion of a suitably positioned glutamic acid-270 residue.

Fig. 5.2   Metal-catalysed formation of cyclic AMP.

Magnesium is necessary for the action of some enzymes which catalyse dehydration and decarboxylation. It also plays a significant role at the β-adrenergic receptor, which consists of the cell membrane-bound enzyme adenyl cyclase in close association with adenosine triphosphate, ATP. Catecholamine responses, such as increased cardiac activity, are mediated by magnesium as a result of complex formation involving its phenolic hydroxyl groups and two oxygen atoms of ATP. This binding facilitates interaction of the positively charged amino group of the hormone with a negative charge on a phosphate oxygen which, as a result, becomes more effectively delocalized. This increases the electrophilic character of the phosphorus and enables intramolecular nucleophilic attack by the 3'-OH group **(5.24)**, resulting in cyclic AMP formation (*see* Fig. 5.2). Protonic dissociation from the 3'-OH group, required for this purpose, is effected by allosteric participation of the imidazole nucleus associated with a histidine residue of adenyl cyclase. Cyclic AMP in turn activates the enzyme phophorylase, which increases the rate of glycogen breakdown enabling the heart to be stimulated followed by the typical physiological actions associated with adrenaline.

5.2   ISOSTERIC MODIFICATIONS IN DRUG DESIGN

5.2.1   Introduction

The concept of isosterism has helped considerably over the years in the search for and design of new drugs. It is a concept which has been useful in the absence of more precise knowledge of how to tailor a chemical structure to produce a required biological effect. The discovery of a compound with promising medicinal activity leads to a search for other structurally closely related compounds, which have improved therapeutic properties and reduced unwanted side-effects. In the past, medicinal chemists have developed a considerable amount of intuition, in this respect, in selecting appropriate structural modifications. Much of this search has been based on isosteric relationships and has led to a fruitful yield of new, improved drugs. This enlightened empirical approach may well be increasingly superseded in future years by a more controlled quantitative evaluation of the contribution of structural modifications to biological activity (*see* Chapter 8).

In its simplest form, isosteric modification involves the replacement of an atom, or group of atoms, in a molecule by another group with similar electronic and steric configuration. Isosterism is an attempt to apply to molecules or molecular fragments the premise that similarities in properties of elements within vertical groups of the Periodic Table are due to identical valence electronic configurations. Thus, two molecules or molecular fragments containing an identical number and arrangement of electrons should have similar properties and are termed isosteres, e.g. CO and N_2, CO_2 and N_2O, CH_2N_2 and $CH_2{=}CO$. Further, the early recognition that benzene and thiophen were alike in many of their properties (*see* Table 5.6) led to the term 'ring equivalents' to describe the interchanging of —CH=CH— and —S—, which distinguishes their structures. The structural

Table 5.6   Boiling points (° C) of benzene and thiophen derivatives

	Benzene	80	Thiophen	84
	methyl-	110	2-methyl-	113
Derivatives	chloro-	132	2-chloro-	130
	acetyl-	200	2-acetyl-	214

resemblance of pyridine to benzene constitutes another pair of ring equivalents, —CH= and —N=. Hydrogens may be ignored in these comparisons, when the respective isosteric pairs are then seen to have similar peripheral electronic arrangements and are of similar size. The idea of such 'equivalents' was extended to a consideration of elements, in the Periodic Table, to which hydrogen atoms were progressively added to give vertical columns of atoms and groups containing identical electronic configurations (*see* Table 5.7). The term, isosteres, was defined as 'atoms, groups or ions in which the peripheral layers of electrons are identical'. Compounds arising from the interchange of such atoms or groups are referred to as 'classical' isosteres.

Table 5.7   Isosterically related atoms and groups

Electronic configurations	2(4)	2(5)	2(6)	2(7)
	=C=	—N=	—O—	—F
		—CH=	—NH—	—OH
			—CH$_2$—	—NH$_2$
				—CH$_3$

The indiscriminate application of these concepts to a wide range of groups may require a consideration of the effect of small atoms such as hydrogen and of differences in the hybridization of outer orbitals which could cause variations in size, shape and polarity of respective molecules. However, since the biological properties of 'classically' related isosteric compounds often turned out to be more similar than their chemical and physical properties, the term 'bio-isosteres' was evolved. This has led to a broadening of the concept in order to recognize 'non-classically' related isosteric features, which may be interchanged in a molecule with retention of some resemblance in steric and local electronic configuration. Thus, modifications in a 'classical' or 'non-classical' sense were expected to yield a product which would pass through membranes to reach a site of action as effectively as a parent drug. At this site, the modified drug might then be able to elicit a similar (or antagonistic) response. Examples of drugs which have evolved from the application of such concepts are best grouped into classical and non-classical modifications respectively.

5.2.2   Classical isosteric modifications

5.2.2.1   *Replacement of univalent atoms or groups*

The analogous groups considered here, —F (or —Cl), —OH, —NH$_2$ and —CH$_3$ are seen in Table 5.7. Progressive modifications of the oral hypoglycaemics have involved the successive replacement of the amino, —NH$_2$, group of carbutamide **(5.49a)** by a methyl, —CH$_3$, or chlorine, —Cl, to give tolbutamide **(5.49b)** and chlorpropamide **(7.70)** respectively (*see* Chapter 7) which possess extended biological half-lives and reduced toxicity.

The development of antagonistic activity when a —OH group of folic acid **(4.25)** is replaced by —NH$_2$ is seen in aminopterin **(4.26)**. Similar antagonistic relationships occur when the 6-OH of inosine **(4.19)** and guanine **(4.21)** is replaced by —SH to give the anticancer drugs, 6-mercaptopurine **(4.35)** and 6-thioguanine **(4.36)**. These contain the tautomeric structures, —N=C(SH)— and —NH—C=S, and act in similar biological systems as their oxygen isoteres. The barbiturates and thiobarbiturates constitute another example (*see* Section 7.3.1) where the latter, due to rapid immobilization in fat, produce a faster and shorter duration of action suitable for intravenously induced anaesthesia.

5.2.2.2   *Interchange of divalent atoms and groups*

Bio-isosterism occurs more frequently between divalent atoms and groups. Steric similarities here are aided by similarities in bond angles (*see* Table 5.8) so that

Table 5.8   Bond angles in divalent atoms and groups

Groups	O	S	NH	CH$_2$
Angles (°)	108±3	112±2	111±3	111·5±3

attached groups are spatially orientated in a like manner. This is borne out in the isosteric relationship of esters and amides. In esters the rotation of C—O—C bonds is restricted by resonance **(5.25)** and aliphatic esters exist, predominantly, in the *cis* configuration **(5.25)** rather than the *trans* **(5.26)**. Studies on amides have

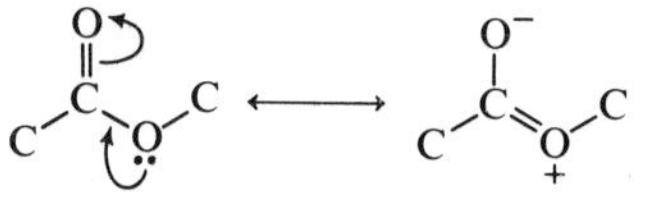

(5.25) 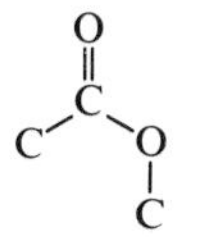   **(5.26)**

also revealed similar planar structures and a predominant configuration **(5.27)**

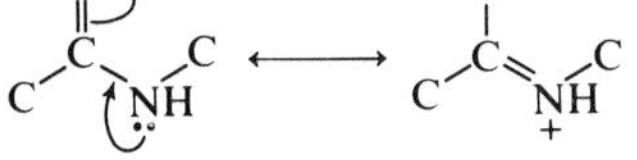

(5.27)

analogous to the *cis* ester. This explains the ability of structurally related esters, e.g. procaine **(5.28)** and amides, e.g. procainamide **(5.29)**, to function as local anaesthetics. Procaine is believed to owe its local anaesthetic activity to an optimum combination of lipid solubility, for transport across the phosphilipid nerve membrane, and polarity for charge-transfer complex formation involving

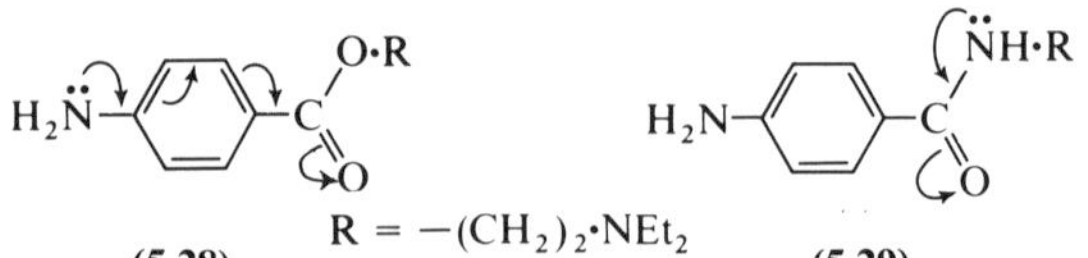

$$R = -(CH_2)_2 \cdot NEt_2$$

(5.28)   **(5.29)**

dipolar C=O and a thiazolinium ion of thiamine pryrophosphate, which has a specific role in nerve conduction.

The local anaesthetic activity of procaine is, however, greater than that of procainamide since, in the former, the dipolar character of the carbonyl group, required for activity, is more pronounced **(5.28)**. In procainamide the amine group resonance, $(+M)$, is offset by the amide resonance so that the magnitude of the C=O dipole is decreased **(5.29)**. Procainamide, however, has found an important role in correcting cardiac arrhythmias. Physiological studies have shown that procainamide is not affected by esterases which catalyse the hydrolysis of procaine. The increased stability of procainamide also permits oral use (*see also* Section 7.3.2.2).

Isosterism between esters and amides explains the mode of action of puromycin which has antibacterial, antitrypanosomidal and anti-tumour activity. Puromycin inhibits protein synthesis in ribosomes by interfering with the utilization of transfer-RNAs (tRNA). In the synthesis of protein, a particular tRNA esterifies a specific amino acid via its terminal adenosine unit, prior to combining with messenger-RNA (mRNA) and aligning with other acylated tRNA units. Puromycin, 3'[α-amino-β-(p-methoxyphenyl)-propionamido]-3'-deoxy-*N,N*-dimethyl-adenosine **(9.7)**, is the amide analogue of the terminal unit of tyrosinyl-tRNA and is taken up by mRNA in place of the latter. This blocks the subsequent formation of a protein peptide chain (*see also* Section 9.3.3).

Interchanges of —O—, —S—, —NH— and —CH$_2$— have been exploited in the development of several drugs. The H$_1$-antihistamine, diphenhydramine **(5.30a)**, has been extensively modified in a non-classical sense (*see* p. 159) after initially replacing the ether oxygen by —NH— **(5.30b)**. Subsequent structural manipulation of **(5.30b)** so as to attach one of the phenyl groups to the imino

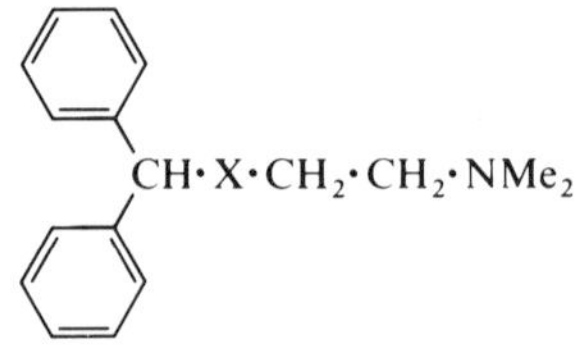

CH·X·CH$_2$·CH$_2$·NMe$_2$

(5.30)   **(a)** = X = O
             (b) = X = NH

nitrogen has led to the potent antihistamine, antergan **(5.31)**. Bulky tricyclic ester groups of anticholinergic spasmolytics (*see* Section 3.3.3) have been modified by interchanging —CH$_2$— for —O—**(3.23b)**. More recently, the substitution of —CH$_2$— by —S— in the side-chain of burimamide **(3.27)** to give metiamide **(3.30a)**, has invoked electronic and conformational effects required for improved H$_2$-antihistaminic activity (*see* Sections 3.4.1, 3.4.2). Further isoteric modification of the thiourea moiety, —NH·C(S)·NH—, in metiamide to guanidino, —NH·C(NH)·NH—, brought the synthesis a stage nearer to cimetidine **(3.30b)**.

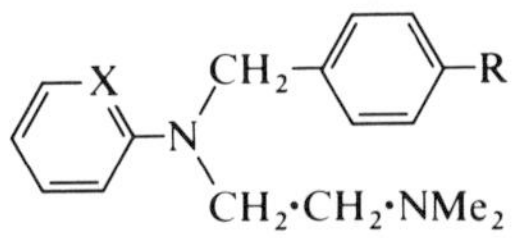

(5.31)   X = CH, R = H
(5.32)   X = N, R = O·Me

The replacement of —S— by —CH$_2$—CH$_2$— in the heterocyclic ring of chlorpromazine **(3.41a)** has led to the development of valuable antidepressant drugs such as imipramine **(3.42)** and amitryptyline **(3.44)**. Further modifications of the resultant 7-membered ring by substitution of —CH$_2$— by —O—, —S— and —NH— have yielded useful psychotherapeutic drugs (e.g. doxepin **(3.46)**).

Ring substitutions of —CH=CH— by —S— or —O— have been very profitable. Replacements of pyridyl rings in sulphonamides in this manner have produced sulphathiazole, sulphafurazole **(4.10)** and sulphamethizole **(4.11)**. Fentanyl citrate **(5.33)** is a potent analgesic, producing surgical analgesia. When administered with a major tranquillizer, it maintains a patient in a calm and indifferent state allowing cooperation with the surgeon. Replacement of phenyl by thienyl **(5.34)** is reputed to yield an analgesic 4500 times as potent as morphine and possessing rapid onset but relatively short duration of action with a high margin of safety.

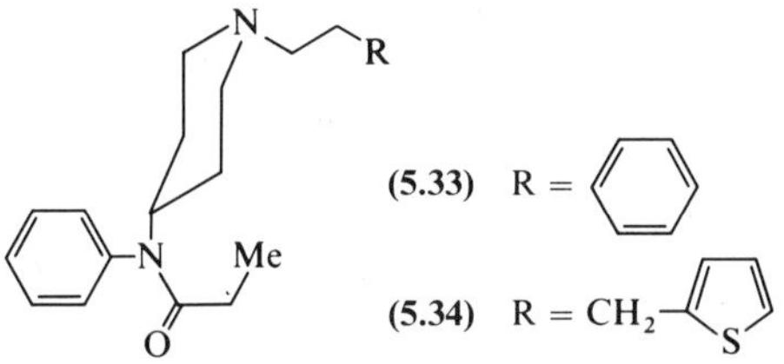

(5.33)   R =
(5.34)   R = CH$_2$—

The interchanging of phenyl with sulphur-, oxygen- and nitrogen-containing heterocyclic rings has also been extensively exploited in the development of semisynthetic penicillins and cephalosporins with broader spectra of activity and greater stability towards β-lactamases (*see* Section 9.5).

5.2.2.3   *Interchange of trivalent atoms and groups*

The substitution of —CH= by —N= in aromatic rings has been one of the most successful applications of classical isoterism. One of the most potent antihistamines, mepyramine **(5.32)**, has evolved from the replacement of a phenyl group in antergan **(5.31)** by pyridyl. The π-electron deficiency of the pyridine nucleus enables the nitrogen electron pair to hydrogen bond with a water molecule, effecting an increase in hydrophilicity which is significant in determining the high level of biological activity. Substitution of the pyridyl amino $-N\overset{\diagup}{\diagdown}$ by $-C\overset{\diagup}{H}$ in mepyramine (and 4-methoxybenzyl by 4-chlorophenyl) produces chlorophen-iramine **(5.35)** valued for its short, powerful action and relative freedom from

(5.35)

sedation, which is an undesirable side-effect of antihistamine drugs. The electron-withdrawing effect of the pyridyl and *p*-Cl phenyl substituents on the $-C\overset{\diagup}{H}$ group promotes formation of an electron-deficient centre, which may determine the mechanism by which bio-receptor interaction occurs.

The substitution of a benzene ring by pyridine has also effected improved activity in the tricyclic antihistaminic and neuroleptic, major tranquillizing, drugs with the introduction of isothipendyl **(5.36)**, cf. promethazine **(5.37)** and pro-thipendyl **(5.38)**, cf. promazine **(5.39)**. Sedative and extrapyramidal effects, respectively, are much reduced.

(5.36)	R = $CH_2 \cdot CH(Me) \cdot NMe_2$,	X = N
(5.37)	R = $CH_2 \cdot CH(Me) \cdot NMe_2$,	X = CH
(5.38)	R = $CH_2 \cdot CH_2 \cdot CH_2 \cdot NMe_2$,	X = N
(5.39)	R = $CH_2 \cdot CH_2 \cdot CH_2 \cdot NMe_2$,	X = CH

Earlier examples of $-N{=}/{-}CH{=}$ substitution are to be found in the sulphonamide antibacterials with the development of sulphapyridine **(4.5)** and sulphadiazine **(4.6)** where the heterocyclic ring confers greater acidity on the sulphonamide group. Similar substitutions in 5-membered rings have yielded sulphonamides renowned for their high solubility in urine (*see* p. 96).

Ring replacement of $-N\overset{\diagup}{\diagdown}$ by $-C\overset{\diagup}{H}$ and its subsequent modification to $\overset{\diagup}{\diagdown}C{=}$ has resulted in a variety of useful drugs. This is seen in the development of psychotherapeutics such as chlorprothixene **(3.43)** and amitryptyline **(3.44)** and the anti-inflammatory, sulindac (clinoril) **(5.40b)**. The excellent anti-inflammatory properties of indomethacin **(5.40a)** are marred by gastrointestinal irritation to the extent of intolerance. Interest in indole derivatives as antirheumatics arose from the possible implication of 5-hydroxytryptamine in the inflammatory process.

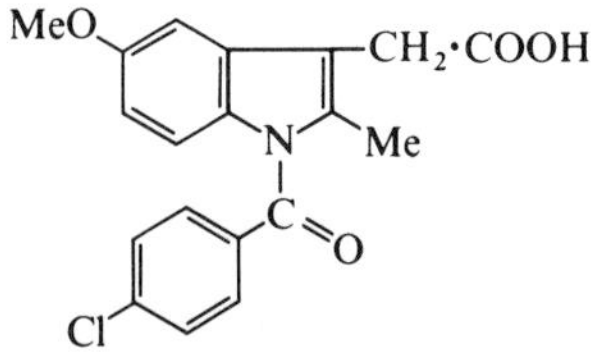

(5.40a) 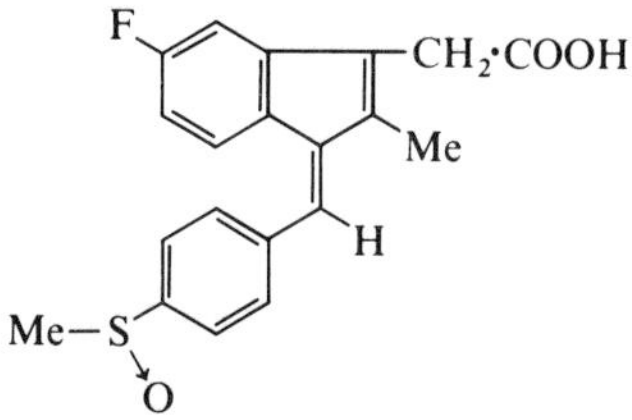   (5.40b)

Modifications of the indole nucleus in indomethacin produced sulindac, whose conformation was shown by X-ray analysis to be similar to indomethacin. The presence of the fluorine atom enhances potency whilst the p-methylsulphinyl group increases solubility and improves pharmacodynamic properties. The methylsulphide (MeS—) metabolite contributes significantly to pharmacological action as a potent inhibitor of prostaglandin synthetase. The methylphenylsulphinyl group also constitutes a chiral centre since in forming the $\overset{+}{S}$—$\bar{O}$ bond there is overlap of p and d orbitals and therefore no requirement for the S and O atoms to lie in one plane as in p-orbital overlap of the C=O double bond. Sulindac is composed of a racemic mixture of D- and L-forms, both of which are equally active.

In a search for histamine H_2-antagonists, extensive isosteric modifications of the imidazole nucleus have been investigated to produce compounds analogous to cimetidine (3.30b). This has recently resulted in the development of a furan derivative, ranitidine (5.41), in which basic properies are retained by substitution

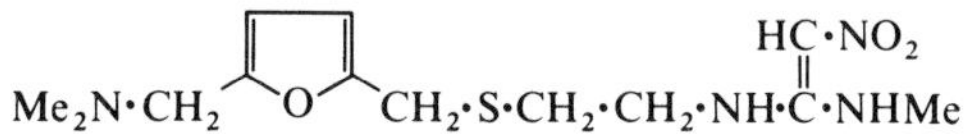

(5.41)

of a dimethyl aminomethyl group on the heterocyclic ring. The substituted guanidino group has also been isosterically modified by utilizing a nitromethenyl moiety to reduce basicity. Preliminary clinical trials have indicated freedom from some side-effects (e.g. gynaecomastia and mental confusion) associated with cimetidine.

5.2.3 Non-classical isosteric modifications

The successful application of classical isosterism to drug design has led to the synthesis of compounds in which the modified molecule bears an isosteric relationship, to the parent structure, which may be interpreted in a wider sense. The resemblance is sometimes more subtle.

5.2.3.1 *Reversal of groups*

Trimeperidine (5.42) is the propanoate ester of a piperidyl alcohol whilst pethidine, meperidine, is an ethyl ester of a piperidyl carboxylic acid (5.43). Thus, the first compound is related to the second by reversal of an ester group.

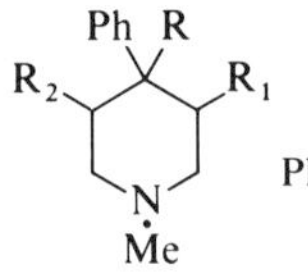

(5.42) R = O·COEt, R$_1$ = R$_2$ = Me
(5.43) R = COOEt, R$_1$ = R$_2$ = H

Care should be taken not to attribute isosterism to the development of drugs when this was not the original guiding principle. It is commonly stated that lignocaine (5.44) represents an extension of the molecular modification of cocaine and other local anaesthetics, e.g. procainamide (5.29) by being a reverse amide. However, it was during an investigation of the plant alkaloid gramine (5.45), that the indole (5.46) was shown to possess local anaesthetic activity. The intermediate (5.47), which preceded ring closure in the synthesis of (5.46), was also active and, from the preparation of a series of analogues, lignocaine was found to be the nearest approach to an ideal local anaesthetic. This also illustrated the usefulness of biologically screening intermediates formed in synthetic routes to medicinal compounds.

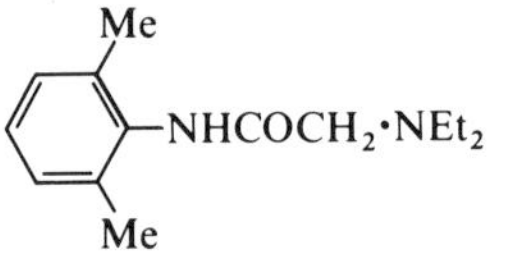

(5.44)

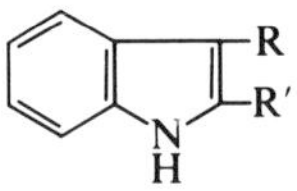

(5.45) R = CH$_2$·NMe$_2$, R′ = H
(5.46) R = H, R′ = CH$_2$·NMe$_2$

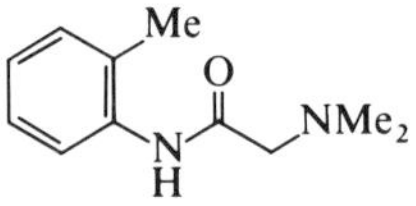

(5.47)

5.2.3.2 Ring opening and closure

Sulphonamide oral hypoglycaemics arose directly from the clinical observation, in 1942, that a sulphathiazole derivative (5.48), which was being used specifically for treating typhoid, lowered the blood sugar almost to a fatal level. It was not until

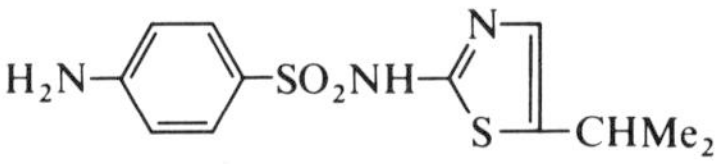

(5.48)

1955 that compounds based on this observation came into use for treating diabetes. Modifications involving opening of the thiazole ring to give a thiourea unit in which =S was ultimately replaced by =O yielded carbutamide (5.49a) which was later replaced by the less toxic tolbutamide (5.49b). More than 12 000 sulphonylureas are reputed to have been synthesized, of which about twenty have

$$R-\text{⟨ ⟩}-SO_2\cdot NH\cdot CONHnBu$$

(5.49) (a) R = NH$_2$
(b) R = Me

been used clinically. Their main effect appears to be in the pancreas through an insulin-releasing mechanism. These have proved a useful and safe oral means of controlling diabetes, being most valuable when the disease commences in adulthood. It is estimated that over five million diabetics throughout the world are taking sulphonylureas orally as a welcome alternative to insulin injections.

The considerable contribution of sulphonamides to medicine may be further illustrated by the development of anti-tubercular thiosemicarbazones **(5.51)**, from the observation that sulphathiadiazole **(5.50)** possessed weak anti-tubercular properties. Although **(5.51)** may be loosely regarded as an open chain analogue of **(5.50)**, it was discovered as a result of biologically screening intermediates in the synthesis of aminothiadiazoles. This was an important discovery since, as early as 1951, thiosemicarbazones were also shown to possess antiviral activity. The substitution of the $=N-NH\cdot CS\cdot NH_2$ group in other nuclei, e.g. 2-oxyindole, led to increased antiviral activity. Thus, methisazone **(5.52)** has remarkable activity in preventing infection by smallpox amongst people who have previously been in contact with fatal cases.

$$H_2N-\text{⟨ ⟩}-SO_2NH-\text{(N-N / S)}$$

(5.50)

$$R\cdot NH-\text{⟨ ⟩}-CH=N\cdot NH-\text{(NH_2 / S)}$$

(5.51)

$$\text{(oxyindole)}N\cdot NH\cdot CS\cdot NH_2$$

(5.52)

Although stilboestrol **(6.22)** may be regarded as a 'ring opened' modification of oestradiol, its discovery was due entirely to a chance observation.

A series of substituted 1,1-diphenyl-3-amino-1-propenes, representing the opening of the central ring in tricyclic antidepressants, have shown promising thymoleptic activity.

A vast number of profitable modifications have evolved from the closure of rings. Thus, the 'tying back' of the aromatic rings of a diphenylmethyl ester **(5.53)** to produce a fluorene analogue **(5.54)** markedly increases anticholinergic spasmolytic activity.

The 'tying back' of basic amino groups has taken many forms. The formation of phenmetrazine **(5.55)** represents an attempt to produce an appetite suppressant lacking the CNS stimulant properties of ephedrine **(5.56)** or amphetamine. Replacement of a terminal N,N-diethylamino group by piperidino exploits the decreasing valency angle at the tertiary nitrogen of the latter so that access of the

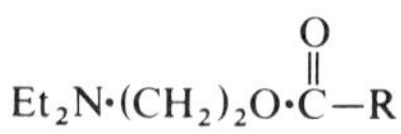

$$Et_2N\cdot(CH_2)_2O\cdot\overset{\displaystyle O}{\overset{\|}{C}}-R$$

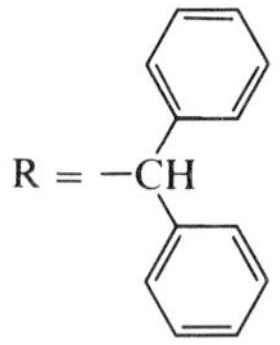

(5.53)   R = —CH (with two phenyl groups)

(5.54)   R = — (fluorene group)

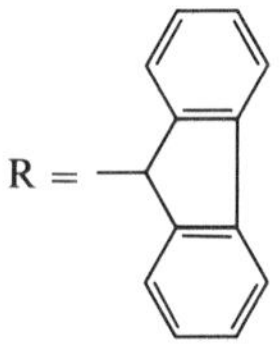

basic group to anionic sites might be improved. This modification often leads to greater potency and is found in the development of major tranquillizers, local anaesthetics, antihistamines and spasmolytics. In the major tranquillizers, the

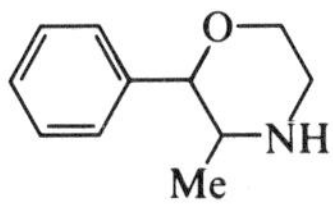

(5.55)

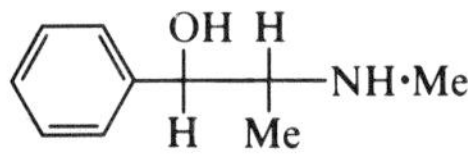

(5.56)

dimethylaminopropyl side-chain has been varied to produce thioridazine (5.57), prochlorperazine and trifluoperazine (3.45); the resultant introduction of additional methylene groups also increases lipophilic properties.

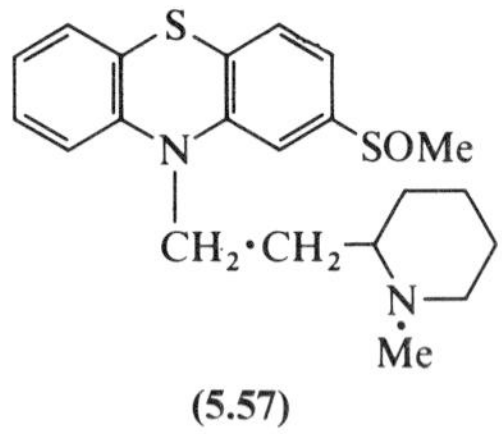

(5.57)

The local anaesthetic, bupivicaine (5.58), has arisen from a similar modification of the side-chain of lignocaine (5.44). The considerably increased lipophilic properties give a product which, when injected between the third and fourth lumbar vertebrae, produces a long lasting spinal anaesthesia.

Several valuable drugs with antihistaminic, motion-sickness preventative and anti-emetic action, e.g. cyclizine (5.59), chlorcyclizine (5.60) and meclozine (5.61),

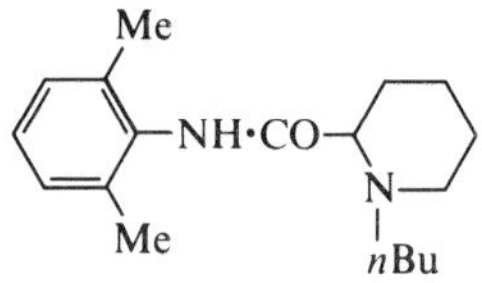

(5.58)

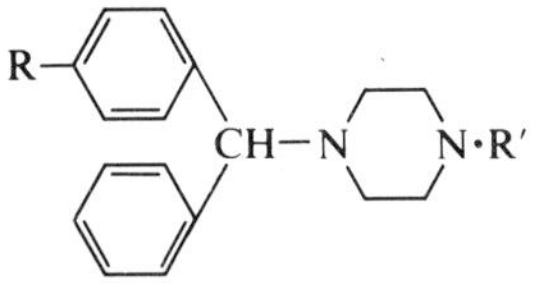

(5.59)   R = H, R' = Me   Me
(5.60)   R = Cl, R' = Me
(5.61)   R = Cl, R' = CH$_2$—

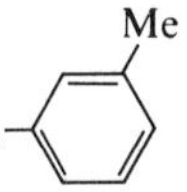

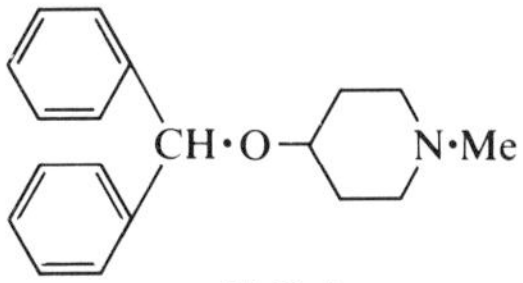

(5.61a)

have evolved from incorporating the two basic groups of the imino derivative (5.30b) of diphenhydramine (5.30a) into a piperazine structure. In a more recent variation of structure, to give diphenylpyraline, the basic side-chain of diphenhydramine is 'tied back' so as to link the benzhydryl ether group with N-methylpiperidine in the 4-position (5.61a). Replacement of the 2-dimethylaminoethyl group of antergan (5.31) by imidazolin-2-ylmethyl to produce antazoline was thought to enhance competition, with histamine, for the H$_1$-receptor.

Improved anticholinergic activity has also been attained by the 'tying back' of alkyl groups attached to basic and quaternary nitrogen atoms, respectively, to produce anti-Parkinsonism agents such as benzhexol (3.24a) and spasmolytics such as poldine (3.23e).

5.2.3.3 Groups with similar polar effects

The correlation of metabolite–antimetabolite relationships in the antagonism of p-aminobenzoic acid by suphonamides (see Section 4.3.1.1) has focussed attention on groups with similar polar effects, e.g. —COOH and —SO$_2$NHR. Thus, the interchange of such groups was pursued in a search for antagonistic or analogous biological effects. The antagonism of nikethamide, (5.62), by pyridine-3-sulphonic acid (5.63) and the simulation of its respiratory stimulant effects by the nitrophenyl analogue (5.64) are further examples. Replacement of CO by SO$_2$ in pethidine, meperidine (5.43), weakens analgesic activity.

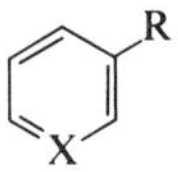

(5.62)   X = N, R = CONEt$_2$
(5.63)   X = N, R = SO$_3$H
(5.64)   X = C—NO$_2$, R = CONEt$_2$

The lack of success in this type of isosteric modification has not discouraged the pursuit of more subtle variations in structures, such as the tetrazole analogues of carboxylic acids. Whilst the acidity of a carboxylic acid (pK$_a$ 4·2–4·4) is related to resonance stabilization of the carboxylate anion (5.65a), the acidity of tetrazole (pK$_a$ 4·9) is attributed to delocalization of the anionic charge over each of the ring nitrogens (5.65b). Although the greater number of canonical forms contributing to the resonance hybrid suggest that resonance stabilization might be more effective

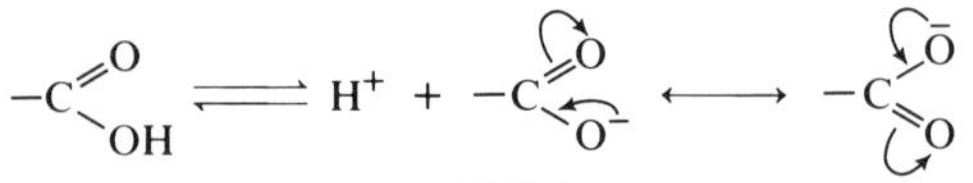

(5.65a)

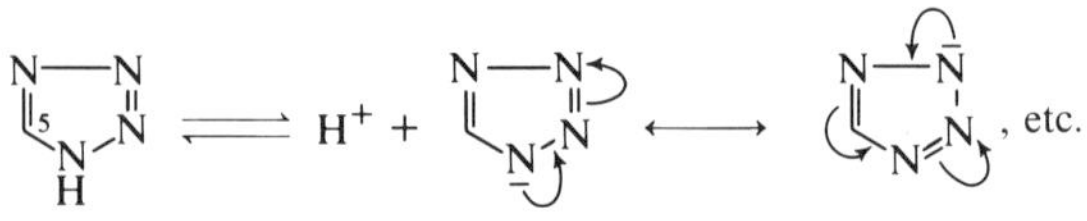

(5.65b)

than in the carboxylate anion, the greater electronegativity of oxygen is an over-riding factor in determining the increased acidity of the carboxylic acid.

In a search for improved antihyperlipidemic agents the tetrazolyl analogue **(5.67)** of nicotinic acid **(5.66)** was found to be three times as active in lowering blood cholesterol.

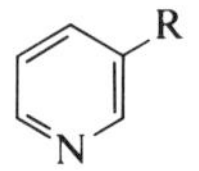

(5.66) R = COOH

(5.67) R =

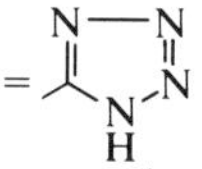

A search for broad-spectrum semisynthetic penicillins revealed that the sub-stitution of hydrophilic groups in the benzylamido side-chain extended their activity to Gram negative bacteria. Thus, α-carboxybenzylpenicillin, carbenicillin **(5.68)**, is active against *Pseudomonas aeruginosa* which is a Gram negative bacteria notable for its general lack of susceptibility to β-lactam antibiotics. Carbenicillin has the added advantage of possessing a sterically hindered acylamino α-carbon, a feature which confers resistance to degradation by β-lactamases. Carbenicillin is not administered orally since the β-carbonyl acid readily decarboxylates in the acidic environment of the stomach to form the further acid-labile benzylpenicillin. The α-(5-tetrazolyl) derivative **(5.69)** represents an attempt to overcome this instability. 3-(5-Tetrazolyl) and 4-(5-tetrazolyl) analogues of penicillins and cephalosporins, respectively, are reported to have potent, broad-spectrum antibac-terial activity.

Classical isosteric replacement of the phenyl ring in carbenicillin to give the α-thien-3-yl analogue, ticarcillin, increases activity against *P. aeruginosa* whilst non-classical isosteric replacement of the α-COOH in carbenicillin by the more strongly acidic —SO$_2$OH increases chemical stability.

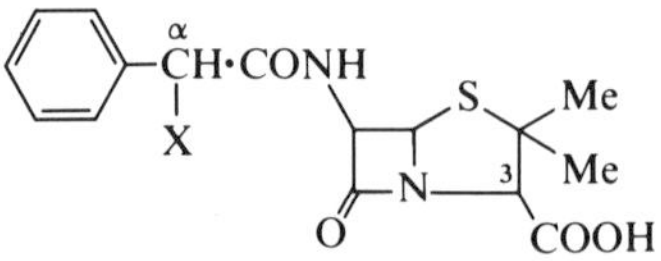

(5.68) X = COOH
(5.69) X = 5-tetrazolyl

The 3-acetoxymethyl side-chain of cephalosporins has been substituted by many structures in attempts to overcome the ease with which this group is metabolically hydrolysed to the less antibacterially active alcohol. Cephamandole is the 3-(1-methyltetrazol-5-ylthiomethyl) analogue which possesses activity against a broad group of Gram negative organisms. (For a fuller account of structure–activity relationships in penicillins and cephalosporins *see* Section 9.5.)

5.3 CHOICE OF ANION (OR CATION) FOR SALT FORMATION

5.3.1 Introduction

A high proportion of synthetic drugs are bases which are usually available as salts of appropriate acids. The most commonly used anions for salt formation are chloride and sulphate. Salts are almost invariably crystalline, more readily purified and generally more stable to oxidation than corresponding bases. Unlike the parent bases, many salts are appreciably water soluble and hence provide a convenient form for preparing sterile aqueous solutions for injection. Salts are also convenient for rapid dissolution from solid dosage forms such as tablets and capsules (*see* Chapter 2).

Sometimes the salts prepared are designed to achieve low water solubility and thus provide preparations of a medicament which, when injected intramuscularly in aqueous suspension, give a depot from which the active drug is slowly leached away. In this way, therapeutic concentrations are maintained for a much longer time when compared with a single injection of a more water-soluble salt.

5.3.2 Factors affecting choice of anion (or cation)

Drug design must take into account several of the above and other factors which may influence the choice of acid for converting a basic drug to a suitable salt for administration by a particular route. These factors may be illustrated by reference to a selection of medicaments.

Adrenaline is formulated as the hydrogentartrate salt for injections, on economic grounds, since the active (−)-isomer is obtained by resolution from a synthetic (±)-mixture using tartaric acid. The dibasic acid also has the advantage of giving rise to acidic salt solutions which assist stability.

Many antihistamines are used in the form of salts with organic acids, e.g. maleate, acid citrate, because hydrohalides may sometimes be difficult to prepare or are hygroscopic or not absorbed effectively. The antihistamines, promethazine (**5.37**) and diphenhydramine (**5.30a**), may be formulated as hydrochlorides or less soluble 8-chlorotheophyllinates (anion, (**5.70**)). The latter produce a more pro-

(5.70)

longed anti-emetic effect and may also partially offset effects of CNS depression. Cyclizine (5.59) hydrochloride is not sufficiently water soluble to be given by injection, so the lactate salt is used to prevent postoperative vomiting. It is administered about 20 minutes before the anticipated end of surgery. Antazoline (*see* p. 159) is usually used as the hydrochloride in tablet form for treating allergies, whilst the more water-soluble methanesulphonate, mesylate, salt is used in preparing solutions for injection.

The major tranquillizer, prochlorperazine (5.71), is formulated as the dimaleate for oral administration but when a more immediate effect is desirable, the highly water-soluble dimethanesulphonate (5.71a) or ethanesulphonate (edysylate) (5.71b) salt is injected. Other alkyl sulphonate salts conferring increased water solubility for injection purposes are benztropine, 3-benzhydryloxytropine,

(5.71) (a) ·2MeO·S·OH
             ‖
             O

(b) ·HO·S·O·CH$_2$·CH$_2$·O·S·OH

mesylate, used for controlling the symptoms of Parkinsonism and pentamidine isethionate, 4,4'-(pentamethylenedioxy)dibenzamidine di(2-hydroxyethane-sulphonate), used for treating African trypanosomiasis.

Salts are sometimes formulated with a view to overcoming bitter taste. Bitterness results from dissolution of a compound in saliva followed by reaction with sensitive receptors for taste. Thus, the normal hydrochloride salts of chlorpromazine (3.41a) and amitryptyline (3.44) which are bitter may be replaced by the much less water-soluble embonates [4,4'-methylene *bis*(3-hydroxynaphthalene-2-carboxylate)] in preparing suspensions for oral medication. Bitterness and the occasional irritation of mucous membranes associated with the analgesic, dextropropoxyphene (3.11) hydrochloride, may be avoided by using the less soluble napsylate, naphthalene-2-sulphonate, salt.

The anti-Parkinsonism drug, biperidine (3.24b), which is usually administered orally as the hydrochloride, may be given intramuscularly or by slow intravenous infusion as the more soluble lactate salt when rapid control of severe cases is necessary. Another preparation formulated for increased water solubility is dinoprost trometamol which is the salt of the acidic prostaglandin F$_{2\alpha}$ with 2-amino-2(hydroxymethyl)propane-1,3-diol. This is intravenously infused in order to stimulate uterine contractions in the induction of labour or in the therapeutic termination of pregnancy.

Relatively insoluble salts are also used for depot therapy when the drug is administered by intramuscular injection. This enables a slow release of the medicament in the bloodstream. Thus, cycloguanyl (4.31) embonate, suspended as fine particles in an oily base, gives protection against malaria when injected on a 3-monthly basis. This dosage form requires vulnerable people living in isolated regions to visit clinics much less frequently. Slow release preparations of penicillin are dependent on an appropriate choice of cation. Benzylpenicillin may be formulated with the bases, *N,N'*-dibenzylethylenediamine or *N*-benzylphen-ethylamine to give benzathine penicillin or benethamine penicillin respectively. These have very low water solubility and may be injected intramuscularly in aqueous suspension to provide a depot from which penicillin is slowly leached by dissociation. Periodic, once or twice weekly, treatment suffices in controlling syphilis. Procaine penicillin, obtained by formulating the acidic benzylpenicillin with the base, procaine, has a solubility of about 0·5% in water and is also injected intramuscularly · in aqueous suspension. Antibacterial concentrations are maintained in the bloodstream for 12–24 hours. The relatively low blood concentrations attained means that these penicillin preparations must be restricted to treating infections due to micro-organisms which are highly sensitive to the antibiotic.

The anticholinesterase, neostigmine (5.72), is formulated as the non-hygroscopic quaternary methobromide in tablets and as the hygroscopic methosulphate for

(5.72)

injection. The choice of quaternizing agents has also been investigated for atropine (3.22a) preparations used, in the form of sprays, as bronchodilators in bronchial asthma. Atropine isopropobromide and ethobromide have been evaluated clini-cally as alternatives to the methonitrate, which was designed to exclude atropine from the CNS (*see* Section 3.3.3).

FURTHER READING

1. Albert A. (1979) Metal-binding substances. In *Selective Toxicity*, 6th ed. London, Chapman & Hall, pp. 385–442.
2. Stenlake J. B. (1979) Metal chelation. In *Foundations of Molecular Pharmacology*: Vol. 2, *The Chemical Basis of Drug Action*. University of London, Athlone, pp. 86–99.
3. Huheey J. E. (1978) Co-ordination Chemistry – theory, structure and mechanisms. In *Inorganic Chemistry. Principles of Structure and Reactivity*, 2nd ed. New York – London, Harper, pp. 332–488.
4. (*a*) Daniels T. C. and Jorgensen E. C. (1977) Physicochemical properties in relation to biological action. Chelation and biological action. (*b*) Schultz H. W. (1977) Surfactants and chelating agents. In Wilson C. O., Gisvold O. and Doerge R. F. (ed.) *Textbook of Organic, Medicinal and Pharmaceutical Chemistry*, 7th ed. Philadelphia – Toronto, Lippincott, (*a*) pp. 50–6, (*b*) pp. 222–46.
5. Fiabane A. M. and Williams D. R. (1977) Principles of bio-inorganic medicine. In *The Principles of Bio-inorganic Chemistry*. London Chemical Society, Monographs for Teachers No. 31, pp. 82–107.

6. Schubert J. (1981) Mixed complex formation: new therapeutic approaches. *Trends Pharmacol. Sci.* **2**, 50–2.
7. Craig P. N. (1980) Guidelines for drug and analogue design. In Wolff M. E. (ed.) *Burger's Medicinal Chemistry*, 4th ed., Part 1. New York – London, Wiley pp. 331–48.
8. Burger A. (1979) Relationships of chemical structures and biological activity in drug design. *Trends Pharmacol. Sci.* **1**, 62–4.
9. (*a*) Anand N. (1980) Sulphonamides and sulphones. (*b*) Hoover J. R. E. and Dunn G. L. (1980) The β-lactam antibiotics. In Wolff M. E. (ed.) *Burger's Medicinal Chemistry*, 4th ed., Part 2, New York – London, Wiley (*a*) pp. 1–40, (*b*) pp. 83–172.
10. (*a*) Shen T. Y. (1981) Non-steroidal anti-inflammatory agents. (*b*) Witiak D. T. and Cavestri R. C. (1981) Inhibitors of the allergic response. (*c*) Tkaman B. H. and Adams H. J. (1981) Local anaesthetics. In Wolff M. E. (ed.) *Burger's Medicinal Chemistry*, 4th ed., Part 3. New York – London, Wiley (*a*) pp. 1206–72, (*b*) pp. 553–622, (*c*) pp. 645–98.

Chapter 6

The chemotherapy of cancer

The chemotherapy of cancer

6.1   INTRODUCTION

About 180 000 new cases of cancer occur each year in the U.K. and the annual number of deaths from cancers of all kinds is about 130 000. This constitutes approximately 20% of all U.K. deaths. The proportion of hospital beds occupied by cancer patients is considerable. Aspects of this disease which still present a formidable challenge to medicinal chemists and clinicians, who need to translate new discoveries into practice, will first be considered.

6.1.1   Nature of the disease

Cancer is a disease of cells characterized by a reduction, or loss of effectiveness, in normal cellular control and maturation mechanisms which regulate multiplication. There are four main features, as described below.

6.1.1.1   *Excessive cell proliferation*

This usually results in the formation of a tumour. Normal adult tissues do not grow – they maintain a steady number of cells. In some tissues, e.g. liver, this is achieved without much proliferation because there is little cell loss. In the bone-marrow, however, a steady number of cells are maintained by a fast rate of cell division balanced by a fast rate of cell loss. Often it requires only a slow rate of proliferation to gradually outgrow normal controlled cellular populations.

6.1.1.2   *Loss of tissue-specific characteristics*

In the early stages of tumour growth cancer cells often resemble the original cells from which they are derived. Later, tumour cells lose the appearance and function of the tissue cells from which they arise.

6.1.1.3   *Invasiveness*

This is the ability to grow into adjacent tissue. The tumour not only expands in size but also infiltrates between surrounding tissue cells. When nerve-endings are affected pain is experienced.

6.1.1.4   *Metastasis*

This is the ability to spread to new sites and establish new cancerous growths. Tumour cells may easily penetrate the walls of the lymphatics and distribute to the draining lymph nodes. Such cells may also invade blood vessels directly since capillaries have weak, thin walls which offer little resistance. A tumour may also spread across cavities from one organ to another, e.g. stomach to ovary. Most patients who die of cancer do so as a consequence of metastasis to vital organs.

At the point of clinical recognition of cancer, curative surgical or radiological treatment is only possible if metastasis from the primary tumour has not occurred. Therefore, early diagnosis is essential. Since about 50% of malignant tumours have metastasized prior to clinical recognition, the condition may be beyond the reach of curative surgery or radiotherapy alone. It is here that systemic chemotherapy has a role to play, often in conjuction with surgery and/or radiotherapy, which will help to reduce the 'total tumour mass'.

6.1.2 Factors influencing the success of chemotherapy

6.1.2.1 *The ability to detect tumours clinically*

Tumours grow by a progressive increase in cell numbers and current techniques are unable to detect in man less than about 10^9 cells, or 1 g of tumour, which may already be widely disseminated. Immunological assay methods are aimed at detection during earlier stages. Symptoms may appear with 10^{10} (10 g) or more cells are present. When the number of malignant cells increases to 10^{12}–10^{13} (1000–10 000 g), death occurs.

6.1.2.2 *The numbers of malignant cells present*

Chemotherapy is most effective when the number of malignant cells is small. Thus, patients with disseminated cancer (e.g. acute leukaemia) may have as many as 10^{12} cancer cells distributed throughout the body. If a given drug is capable of killing 99·9% of these cells, without intolerable toxicity to the host, then this would effectively reduce the number of cells to 10^9 (i.e. 3 'log kills'). Clinically, this would result in symptomatic improvement but would otherwise be ineffective. A better result would be obtained if a drug killed 99·9999% of cancer cells – affording a reduction from 10^{12} to 10^6 cells (i.e. 6 'log kills'). However, a 6 'log kill' reduction in tumour cells would only constitute a cure if the initial tumour mass was small, i.e. if the patient had fewer than 10^6 tumour cells. A 6 'log kill' would then reduce the number of cells to zero. Thus, the dose of cytotoxic drug is adjusted to the limits tolerated in order to achieve maximum 'log-kill'. The interval between doses must be such that the rate of tumour regrowth does not exceed tumour kill. Treatment must be continued until clinical evidence of cancer disappears (clinical regression).

6.1.2.3 *The cell cycle*

Most progress in cancer chemotherapy has been in treating various leukaemias, lymphomas and other virulent conditions such as choriocarcinoma. The greater sensitivity to drugs in these instances is a consequence of most of the cells in the cancer population being 'in cycle', i.e. continuously undergoing or preparing for mitosis. Cells in cycle are more sensitive to all types of cytotoxic agents than are resting cells. In slower growing solid tumours, which resist chemotherapy, most of the cells are in the resting (G_0) stage. However, chemically reactive drugs such as the nitrogen mustards (see Section 6.2.1) and DNA intercalators, e.g. actinomycin, adriamycin (see Section 3.5.3), are more effective against resting cells than are the antimetabolites (see Section 4.3).

6.1.3   Difficulties encountered in chemotherapy

6.1.3.1   *Preclinical testing*

The ideal preclinical testing of drugs has not been achieved. Experimental animal models have no sure correspondence to tumours in humans. Toxicity, not even detected in rodents, may be so serious in man as to prevent clinical use. This is a consequence of variations in drug metabolism from species to species. Despite these problems, most of the drugs used clinically, with the exception of hormones, were introduced as a result of activity previously demonstrated in animal tumours. However, hexamethylmelamine, 2,4,6-tris(dimethylamino)-1,3,5-triazine, is an example of a drug possessing activity against human carcinomas of the bronchus, ovary and breast but previously exhibiting only minimal activity when tested against rodent tumours.

6.1.3.2   *Accessibility of diseased cells*

The accessibility of tumour cells to a drug varies. Whilst a large tumour has a failing blood supply, due to a diminishing rate of growth, a small tumour will have a good blood supply and be more susceptible to drug action. This further emphasizes the greater sensitivity to chemotherapy of small metastases.

6.1.3.3   *Drug resistance*

The development of drug resistance may seriously interfere with treatment. Here, an initial preferential cytotoxic action against a tumour will be followed, after each treatment, by a rapid recovery in tumour growth. Drug resistance has been observed in such drug-sensitive tumours as carcinoma of the breast, choriocarcinoma and lymphoblastic leukaemias. This effect has been overcome in several tumours by treating with a combination of different cytotoxic agents (see Section 6.7).

6.1.3.4   *Sanctuary sites*

The occurrence of sanctuary sites in the body, where malignant cells may reside, renders these cells inaccessible to drugs. Thus, a previous assessment of complete remission in the treatment of lymphoblastic leukaemia in children may be followed years later by relapse due to the presence of residual tumour cells in the brain which had eluded chemotherapy. The testes are another sanctuary site for leukaemic cells.

6.1.3.5 *Selective toxicity*

The chemotherapy of cancer still awaits the discovery of fundamental biochemical differences between normal cells and tumour cells. This could then enable a rational approach to drug design to replace the enlightened empirical manner by which many of present day drugs have evolved. Apart from discovering that some lymphoid malignancies are dependent on an exogenous supply of asparagine, extensive biochemical investigations of tumour cells have so far uncovered only quantitative differences between cancer and normal cells. Thus, a greater proportion of lymphoma cells are in cycle compared with normal bone-marrow cells (*see* below).

The low selectivity of action of anticancer drugs presents a major problem. Their main cytotoxic effect is on the most rapidly dividing cells but, in the majority of tumours, the rate of cell division is in fact slower than that of normal bone-marrow, gut and skin epithelium or mucosa of the mouth. This explains the pattern of serious side-effects, accompanying chemotherapy, which are dose-limiting in practice.

The toxic side-effects in the bone-marrow have been limited by exploiting cell kinetic differences between normal stem cells and tumour stem cells. Stem cells constitute the smallest, yet most important, compartment in a proliferating system. Stem cells are capable of an indefinite number of divisions and are responsible for maintaining the integrity and survival of a cell population. Thus, the observed increased percentage kill of lymphoma cell populations compared with normal stem cells was explained by the discovery that only 20% of bone-marrow stem cells are in active cycle at any one time – the remaining 80% being in the resting (G_0) phase. Further studies revealed that when the dividing marrow stem cells are reduced by cytotoxic therapy it takes 3–4 days for the remaining stem cells to move from G_0 into active cycle. Translated into clinical practice, this means that very high doses of drugs may be given for 24–36 hour periods, interspersed with adequate recovery intervals.

Studies of the cell kinetic pattern of tumour growth have suggested a classification of cytotoxic agents on the basis of their ability to reduce the stem cell population in normal bone-marrow and lymphoma cells in mice. Three classes of anti-tumour agents are distinguished:

(i) Class 1. Non-cell-cycle-specific agents which kill cells whether they are dividing or not, e.g. nitrogen mustard.

(ii) Class 2. Cell-cycle-phase-specific agents which kill cells only in one phase of the cell cycle, such as the S phase (during the period of DNA synthesis), e.g. 6-mercaptopurine, cystosine arabinoside, methotrexate; or the M phase (during mitosis), vinblastine, vincristine.

An increased dose of these drugs will not kill more bone-marrow stem cells beyond those killed by the initial dose.

(iii) Class 3. Cell-cycle-specific agents which kill cells at all phases of the cell cycle, e.g. cyclophosphamide, 5-fluorouracil, actinomycin D, melphalan, chlorambucil, BCNU, CCNU, *cis*-platinum, daunorubicin.

These increase the kill of bone-marrow stem cells with increasing dose.

In both Classes 2 and 3 there is a maximum selective kill of malignant stem cells but in periodic high dosage forms of drug administration there should be a proportional reduction in the amounts of Class 3 agents used.

With a few exceptions, such as the cumulative toxicities associated with adriamycin (cardiac), bleomycin (pulmonary) and *cis*-platinum (renal), the common toxicities of anticancer drugs are usually reversible within 2–3 weeks. Mucositis (associated with actinomycin D, adriamycin, bleomycin, methotrexate, 5-fluorouracil and daunorubicin) is reversible over a period of 5–10 days, reflecting the rapid recovery phase of normal tissues. Nausea and vomiting, which accompanies certain drugs, may be partially overcome with anti-emetics.

6.1.4   Chemotherapeutic agents

The beginnings of cancer chemotherapy may be traced back to the 1940s with the introduction of stilboestrol phosphate for treating cancer of the prostate gland. This was followed by the use of nitrogen mustards to induce remissions in malignant lymphomas and folic acid antagonists (*see* Section 4.3.2) to treat childhood leukaemias. Currently there are some 30–40 anticancer drugs in clinical use whilst the annual literature in cancer chemotherapy has more than doubled in the past 5 years.

Although cytotoxic drugs may be classified in several ways, the medicinal chemist prefers to divide them into various groups dependant on their probable mode of action at the cellular (molecular) level. The antimetabolites (*see* Sections 4.3.2, 4.3.3, 4.3.4) which exert their action by enzyme inhibition and the antitumour antibiotics which intercalate with DNA (*see* Section 3.5.3) have previously been described. Another group of drugs, owing their anticancer activity to inhibition of the normal functioning of DNA, are the biological alkylating agents.

6.2   BIOLOGICAL ALKYLATING AGENTS

Members of this class react with the DNA twin helix, inhibiting its ability to unwind prior to replication and cell division. The role of DNA in the synthesis of essential proteins is also impaired. These actions follow from the ability of the biological alkylating agents, under physiological conditions, to alkylate certain nucleophilic, electron-excessive groups such as carboxylate and phosphate anions, thiolate groups of proteins and the basic nitrogen atoms of DNA nucleotides.

6.2.1   Nitrogen mustards

The first of the aliphatic alkylating agents to be introduced clinically was mustine hydrochloride. Nitrogen mustard (mustine, mechlorethamine, chloromethine), di-

(2-chloroethyl)methylamine **(6.1a)**, was discovered in the course of work on potential war gases during World War II. Mustine was found to depress the white blood cell count and this suggested its use for treating certain leukaemias. The term nitrogen mustard indicates its isosteric relationship to mustard gas **(6.1b)**. The high chemical reactivity of the nitrogen mustards and their ability to attack a wide range of nucleophilic centres, result in a number of toxic side-effects. The drugs affect all fast growing cells, including the healthy cells of the bone-marrow, tongue and intestines. They do, however, show a small selectivity largely confined to the bone-marrow, bloodstream and lymphatics.

$$X \overset{\displaystyle CH_2 \cdot CH_2 Cl}{\underset{\displaystyle CH_2 \cdot CH_2 Cl}{<}}$$

(6.1a)   X = Me·N
(6.1b)   X = S

Mustine is still clinically used for treating lymphadenoma (Hodgkin's disease). The hydrochloride salt must be supplied in the dry state, as it is hygroscopic, absorbing water to give the inactive hydroxy form. It is dissolved in water immediately before injection as a fast flowing intravenous saline infusion. Since it is also highly vesicant, it is washed out of the vein as soon as is practicable. Although much of the dose becomes hydrolysed, sufficient reaches the tumour cells to produce a powerful effect. This treatment has kept patients in fair health for many years. When combined with vinblastine (*see* Section 6.3) and procarbazine **(6.15)** remission rates of 80% and 5 years survivals of 75% have been experienced. Further, since alkylation proceeds rapidly after administration, mustine has proved valuable in combating life-threatening situations due to the growth of some solid tumours.

The aromatic nitrogen mustards were introduced in the 1950s and are milder alkylating agents which may be taken orally. They reach their target sites before being dissipated extensively by side-reactions. Chlorambucil **(6.2)**, one of the slowest acting and least toxic of the nitrogen mustards, is effective in chronic lymphocytic leukaemia, malignant lymphomas and carcinoma of the breast and ovary. Like mustine hydrochloride, it is often administered in conjunction with other drugs such as vinblastine and procarbazine which increase the remission rates.

Melphalan (phenylalanine mustard **(6.3)**) was synthesized with the aim of attaching a nitrogen mustard group to an amino acid residue, which could facilitate selective uptake by the tumour cell where rapid protein synthesis was proceeding. Since the nitrogen mustard derivative of D-phenylalanine is much less

$$R \overset{}{-\!\!\!\bigcirc\!\!\!-} N \overset{\displaystyle CH_2 \cdot CH_2 Cl}{\underset{\displaystyle CH_2 \cdot CH_2 Cl}{<}}$$

(6.2)   R = HOOC·CH_2·CH_2·CH_2—
(6.3)   R = HOOC·CH·CH_2—
                              |
                             NH_2

active than the L-form, it has been suggested that melphalan is conveyed into cells by the L-phenylalanine active transport mechanism (*see also* Section 1.2.2.2). Melphalan has been widely used in selected tumours such as multiple myeloma, breast and ovarian carcinoma and in the rare condition of macroglobulinaemia.

6.2.1.1 *Mode of action*

Under physiological conditions, the aliphatic nitrogen mustards readily form cyclic aziridinium (ethyleneiminium) ions, with the elimination of chloride ion, as a result of intramolecular catalysis involving neighbouring group participation. The resultant positive charge on the nitrogen is delocalized over the two adjacent carbon atoms to give a cation which, although stabilized in aqueous biological fluids, is highly strained and able to react readily with a nucleophilic group believed to be the N-7 atom of a guanine residue of DNA. The second $\beta(2)$-chloroethyl group then alkylates, by a similar mechanism, a further guanine residue on the other strand so that the twin-stranded helical DNA structure becomes crosslinked (*see* Figs. 6.1 and 6.2). Such alkylations by aliphatic mustards resemble an S_N2 process since the rate-controlling step is the bimolecular reaction of the cyclic iminium ion with the nucleophile and involves simultaneous bond-forming and bond-breaking. The preceding step, involving iminium ion formation, is a fast unimolecular process. In practice it may not be possible to draw sharp distinctions between the involvement of S_N1 and S_N2 mechanisms.

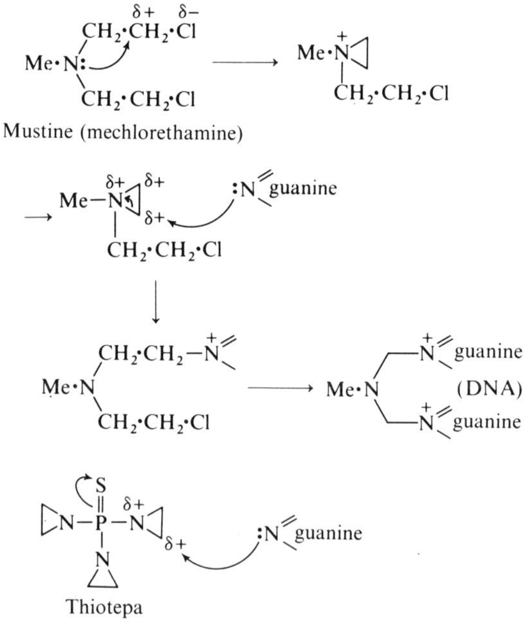

Fig. 6.1   Alkylation of DNA by aliphatic nitrogen mustards.

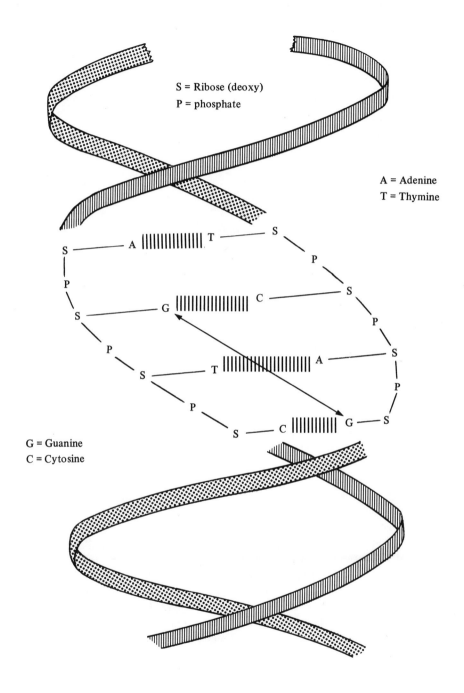

Fig. 6.2   Cross-alkylation of DNA by nitrogen mustard (↔).

Aziridines (ethyleneimines) as such are used as alkylating agents although ring-opening reactions of the unprotonated cyclic form with nucleophiles are slower than the corresponding iminium analogues. Their activity is however enhanced by electron-withdrawing groups which generate an electron deficiency on the ring carbons atoms. Thus, thiotepa (*see* Fig. 6.1) has been used in the treatment of carcinoma of the breast and ovary. The drug may be injected intramuscularly, intravenously or introduced directly into a tumour mass by intrapleural or peritoneal infusion. Recently, a carbamyl substituted benzoquinone moiety has been employed to activate aziridine groups (6.4).

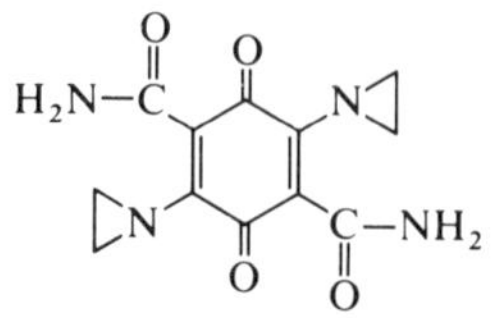

(6.4)

Aromatic nitrogen mustards are not sufficiently strong bases to form cyclic iminium ions since the nitrogen electron pair is delocalized by interaction with π electrons (+M effect) of the aromatic ring. Alkylation proceeds via an S_N1 mechanism with formation of a carbonium ion, due to fission of a covalent bond, as the rate-determining step (*see* Fig. 6.3). S_N2 characteristics have also been ascribed to this alkylation where the rate is controlled by interaction of a cyclic iminium ion and a nucleophile. Whichever mechanism predominates, the resultant effect is cross-alkylation of the guanine residues of the twin strands of DNA.

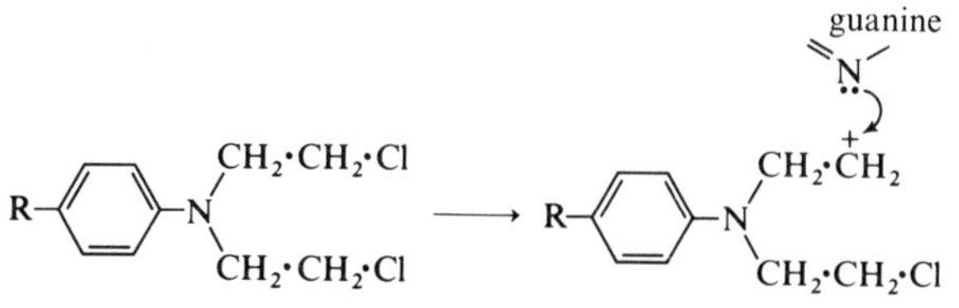

Fig. 6.3   Alkylation of DNA by aromatic nitrogen mustards.

The consequences of DNA crosslinking are manifold: (*a*) the critical base sequence, which provides a genetic code for the synthesis of the cell's proteins, may be spatially disoriented; (*b*) interference occurs with the unwinding of the twin strand which is a necessary prerequisite for replication prior to cell division; (*c*) the crosslinked *bis*-guaninium complex is susceptible to an enzymic (ribonuclease) mediated nucleophilic attack which causes deletion of the *bis*-purinylalkyl complex and scission of the DNA strands (*see* Fig. 6.4). The resultant miscoding of purine and pyrimidine bases interferes with replication and transcription (and hence protein synthesis).

Resistance to alkylating agents may arise due to the increased activity of enzymes involved in DNA repair which also results in excision of alkylated bases. Rapidly proliferating cells are believed to be more sensitive to DNA crosslinking

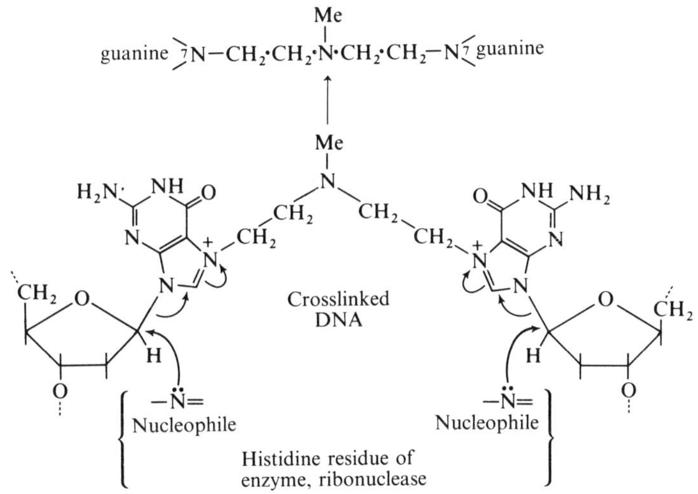
Me
guanine ⁷N—CH₂·CH₂·N·CH₂·CH₂—N⁷ guanine
Me
Crosslinked DNA
Nucleophile
Nucleophile
Histidine residue of enzyme, ribonuclease

Fig. 6.4 Deletion of *bis*-guaninium complex from cross-alkylated DNA.

than resting cells since the former fail to repair DNA before the damage becomes irreversible during the next DNA synthesizing cycle.

More recent developments with alkylating agents involve linking them to steroidal hormones. Since some tumour cells have specific hormone receptors, it was considered that such structural modifications would aid selectivity. Two such clinically available hormonal alkylating agents are estramustine phosphate (estractyl **(6.5)**) possessing activity in prostatic cancer, and prednimustine **(6.6)**, used for lymphocytic leukaemia.

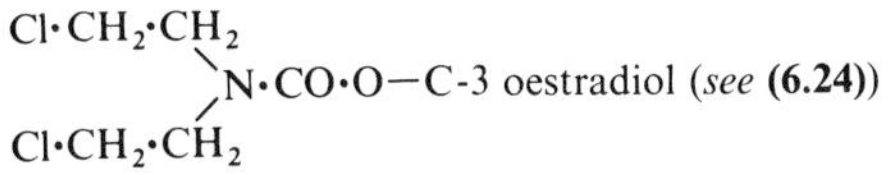
Cl·CH₂·CH₂
N·CO·O—C-3 oestradiol (see (6.24))
Cl·CH₂·CH₂

(6.5)

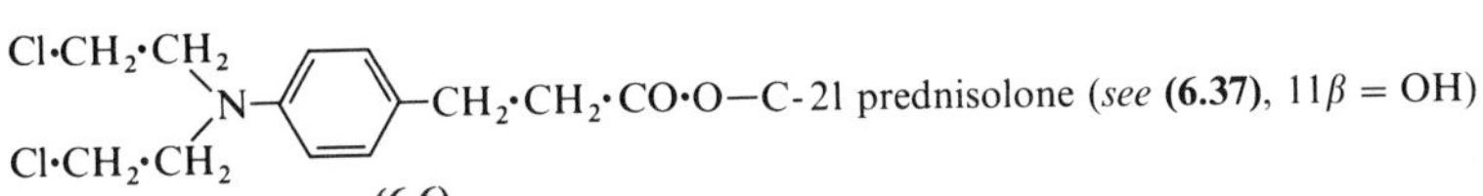
Cl·CH₂·CH₂
N
Cl·CH₂·CH₂
CH₂·CH₂·CO·O—C-21 prednisolone (see (6.37), 11β = OH)

(6.6)

6.2.1.2 *Latent activity*

The nitrogen mustards hitherto described react, as soon as introduced into the bloodstream, by alkylating plasma proteins. Drugs with latent activity enable more selective action towards the tumour. This has sometimes been achieved by manipulation of electron densities within a molecule. An early example of such an approach is found in nitromin **(6.7)** where the availability of the nitrogen lone pair, required for iminium ion formation, is blocked by *N*-oxide formation. Reduction *in vivo* was believed to activate the drug.

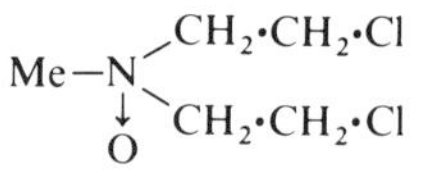

$$Me-N \overset{\downarrow}{\underset{O}{\big\langle}} \overset{CH_2 \cdot CH_2 \cdot Cl}{\underset{CH_2 \cdot CH_2 \cdot Cl}{}}$$

(6.7)

A considerable number of phosphamide mustards were produced as contenders for hydrolysis by phosphoramidases reputed to be concentrated in tumour tissues. The most successful of these was cyclophosphamide (6.8) in which the electron-withdrawing P=O group prevents cyclization of the nitrogen mustard by decreasing the availability of the nitrogen lone pair. Later it was shown that activation was

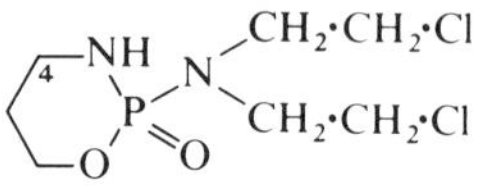

$$\left\langle \overset{NH}{\underset{O}{\big|}} \overset{}{P} \overset{}{\underset{O}{\big\|}} N \overset{CH_2 \cdot CH_2 \cdot Cl}{\underset{CH_2 \cdot CH_2 \cdot Cl}{}} \right.$$

(6.8)

not due to hydrolysis within the tumour but to liver microsomal oxidation. The products formed by loss of acrolein from the 4-hydroxylated derivative include phosphoramide mustard and normustine, both of which may be the active forms due to restoration of their ability to form ethyleneiminium ions (*see* Section 7.2.4.1). The slow rate of *in vivo* hydroxylation of cyclophosphamide in man has led to the synthesis of a 4-hydroperoxy derivative which spontaneously yields the 4-hydroxy intermediate after administration. Cyclophosphamide has a wide spectrum of activity which spans malignant lymphomas, lymphoblastic leukaemia, carcinomas of the bronchus, breast and ovary and various sarcomas.

6.2.2 Nitrosoureas

The nitrosoureas are alkylating agents of more recent origin. Advantages over other cytotoxic drugs lie in their activity towards tumour and leukaemic cells in the brain and cerebrospinal fluid – the so-called sanctuary sites. The screening of a large number of nitrosoureas established the structural unit for optimal activity to be a 2-chloroethyl-N-nitrosoureido group. Two clinically useful drugs are carmustine, N,N'-*bis*(2-chloroethyl)-N-nitrosourea, BCNU, (6.9) which is intravenously administered, and lomustine, N-(2-chloroethyl)-N'-cyclohexyl-N-nitrosourea, CCNU, (6.10), which is administered orally.

Activity cannot be related to cyclic iminium ion formation since availability of the required electron pair on an amide nitrogen is much decreased. Although the mechanism of action has not been firmly established it is likely that alkylation of

$$Cl \cdot CH_2 \cdot CH_2 \cdot \underset{NO}{\overset{|}{N}} \cdot CO \cdot NHR$$

(6.9)   R = —CH$_2$·CH$_2$·Cl

(6.10)   R = —⬡

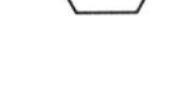

nucleic acids proceeds via generation of a chloroethyl carbonium ion whilst carbamoylation of amino groups of proteins occurs via an alkyl isocyanate (*see* Fig. 6.5).

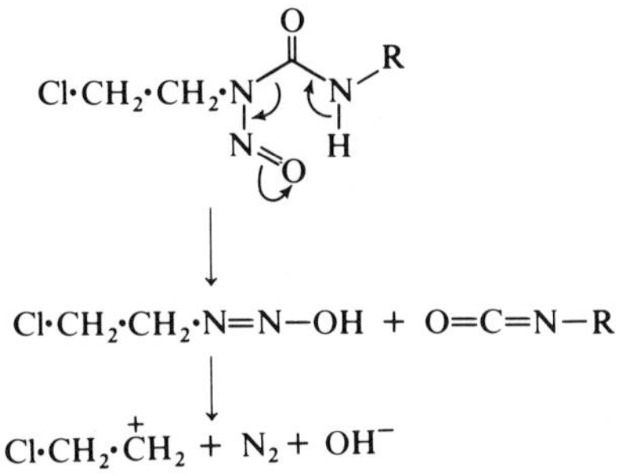

$$Cl\cdot CH_2\cdot CH_2\cdot N=N-OH + O=C=N-R$$

$$Cl\cdot CH_2\cdot \overset{+}{C}H_2 + N_2 + OH^-$$

Fig. 6.5 2-Chloroethyl-*N*-nitrosoureas – alkylation mechanism.

Although their lipophilic properties render them particularly suitable for treating intracerebral tumours, BCNU and CCNU are also active in malignant lymphomas, carcinomas of the breast, bronchus and colon. Carcinoma of the gastrointestinal tract, which is notably intractable to drug treatment, also responds to the nitrosoureas.

The discovery of anticancer activity in the naturally occurring nitrosourea, streptozotocin (6.11) led to the synthesis of a β-chloroethyl analogue, chlorozotocin (6.12) which possessed antileukaemic activity accompanied by reduced bone-

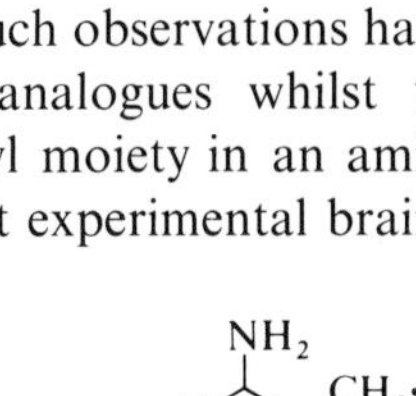

(6.11) R = Me
(6.12) R = —CH_2·CH_2Cl

marrow toxicity. Such observations have initiated the preparation of other mono- and disaccharide analogues whilst the substitution of the 2-chloroethyl-*N*-nitrosoureidomethyl moiety in an aminopyrimidine ring (6.13) has provided an active agent against experimental brain tumours.

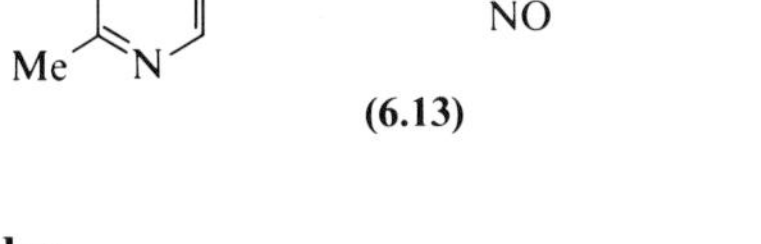

(6.13)

6.2.3 Triazenoimidazoles

Dacarbazine, 5-(3,3-dimethyl-1-triazenyl)imidazole-4-carboxamide, DTIC, (6.14) was originally developed as an inhibitor of purine biosynthesis and is one of several

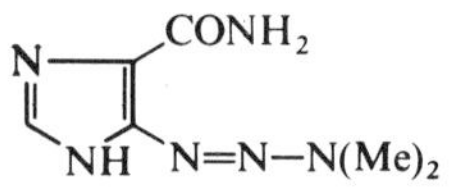

(6.14)

triazenes which have been evaluated clinically. It has a wide spectrum of activity including malignant lymphomas, melanomas and sarcomas. Combinations with adriamycin (*see* Section 3.5.3), bleomycin (*see* Section 6.5) and vinblastine (*see* Section 6.3) have been employed. Since the triazene is liable to photochemical decomposition, the infusion bottle must be protected with a cover during intravenous administration. Irritant properties also preclude contact with skin and mucous membranes.

Anticancer activity stems from demethylation to give 5-amino-imidazole-4-carboxamide and a transient methyl diazonium ion which has been shown, by radioactive labelling, to methylate guanine in position 7 (*see also* Section 7.2.4.2 for alternative explanation).

6.2.4   Hydrazine derivatives

Procarbazine, N - (1 - methylethyl) - 4 - [(2 - methylhydrazino) methyl] - benzamide, (6.15) is a hydrazine derivative, first synthesized as a monoamine oxidase inhibitor but later shown to be active in lymphomas and carcinoma of the bronchus. Cytotoxic activity is probably due to metabolic products amongst which, methyl-diazene, $MeN{=}NH$, is a source of methyl radicals capable of methylating guanine residues of DNA.

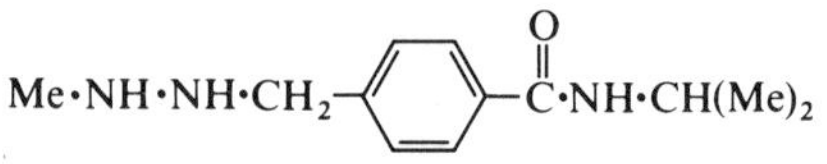

(6.15)

6.2.5   Methanesulphonic esters

In a homologous series of alkyl dimethanesulphonates the most active was found to be the butane analogue, busulphan, 1,4-di(methanesulphonyloxy)butane (6.16). The administration of this ester is not accompanied by nausea or vomiting, which is common to many other drugs, and is consequently more acceptable to patients.

$$MeSO_2{\cdot}O{\cdot}(CH_2)_4{\cdot}O{\cdot}SO_2Me$$
(6.16)

It is highly effective in chronic granulocytic leukaemia when patients are main-tained symptom free during their illness. Unfortunately, it has a profound toxic effect on granulocytes and megakaryocytes which requires careful monitoring.

The mode of action as a tumour inhibitor has been revealed by the preparation of unsaturated analogues of known stereochemistry. Thus, the corresponding butyne and *trans*-butene derivatives were inactive whilst the *cis*-butene derivatives

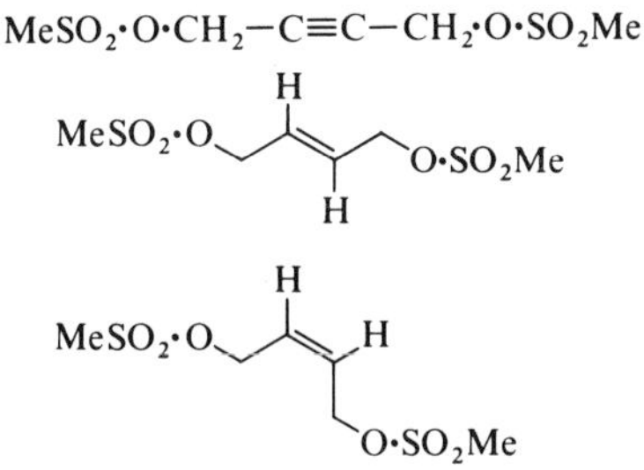

$$MeSO_2 \cdot O \cdot CH_2 - C \equiv C - CH_2 \cdot O \cdot SO_2Me$$

(6.17)

retained activity (6.17). This indicated that the activities of the *cis*-analogue and the saturated flexible busulphan depended on their ability to form a cyclic derivative by 1,4-bisalkylation of a suitable nucleophilic group. The isolation of an urinary metabolite (6.18) suggested that the site of alkylation was a cysteine

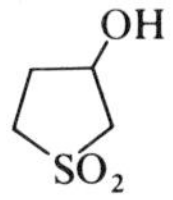

(6.18)

residue in protein from which sulphur was stripped (*see* Fig. 6.6). The methanesulphonate moiety provides an excellent leaving group in an S_N2 type alkylation reaction. Other methanesulphonates, which have been clinically tested, are nitrogen mustard analogues where β-chloroethyl groups have been replaced by sulphonate esters.

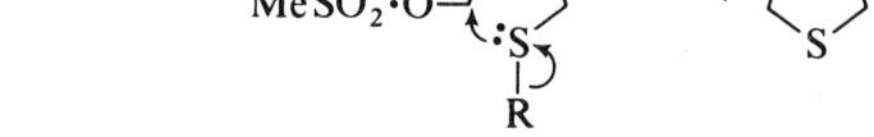

Fig. 6.6   Busulphan – alkylation of thiol group.

Recently, 1,4-di(7-guanyl)butane has been identified as a product of reaction between busulphan and DNA. This suggests that busulphan may also act as a crosslinking agent in effecting its cytotoxic activity.

6.3   PLANT PRODUCTS

For many centuries, medical treatment has relied to a large extent on the use of plants. In 1973, in the U.S.A., it was estimated that 25% of total prescriptions

Table 6.1   Pharmacologically active natural products from plants

Pharmacological activity	Natural product
Central nervous system	Reserpine, Caffeine, Picrotoxin Strychnine
Analgesic	Morphine, Codeine
Local anaesthetic	Cocaine
Autonomic nervous system	
cholinergic	Physostigmine, Pilocarpine
cholinergic blocking	Atropine, Hyoscine
adrenergic	Ephedrine
adrenergic blocking	Ergotamine
ganglionic blocking	Nicotine
Anti-inflammatory	Colchicine
Muscle relaxant	Tubocurarine
Cardiovascular	
vasodilators	Papaverine, Theophylline
hypotensive	Reserpine
cardiotonic	Digoxin
anti-arrhythmic	Quinidine
anti-coagulant	Coumarin
Cathartic (purgative)	Anthroquinones
Anticancer	Vinca alkaloids, Bruceolides
Chemotherapeutic	
antimalarial	Quinine
antiamoebic	Emetine
Anthelmintic	Santonin

issued could be accounted for by plant products. Natural products in current use possess nearly every conceivable type of biological activity (*see* Table 6.1). The discovery of a vegetable extract of medicinal benefit leads to the isolation of the active principle and its subsequent chemical characterization. Once this has been established, the synthesis of analogues retaining the essential structural features for improved therapeutic activity becomes possible. Several such examples of drug development have been described in other chapters. The unequivocal success of this approach has led to a search for anti-tumour activity from natural sources.

It is estimated that the number of species of higher plants on earth may be as great as 500 000. Only about 10% of these have been investigated pharmacologically for the active principles. In 1975 alone, some 300 compounds isolated from plants were reported to possess biological activity in some test system. Occasionally plants are selected on the basis of a knowledge of compounds thought to be present, whilst other plants have been investigated on the basis of folk-lore uses. Compounds are isolated and subjected to a whole series of pharmacological tests. In an ambitious programme carried out by the National Cancer Institute at Bethesda in the U.S.A., plants are taken on a random basis for extraction and testing against *in vitro* tumour systems. A number of novel chemical structures with anticancer activity has been characterized in spite of the absence of preconceived ideas about the type of compounds which might be found. Since 1960 over 20 000 species of plants have been screened and the activity of some 78 000 extracts have been assessed against experimental animal tumours. By 1975, over 1000 species had been found to possess activity against one or more test tumours.

As a result of such investigations two alkaloids – vinblastine and vincristine – which occur as minor constituents of the Madagascar periwinkle (*Vinca rosea*) have been isolated and have subsequently found an important role in cancer chemotherapy. The previously suspected hypoglycaemic properties of infusions of the plant were not confirmed in practice since no drop in blood sugar was detected but a drop in the white blood cell count was pronounced.

The two *Vinca* alkaloids have complex chemical structures which are closely similar (*see* Fig. 6.7). Vincristine is more widely used than vinblastine but the plant

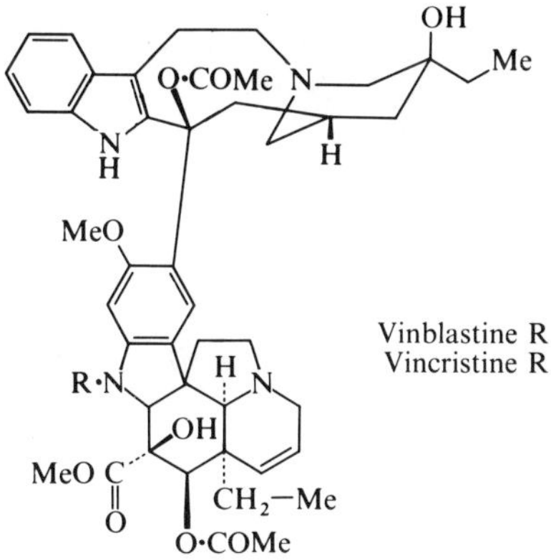

Vinblastine R = Me
Vincristine R = —C·H
                     ‖
                     O

Fig. 6.7   Vinca alkaloids.

produces the latter in a hundred-fold greater quantity. Fortunately, vinblastine may be converted to vincristine by a simple chemical step involving the conversion of a methyl group to a formyl group. Furthermore, since these *Vinca* alkaloids have proved so useful in therapy, efforts are being directed towards synthesizing new derivatives for clinical appraisal. Early indications suggest that superior activity may be forthcoming from this work. The synthesis of vinblastine itself, was reported in 1979. Cell culture fermentation techniques, utilizing plant enzymes, may also be a future source of these alkaloids. It has also been found that compounds representing the two halves of the structure of the dimeric *Vinca* molecules occur in much higher proportions in the plant extract and the possibility of linking these in the correct positions, with the same stereochemistry, has become experimentally feasible.

The *Vinca* alkaloids are cell-cycle-specific agents which block mitosis with metaphase arrest. Their cytotoxic effects appear to result from binding to the microtubules. Damage to the mitotic spindle apparatus ensues and this prevents the chromosomes from travelling out to form daughter cell nuclei.

Vinblastine sulphate is included, on a weekly basis, in several drug regimens for

treating Hodgkin's disease, disseminated carcinoma of the breast, choriocarcinoma and testicular carcinoma. Despite its close similarity in structure to
vinblastine, vincristine sulphate has a different spectrum of anti-tumour activity
and side-effects. Several drug combinations include the alkaloid for treating acute
lymphoblastic leukaemia, myeloblastic leukaemia, Wilms' tumour of childhood,
rhabdomyosarcoma, neuroblastoma, retinoblastoma, soft tissue sarcomas and disseminated cancers of the breast, testes, ovaries and cervix. Although neurotoxicity
may be pronounced, relatively slight toxicity to the bone-marrow renders it suitable for combination with drugs causing greater bone-marrow depression.

Podophyllotoxin is another example of a natural product possessing anticancer
activity. This is an extract from the American mandrake rhizome which has been
shown to inhibit cell division by binding to the mitotic spindle. A semisynthetic
glucoside of epipodophyllotoxin, etoposide, has recently been introduced clinically
for treating small cell bronchial carcinoma. It is claimed to be one of the most
active compounds yet tested against this particular type of lung cancer. Other
semisynthetic derivatives, such as podophyllic acid ethyl hydrazide, have been
prepared and tested on selected tumours. These appear to have a more direct effect
on DNA, inducing single strand cleavage. Activity has been reported in some
leukaemias and lymphomas, oat cell carcinoma of the bronchus and in malignant
teratomas.

Another alkaloid, ellipticine (6.19), has received attention in recent years. The
preparation of various derivatives has indicated the importance of a 9-hydroxy
substituent (6.20) for improved anticancer activity.

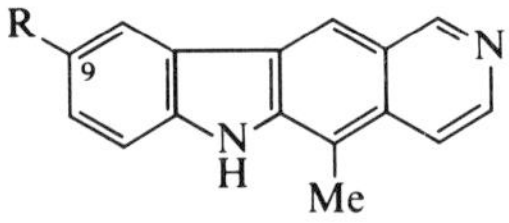

(6.19)   R = H
(6.20)   R = OH

A group of bitter tasting compounds belonging to a series described as the
bruceolides currently show promise as anti-tumour agents. These are isolated in
small yield from species of *Brucea* (Simaroubacaea) and show a wide range of
activity against a number of test systems including lymphocytic leukaemia in mice,
Lewis lung carcinoma and melanocarcinoma. The natural products constitute a
series of esters based on the parent bruceantinol of which the active compounds are
α,β-unsaturated esters (Fig. 6.8).

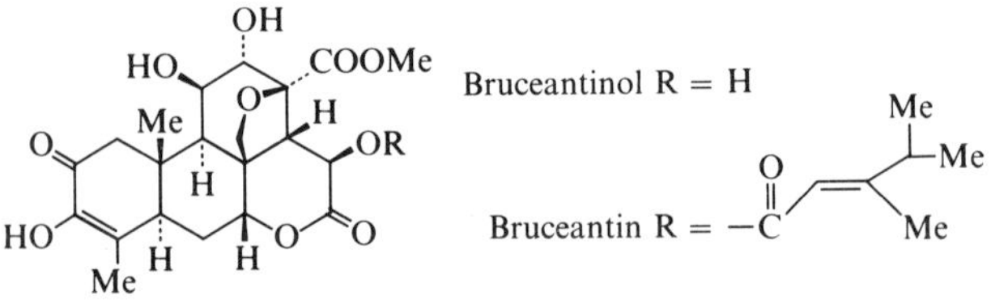

Bruceantinol R = H

Bruceantin R = —C(=O)CH=C(Me)(CH(Me)Me)

Fig. 6.8   Bruceolides.

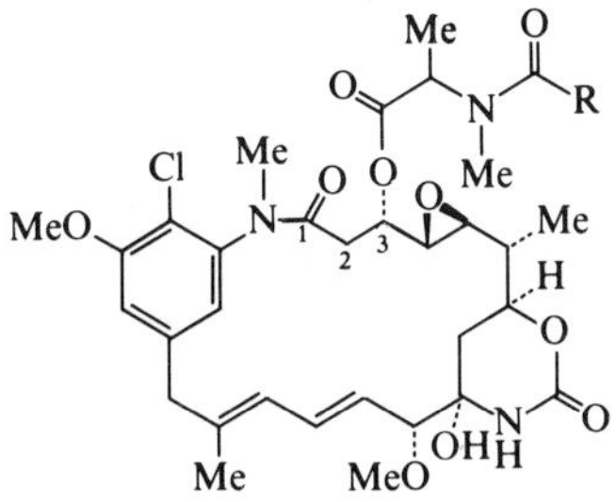

Maytansine R = Me

Fig. 6.9   Maytansinoids.

Other compounds with potent antileukaemic activity are the maytansinoids (Fig. 6.9) isolated from a Kenyan shrub, *Maytensus ovatus*. Their preclinical evaluation is particularly encouraging. This group of ansamacrolides are the first to possess carbinolamide, epoxide and aryl halide functional groups. Ten maytansinoids have been isolated and it has been demonstrated that, for activity, the ester group at C-3 is essential. However, this need not necessarily be an amino acid residue, since the acetate also exhibits activity.

6.4   ENZYMES

The discovery that some lymphoid malignancies were dependent on an exogenous supply of asparagine coupled with the observation in 1953 that guinea-pig serum, containing L-asparaginase, caused regression of certain types of rat and mouse tumours, was hailed as a milestone in cancer research. This was the first evidence of a significant biochemical difference between malignant and normal cells.

The difficulty presented by the enormous quantities of guinea-pig serum required, as a source of the enzyme, was overcome in 1965 by the large scale production of L-asparaginase from bacterial, *E. coli*, sources. The enzyme is not myelosuppressive (bone-marrow depressive) but it can cause liver damage. Its use is confined to acute lymphoblastic leukaemia and lymphomas.

Anaphylaxis and immunological problems associated with L-asparaginase from *E. coli* sources have recently been overcome by using samples of the enzyme isolated from *Pseudomonas geniculata*. Polymers produced by binding the enzyme to dextrans may show increased anti-tumour activity. More recently, a succinylated *Acinetobacter* glutaminase–asparaginase has been prepared, possessing increased plasma half-life (as a result of acylation of free amino groups) and clinical activity towards leukaemias and lymphomas in children.

6.5   ANTIBIOTICS

Anti-tumour antibiotics, which owe their activity to intercalation with DNA, were previously described in Section 3.5.3. The bleomycins constitute an important and relatively new group of clinically active cytotoxic agents. Bleomycin sulphate consists of the sulphate of a mixture of glycopeptide bases (A2 and B2) obtained by the growth of *Streptomyces verticillus*. The various bleomycins have individual molecular weights in the region of 1550. They are copper bonded and essentially consist of a glycopeptide structure with one imidazolyl, one pyrimidinyl and a dithiazolyl group attached at separate points on the peptide chain (Fig. 6.10).

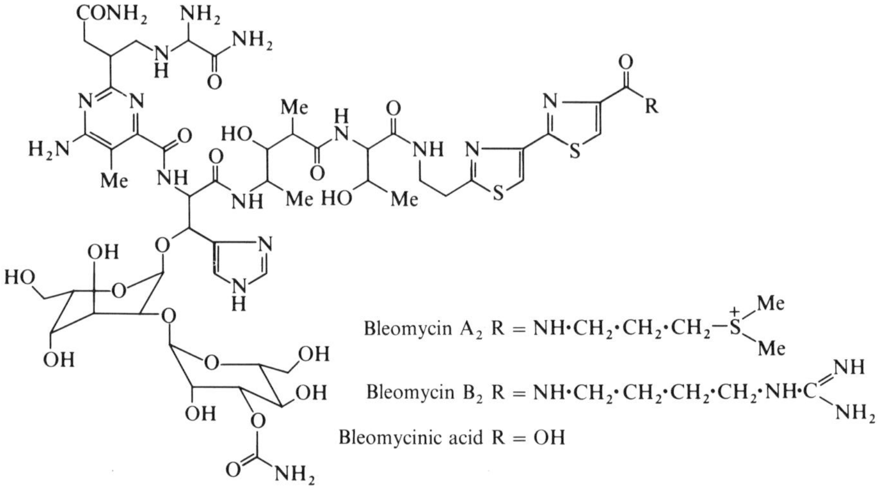

Bleomycin A$_2$ R = NH·CH$_2$·CH$_2$·CH$_2$-S$^+$$\langle$Me / Me

Bleomycin B$_2$ R = NH·CH$_2$·CH$_2$·CH$_2$·CH$_2$·NH·C$\langle$NH / NH$_2$

Bleomycinic acid R = OH

Fig. 6.10   Bleomycins.

The bleomycins have attracted interest because they tend to be selectively concentrated in squamous cells and are therefore suitable for inclusion in regimens for treating tumours of this cell type in the head, neck and genitalia. Bleomycin sulphate has also been used in Hodgkin's disease and testicular carcinomas. It may be given intravenously, intramuscularly or subcutaneously. Unlike most anticancer drugs, it is only slightly myelosuppressive and dose-limiting toxicity is confined to the skin, mucosa and lungs. Enzymes in most other tissues rapidly deactivate the bleomycins, probably as a result of deamination or peptidase activity. A carboxylic acid derivative, bleomycin acid (*see* Fig. 6.10), has been prepared and the substitution of various amino moieties in this molecule has enabled the synthesis of over 100 analogues. Pepleomycin is a recently reported derivative with considerable less tendency to cause pulmonary fibrosis.

Cytotoxic activity is probably due to spanning by the bleomycin molecule across diester bonds of the ribophosphate skeleton of DNA strands. This binding, which may also be reinforced by sulphur linkages, results in single strand scission about the 3',5'-diphosphate linkage **(6.21)**. It is also possible that bleomycin impairs repair of chain scission so that progressive degradation of the DNA chain occurs. Chelation with metal ions (*see* Section 5.1.4) may also play a part in the fragmentation of DNA by the glycopeptide.

$$-dR-O-\underset{\underset{O}{\overset{O^-}{\underset{\|}{|}}}}{P}-O-\overset{3'}{\Big\langle}\overset{\text{base}}{\underset{\overset{5'}{CH_2}-O-\underset{\underset{O}{\overset{O^-}{\underset{\|}{|}}}}{P}-O-dR-}{O}\Big\rangle$$

(dR = deoxyribose)

(6.21)

6.6 HORMONES

6.6.1 Introduction

It has long been recognized that tumours derived from tissues which are hormone dependent are themselves dependent on the same hormone. This has been demonstrated by the remissions seen in premenopausal breast cancer following ovariectomy and in prostatic cancer following orchidectomy. This observation that the development of certain tumours may be influenced by manipulation of endogenous hormonal levels has led to exogenous hormonal therapy for treating carcinoma of the breast, prostate, thyroid and uterus. Eventually all hormonal-sensitive tumours become resistant, although remissions of several years' duration have occurred.

Hormones which are important in cancer chemotherapy are produced in the hypothalamus, anterior pituitary, adrenals and gonads. The hypothalamus pro-duces polypeptide hormones which pass to the anterior pituitary to effect production and release of complex protein hormones, which in turn stimulate the adrenal glands to produce corticosteroids and the ovary and adrenal glands to release oestrogens and androgens.

Hormonal agents which favourably influence the course of some cancers were originally introduced clinically for other purposes. Thus, knowledge of hormonal chemotherapy of cancer is largely of clinical origin.

6.6.2 Oestrogens

The main role of oestrogen therapy has been in recurrent breast carcinoma in postmenopausal women and in metastatic prostatic cancer. In premenopausal patients the ovaries are actively producing circulating oestrogens so that ovariec-tomy or radiotherapy is usually adopted to curtail hormone production in metastatic breast cancer. However in postmenopausal women, the administration of oestrogens in high doses causes tumour regression probably by inhibiting pituitary secretion of prolactin which, in excess, may promote tumour growth. The study of tissues normally receptive to oestrogens has revealed the presence of specific receptor proteins in the cellular cytoplasm. Oestrogens bind with this protein to give an oestrogen–receptor complex which enters the cell nucleus to affect a specific site in the chromosomes. The aromatic ring of the oestrogen in all probability provides a region of high electron density for protein binding. The oestrogen–receptor complex stimulates RNA synthesis, which in turn promotes protein formation. Recent work on oestrogen receptor assays have aided in the selection of patients who are likely to respond to hormonal therapy.

Naturally occurring oestrogens are unsuitable for therapy since they are rapidly metabolized by the liver. The synthetic oestrogens commonly used are stilboestrol **(6.22)**, 17α-ethynyloestradiol **(6.23)** and esters of 17β-oestradiol **(6.24)**. 17α-Ethynyloestradiol is the most potent, since substitution of the ethynyl group retards its metabolism, whilst stilboestrol is the most widely used.

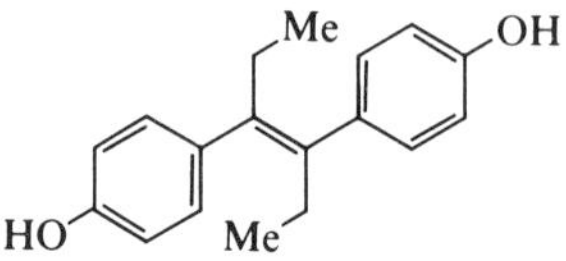

(6.22)

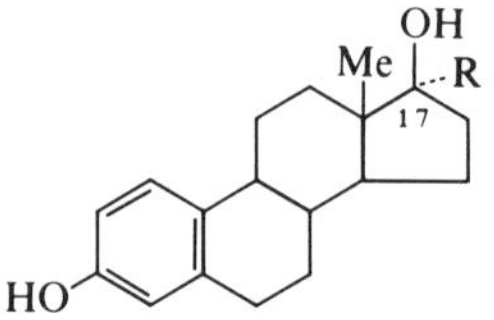

(6.23) R = —C≡CH
(6.24) R = H

Studies into the problems of fertility and birth control in the 1960s led to the discovery of synthetic hormones which have proved valuable in treating late breast cancer. These have an antioestrogenic action by competitively binding to oestrogen receptors in tumour cells, thus inhibiting translocation of the oestrogen–receptor complex to the nucleus. Several antioestrogens are related structurally to the strongly oestrogenic chlortrianisene **(6.25)**, the most widely used being clomiphene **(6.26)** and tamoxiphen **(6.27)**. The antioestrogenic activity of clomiphene is associated with the *trans* ($C_6H_4 \cdot O(CH_2)_2NEt_2/Cl$) isomer. These oestrogen antagonists are deemed more suitable for older patients and cause less fluid retention and hypercalcaemia than ethinyloestradiol.

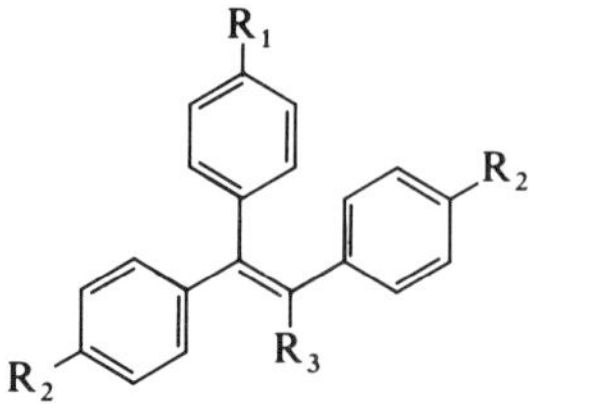

(6.25) $R_1 = R_2 = $ —OMe, $R_3 = $ Cl
(6.26) $R_1 = $ —O(CH$_2$)$_2$N(Et)$_2$, $R_2 = $ H, $R_3 = $ Cl
(6.27) $R_1 = $ —O(CH$_2$)$_2$N(Me)$_2$, $R_2 = $ H, $R_3 = $ Et

Oestrogens have also been widely used in treating prostatic cancer. A majority of patients obtain subjective relief of pain from bone metastasis and occasionally tumour regression occurs. However, there is no great impact on survival. Oestrogens have a similar effect to orchidectomy. They may act by inhibiting gonadotrophin release from the pituitary and consequently reduce androgen secretion in the testes. Alternatively they may antagonize the effects of androgens on tumour cells. Ethinyloestradiol rather than stilboestrol may be preferred for treatment although chlorotrianisene has a more prolonged action, being slowly converted in the liver to the active compound.

6.6.3   Progestogens

The main role of progestogens is in the treatment of advanced endometrial carcinomas, which may result from the long continued action on the endometrium of oestrogens in the absence of progesterone. Progestogens may either inhibit this action or have a direct effect on the tumour. Progesterone itself is not used clinically, since synthetic analogues are more potent. Synthetic progestational derivatives fall into two main groups. Those related to 17α-hydroxyprogesterone include 17α-hydroxyprogesterone hexanoate (6.28) for intramuscular injection, medroxyprogesterone acetate (6.29), megestrol acetate (6.30a) and chlormadinone acetate (6.30b). Methyl substitution at C-6 inhibits metabolic oxidation at this

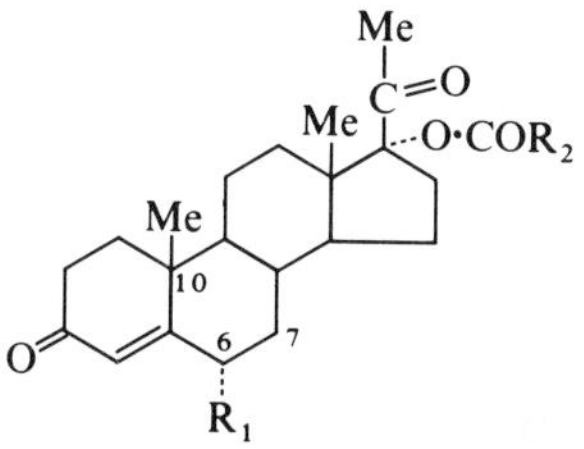

(6.28) R_1 = H, R_2 = —$(CH_2)_4$Me
(6.29) R_1 = R_2 = Me
(6.30a) R_1 = R_2 = Me; 6,7-ene
(6.30b) R_1 = Cl, R_2 = Me; 6,7-ene

position, giving a 50-fold increase in potency over progesterone. The second group of derivatives are related to 19-nortestosterone and testosterone and include norethisterone acetate (6.31) and dimethisterone, 6α,21-dimethylethisterone (6.32). Replacement of the C-10 angular methyl group by hydrogen in norethisterone facilitates binding of the β-face of the molecule to a receptor surface, thus explaining the substantial increase in potency.

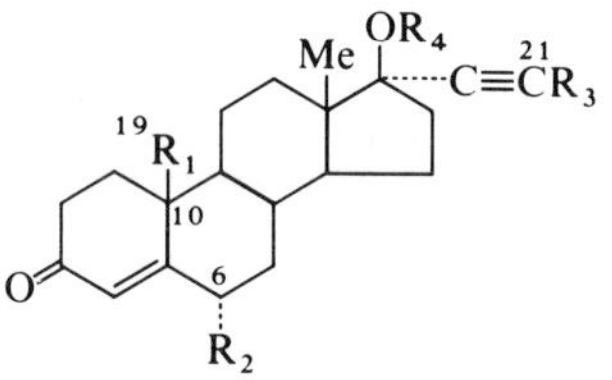

(6.31) R_1 = R_2 = R_3 = H, R_4 = COMe
(6.32) R_1 = R_2 = R_3 = Me, R_4 = H

Newer antiandrogenic progesterone derivatives such as cyproterone acetate (6.33) have shown favourable responses in advanced prostatic cancer with the advantage of being non-feminizing. Cyproterone is believed to competitively inhibit the binding of dihydrotestosterone, the reduction product of testosterone at

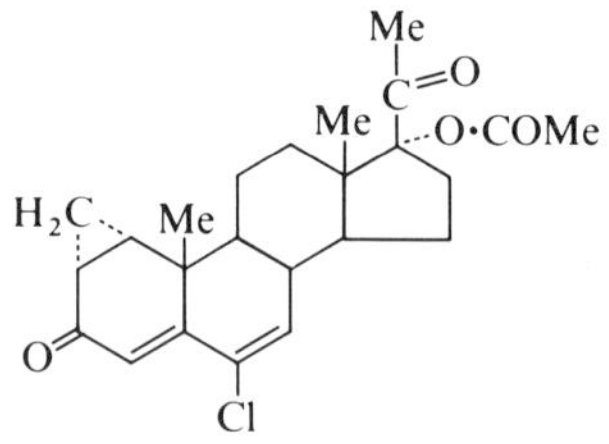

(6.33)

the cellular level, to a cytoplasmic receptor protein which initiates a sequence of steps similar to the oestrogen–receptor complex previously described.

6.6.4 Androgens

The main therapeutic use of androgens is in carcinoma of the breast. A few years after testosterone was isolated its esters were reported to be beneficial for treating recurrent forms of breast cancer. Testosterone propionate (6.34) became a standard for evaluating other androgens subsequently developed in attempts to decrease undesirable masculinizing effects and hypercalcaemia. A number of derivatives have groups substituted in the 17α-position, such as 17α-methyltestosterone (6.35) and the more active fluoxymesterone ($11\beta,17\beta$-dihydroxy-9α-fluoro-17α-methylandrost-4-en-3-one). These have the advantage of being absorbed orally. Although some virilization occurs, even with more recent synthetic androgens, their anabolic properties promote protein synthesis and bone-marrow stimulation in wasted patients. The much decreased androgenic, but similar anabolic potency of 19-nortestosterone (cf. testosterone), has led to the development of 17α-ethyl-19-nortestosterone phenylpropionate (6.36) and de-canoate where esterification prolongs anabolic activity. Another derivative with similar response and regression rates as testosterone propionate, but with reduced virilizing properties, is 2α-methyldihydrotestosterone propionate (dromostanolone propionate, masteril).

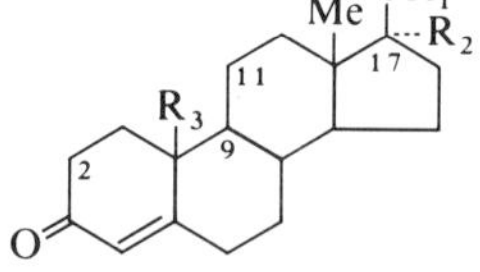

(6.34) $R_1 = COEt$, $R_2 = H$, $R_3 = Me$
(6.35) $R_1 = H$, $R_2 = R_3 = Me$
(6.36) $R_1 = CO(CH_2)_2C_6H_5$, $R_2 = Et$, $R_3 = H$

Androgens may induce breast cancer regression either by blocking oestrogenic receptors in the tumour or by reduction of pituitary gonadotrophic levels with resultant low oestrogen secretion. The most likely explanation is one of direct action on cancer cells, whilst their anabolic activity repairs the structure of stomal and epithelial tissues.

6.6.5   Corticosteroids

As early as the 1930s, it was noted that inadequate adrenal secretion caused increased development of lymphoid tissue. Since administration of adrenocortico-trophic hormone (ACTH) led to diminution of this tissue, it was used for treating lymphatic leukaemia. Subsequent trials with the natural corticosteroids (cortisone and hydrocortisone) produced remissions in lymphocytic leukaemia and lymphomas. The later synthetic glucocorticoids, prednisone **(6.37)** and prednisolone

(6.37)

(6.37, 11 β-OH), were found to be equally effective with less disturbance of electrolyte balance and water retention. These synthetic compounds are now firmly established in treating acute lymphoblastic leukaemia and malignant lymphomas.

The glucocorticoids appear to have a direct cytotoxic action in their antilymphocy-tic effect. Prednisone is believed to act at an early stage in the cell cycle, inhibiting the synthesis of DNA. This may be due to suppression of both protein synthesis and the activity of RNA polymerase. These actions are more apparent in lymphoid cells due to a specific binding of glucocorticoids to lymphatic tissue. Prednisone is now a frequent component of combination chemotherapy for treating lymphocytic leukaemia.

Glucocorticoids have also been used for treating metastatic breast cancer since they suppress the adrenal and pituitary glands with decreased oestrogen production. However, the main benefit of corticosteroid therapy here is due to an anti-inflammatory action which relieves pain from bone metastasis, shortness of breath from lung metastasis and raised intracranial pressure from cerebral metastasis.

Glucocorticoids are helpful in the control of complications associated with malignant disease, such as hypercalcaemia (commonly occurring in breast cancer and accompanying oestrogen therapy) and cerebral oedema resulting from brain tumours.

More powerfully anti-inflammatory corticosteroids also find a place in cancer chemotherapy. Thus, dexamethasone **(6.38)** and triamcinolone **(6.39)** may be used for CNS metastasis causing raised intracranial pressure over a period of radio-therapy. Anti-inflammatory properties have been enhanced at the expense of gluco- and mineralocorticoid properties by the substitution of 9α-halogen, 16α-methyl and 16α-hydroxyl groups.

Anti-inflammatory fluorocorticosteroids have also been useful in the control of the intractable non-malignant skin disease, psoriasis, where excessive cells (result-ing from overproduction of dihydrofolate reductase) are shed periodically from epidermal lesions. In the treatment of this condition, the 9α-fluoro substituent enhances the lipid solubility of the corticosteroid for penetration of the stratum corneum and subsequent action on the squamous cell layer of the epidermis. Other synthetic analogues have been synthesized with a view to further increasing lipid solubility by esterification of either C-21 hydroxyl (fludrocortisone acetate) or C-17 hydroxyl (betamethasone valerate (6.40)) groups. The latter type of compound may, unfortunately, undergo deactivation at physiological pH due to C-17/C-21 transesterification. This has been overcome, however, either by substituting a chlorine atom for the —OH group on C-21, yielding the powerful anti-inflammatory clobetasol 17-propionate, or by converting to the diester betamethasone 17,12-dipropionate. Another analogue, fluocinolone (6.41), has an additional fluorine atom substituted at C-6. Conversion of the two α-hydroxyl groups at C-16 and C-17 to a ketal, as in fluocinolone and triamcinolone acetonides, is a further means of ensuring adequate lipophilicity for local (epidermal) anti-inflammatory activity, free from undesirable systemic absorption.

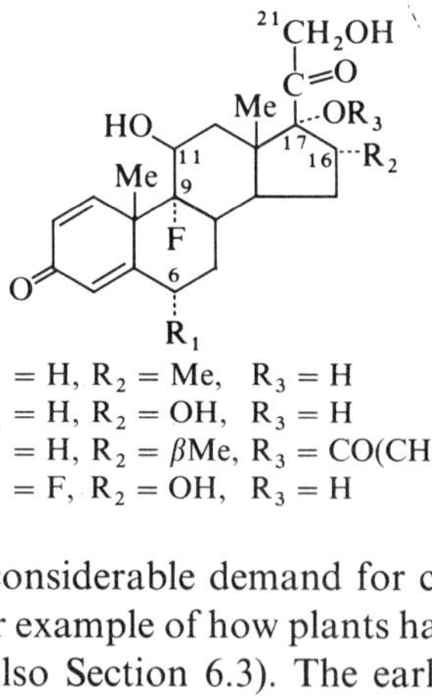

(6.38) $R_1 = H$, $R_2 = Me$, $R_3 = H$
(6.39) $R_1 = H$, $R_2 = OH$, $R_3 = H$
(6.40) $R_1 = H$, $R_2 = \beta Me$, $R_3 = CO(CH_2)_3 \cdot Me$
(6.41) $R_1 = F$, $R_2 = OH$, $R_3 = H$

The manner in which the considerable demand for corticosteroids in medicine has been met provides another example of how plants have contributed to progress in medicinal chemistry (see also Section 6.3). The early animal sources of these compounds, such as cholesterol and bile acids, have now been replaced by steroidal sapogenins as starting materials in their economic production. Research at the Syntex Organization revealed that diosgenin (6.42), obtained from the Mexican yam dioscora, could provide an excellent source of synthetic steroidal compounds. The closely related hecogenin (6.43), obtained from the sisal plant *Agave sisalana*, has also proved useful as a starting material not only for cortisone but also for the 16-β-methyl analogues of corticosteroids.

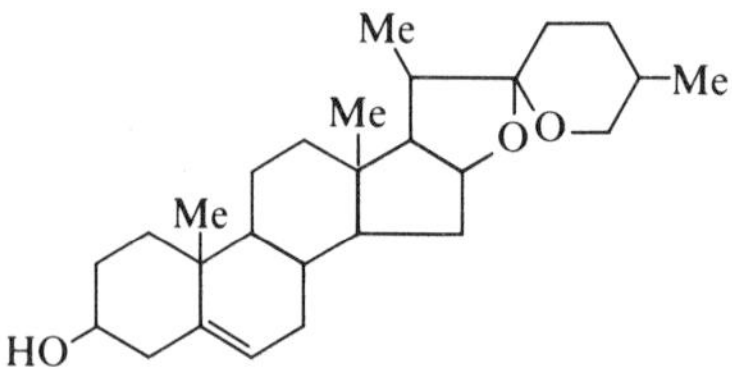

(6.42)

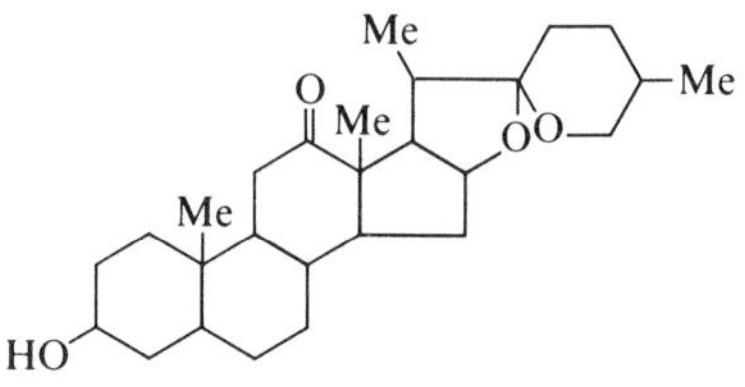

(6.43)

6.7   COMBINATION CHEMOTHERAPY

Most attempts at treating tumours with single agents have been disappointing. A single drug kills the proportion of cells which are sensitive to it and leaves the resistant fraction still dividing. The brevity of response to a single drug led to the introduction, in 1960, of a combination of drugs for treating testicular tumours. Since then the principle has been rapidly extended to other types of cancer. Each drug included in a particular combination should be active as a single agent and have different toxic (dose-limiting) side-effects. Multiple drug therapy also enables attack at multiple sites associated with the synthesis or function of essential biological macromolecules. The successful application of this technique to the treatment of acute lymphoblastic leukaemia is illustrated by the comparative response rates of single agents and various combinations:

Drugs	Complete bone-marrow remissions (%)
Methotrexate (M, see Section 4.3.2.1)	22
Mercaptopurine (MP, see Section 4.3.3)	27
Prednisone (P, see Section 6.6.5)	63
Vincristine (V, see Section 6.3)	57
Daunorubicin (D, see Section 3.5.3)	38
P, V	90
P, V, M, MP	94
P, V, D	100

A variety of combination schedules, using different drugs and doses, are now available and are accepted as superior to single drug therapy in the treatment of many types of cancer.

It is also considered that many cancers may be already disseminated at presentation or clinical detection so that chemotherapy is commenced concurrently with local treatment (e.g. radiotherapy, surgery). The micrometastases associated with the primary tumour are very sensitive to chemotherapy since they have a good blood supply facilitating drug access, a low concentration of competitive metabolites and less chance of developing drug resistance. The drugs and drug combinations used should only be those previously shown to be effective in the advanced state of the same disease. Such 'adjuvant chemotherapy' has been applied successfully in a number of carcinomas.

6.8   SUMMARY

The clinical impact of cancer chemotherapy, employing combination and adjuvant techniques, has been dramatic in the following drug-sensitive tumours:

Acute lymphoblastic leukaemia
Hodgkin's disease
Histiocytic lymphoma
Wilm's tumour

Burkitt's lymphoma
Embryonal rhabdomyosarcoma
Teratomas (testicular tumours)
Retinoblastoma
Ewing's sarcoma
Choriocarcinoma

Although these constitute only about 7% of all cancers, a varying proportion of patients are enabled to achieve a normal lifespan. Some of the more common tumours, accounting for about 25% of all cancers, fall into a group which are relatively drug sensitive:

Breast carcinoma
Ovarian carcinoma
Acute myeloid leukaemia
Chronic lymphocytic leukaemia
Multiple myeloma
Prostatic cancer
Neuroblastoma
Lymphocytic lymphomas
Osteosarcomas
Squamous cell carcinoma of the head and neck

In this group, chemotherapy can effect an improved survival in a proportion of patients.

A third group, representing about 50% of all cancers, respond only to some extent to chemotherapy offering no clearly demonstrated useful improvement in survival. A further group of tumours represent those for which drugs have either not been evaluated or for which drugs do not produce a response.

There is no sign yet of a 'magic bullet' being produced for cancer chemotherapy and it is more likely that advances will come from the more enlightened use of existing drugs so that better systemic therapy will be evolved to combat the metastatic complications from which the majority of cancer patients now die.

A recent attempt to overcome the problem of non-selectivity of action employed the technique of 'arterial chemoembolization'. Thus, a saline suspension of mitomycin C, contained in microcapsules, given by infusion into an artery supplying the tumour, enabled the drug to be taken directly to the tumour site where the capsules disintegrated to slowly release their contents. Smaller arteries were occluded to prevent clearance of the drug.

The belief, held by many, that several cancers may be virally induced has led to the occasional inclusion of an antiviral agent such as virazol (see p. 107) or cytosine arabinoside (see p. 106), in combination chemotherapy. Such considerations have also aroused interest in the possibility of utilizing interferon, which has a broad spectrum of antiviral activity, for treating cancer.

6.9 INTERFERON (see also Section 9.8.2.1)

Interferon was discovered in 1957 by scientists at the National Institute for Medical Research, U.K. It is a glycoprotein which is induced in response to viral infections and is effective only in species in which it is produced. It was first investigated as an antiviral agent and this activity is being further examined in chronic hepatitis B and in viral infections associated with immunosuppressed patients.

Interest in the anticancer activity of interferon first arose due to encouraging results obtained in Sweden whilst treating oesteogenic sarcoma and myelomatosis. More recently (1981) doctors in Yugoslavia, using human leucocyte interferon preparations injected directly into the tumours, have reported substantial or total remission for cancer of the head and neck. Although the mechanism of anti-tumour activity is not known, they suggest that a direct effect on malignant cells or stimulation of the host's immune system may be responsible.

The Medical Research Council will coordinate U.K. trials firstly in myeloma-tosis, a common bone-marrow tumour, for which no adequate treatment exists at present. The study will then be extended to patients with different forms of cancer. All animal investigations have been completed so that toxicity tests and controlled trials may begin by injecting interferon into or near localized tumours.

It has proved difficult to make interferon in sufficient quantities for trials, since human tissue culture methods have needed to be developed. At least three types of interferon are known – leucocyte, fibroblast and type II immune. Most initial studies on antiviral properties have been done with leucocyte interferon produced from white cells. Fibroblast and lymphoblastoid interferon are produced in tissue culture, although recombinant DNA techniques may ultimately be cheaper. The product to be tested in the U.K. will be obtained from human lymphoblastoid cell cultures.

In 1980, researchers at Upjohn showed that a new group of 6-phenylpyrimidine derivatives caused the body to produce interferon. The American Association for Cancer Research has demonstrated that the same drugs protect animals against viruses and also improve their defences against tumour cells. Studies in humans are yet to be done. It has also been suggested that interferon stimulates prostaglandin synthesis and this may help to explain how interferon inhibits cell growth.

A new system of nomenclature for interferon has been devised by an inter-national group of scientists. The group indicate that 'to qualify as an interferon a factor must be a protein which exerts virus non-specific, anti-viral activity at least in homologous cells through cellular metabolic processes involving synthesis of both RNA and protein'. The preferred abbreviation for interferon is IFN. Each interferon is then designated by the animal of origin, e.g. human HuIFN, murine MuIFN, bovine BovIFN. The interferons are next classified into types according to antigen specificities, e.g. α β, and γ, which correspond to previous designations of leucocyte, fibroblast and type II immune, respectively. It was thought that previous type names were misnomers as both leucocytes and fibroblasts can produce each of the two types, α and β, of interferon. If other classes are discovered they will be designated δ, ε, etc. α and β interferons are usually stable in acid media whilst γ interferons are acid-labile. Properly documented differences in molecular size appear to be useful parameters until more stringent criteria such as amino acid sequence and monoclonal antibodies are forthcoming. Molecular weight desig-nations are indicated as HuIFN-α (18 K), MuIFN-β (39 K), etc.

Interferon preparations may contain more than one type of interferon. Thus, interferons derived from human lymphoblastoid cells and those derived from murine fibroblasts contain both IFN-α and IFN-β. Interferons presently employed in clinical trials are either HuIFN-α or HuIFN-β or admixtures of both.

FURTHER READING

1. Albert A. (1979) *Selective Toxicity*, 6th ed. London, Chapman & Hall.
2. Calman K. C., Smyth J. F. and Tattersall H. N. (1980) *Basic Principles of Cancer Chemotherapy*. London – Basingstoke, Macmillan.
3. Carter S. K., Sakurai Y. and Umezawa H. (eds.) (1981) *New Drugs in Cancer Chemotherapy*. Berlin – Heidelberg – New York, Springer–Verlag.
4. Carter S. K., Bakowski M. T. and Hellman K. (1981) *Chemotherapy of Cancer*. 2nd ed. New York, Wiley.
5. Rosowsky A. (ed.) (1979) *Advances in Cancer Chemotherapy*. New York – Basel, Marcel Dekker.
6. Pratt W. B. and Ruddon R. W. (1979) *The Anti-cancer Drugs*. Oxford, Oxford University Press.
7. Stenlake J. B. (1979) Biological alkylating agents. In *Foundations of Molecular Pharmacology*: Vol. 2, *The Chemical Basis of Drug Action*. University of London, Athlone, pp. 82–6.
8. Montgomery J. A., Johnston T. P. and Fulmer Shealy Y. (1980). Drugs for neoplastic diseases. In Wolff M. E. (ed.) *Burger's Medicinal Chemistry*, 4th ed., Part 2. New York, Wiley, pp. 595–670.
9. Phillipson J. D. (1979) The search for new drugs from plants. *Pharm. J.* **222**, 310–12.
10. Smith F. R. (1967) The contribution of plants to medicinal chemistry. *Pharm. J.* **198**, 489–96.
11. Holcenberg J. S., Borella L. D., Camitta D. M. and Ring B. J. (1979) Human pharmacology and toxicology of succinylated *Acinetobacter* glutaminase-asparaginase. *Cancer Res.* **39**, 3145–51.
12. Hollstein U. (1980) Non-lactam antibiotics – bleomycins. In Wolff M. E. (ed.) *Burger's Medicinal Chemistry*, 4th ed., Part 2. New York, Wiley, pp. 251–3.
13. Wolff M. E. (1981) Anti-inflammatory steroids. In Wolff M. E. (ed.) *Burger's Medicinal Chemistry*, 4th ed., Part 3. New York, Wiley, pp. 1273–311.
14. Interferon nomenclature (1980) *Nature (London)*, **286**, 110.
15. Cordes E. H. (1981) The human interferons. In Hess H.-J. (ed.) *Annual Reports in Medicinal Chemistry*, Vol. 16. New York – London, Academic Press, pp. 229–41.
16. Struck R. F. (1980 and 1981) Antineoplastic agents. In Hess H.-J. (ed.) *Annual Reports in Medicinal Chemistry*, Vol. 15 and 16, New York – London, Academic Press, pp. 130–8 (1980), pp. 137–47 (1981).

Chapter 7

Relationship of drug metabolism to drug design

Relationship of drug metabolism to drug design

7.1 PRO-DRUGS

Many instances are known of drugs which are metabolized by the body to metabolites which possess the activity of the drug, the parent drug itself being an inactive precursor. Such precursors have been termed pro-drugs. The discovery that the activity of a drug is due to a metabolite sometimes leads to introduction of the metabolite itself into therapy. The reasons for this may be either that the metabolite is less toxic or has fewer side-effects than the pro-drug, or that generally the metabolite reduces the variability of the clinical response within the population due to different metabolizing powers of individuals, especially in the disease state.

One of the first drugs used clinically and later found to be a precursor was arsphenamine **(7.1)** used by Ehrlich for the treatment of syphilis. Later work by Voegtlin showed that arsphenamine owed its activity against the syphilis organism to the metabolite oxophenarsine **(7.2)**. Oxophenarsine later replaced arsphenamine

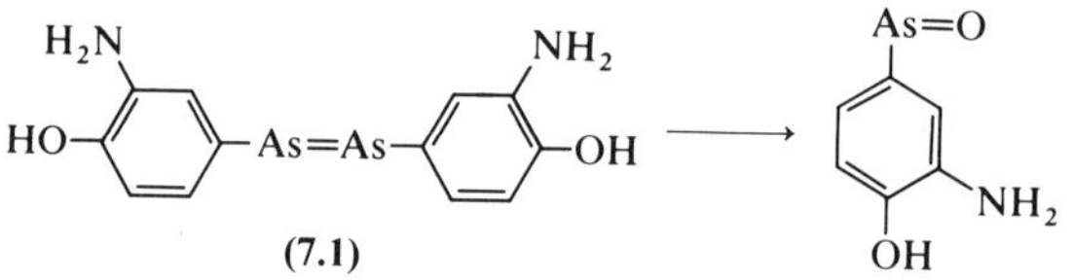

(7.1)

(7.2)

in therapy since it was less toxic at the dose required for effective treatment. The discovery of the azo dye prontosil **(7.3)** by Domagk in 1935 marked the advent of present day sulphonamide therapy. Prontosil is inactive against micro-organisms *in vitro* but active *in vivo*. The discovery that prontosil was a precursor and that the active form was a metabolite, *p*-aminobenzenesulphonamide **(7.4)**, directed research for therapeutically superior sulphonamides away from dyes and towards the modification of the aminobenzenesulphonamide molecule which led to the wide range of sulphonamides that are now available for treatment (*see* Section 4.3.1).

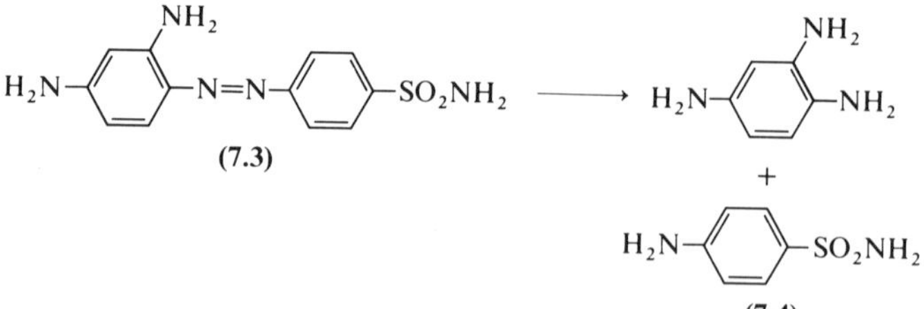

(7.3)

(7.4)

196

The antimalarial drugs pamaquin **(7.5)** and paludrine **(7.7)** are both converted by the body to active metabolites against forms of the malarial parasite. Pamaquin is dealkylated and oxidized to the quinone **(7.6)** which has 16 times the *in vivo* activity of the parent compound. Paludrine is metabolized by ring closure to the active dihydrotriazine **(7.8)**. There is a clear structural relationship between the dihydrotriazine **(7.8)** and the active antimalarial drug pyrimethamine **(7.9)** which has a similar action to paludrine. The dihydrotriazine (cycloguanyl **(7.8)**) is used as the insoluble embonate (pamoate) salt and a single intramuscular injection of a suspension in an oily base provides protection against malarial infection for several months.

The once used hypnotic, chloral hydrate, is metabolized in man to trichloro-ethanol and its glucuronide and also to trichloroacetic acid. The depressant effect of therapeutic doses of chloral hydrate is now considered to be entirely due to trichloroethanol. This knowledge led at that time to the use of trichloroethanol acid phosphate (trichlofos **(7.10)**) in place of chloral hydrate for patients where the latter was found to be either unpalatable due to its objectionable taste or because of gastrointestinal irritation.

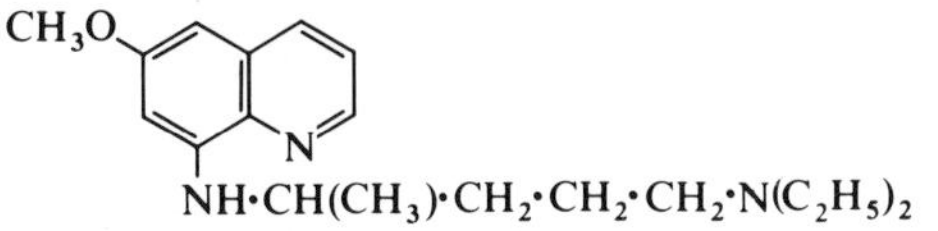

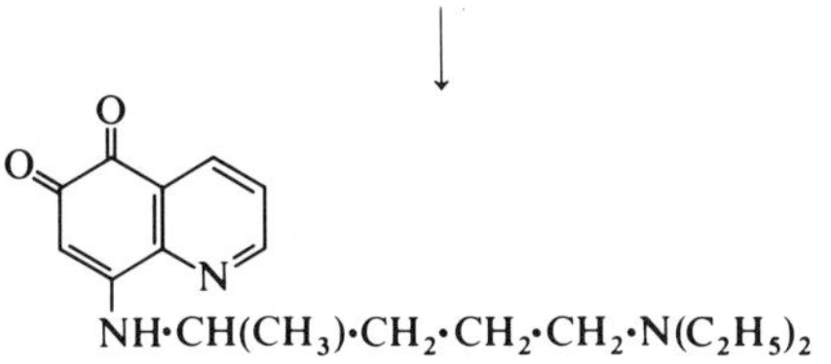

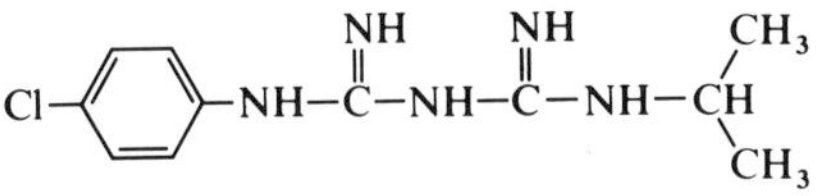

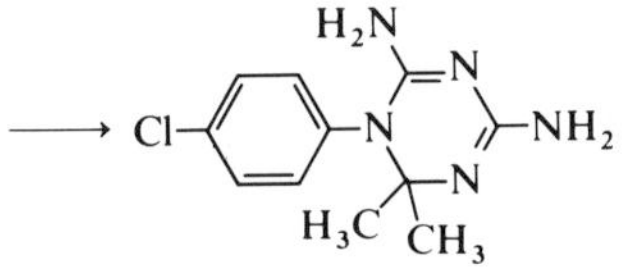

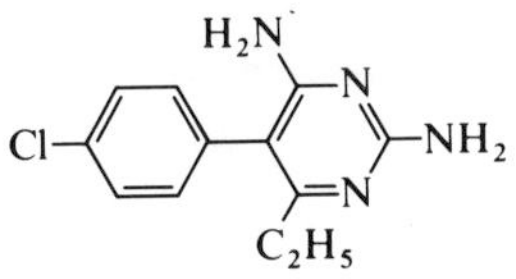

Methsuximide **(7.11)**, an anti-epileptic drug, is demethylated in the body to the active form and at the steady state the metabolite is present at a 700-fold greater concentration than the parent drug. Anti-epileptic activity has been correlated with the plasma concentration of the metabolite. In a similar manner

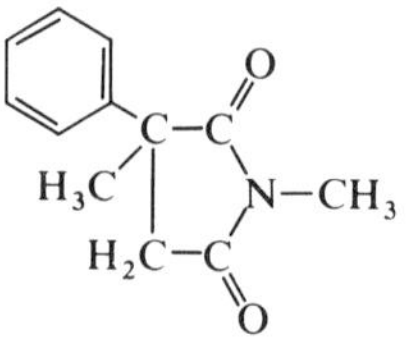

(7.11) 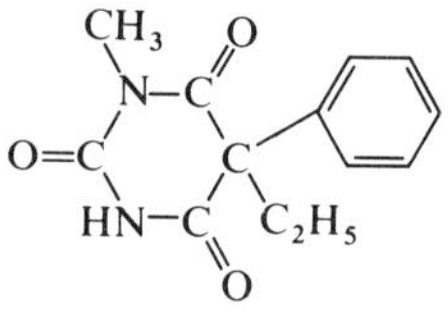 (7.12) 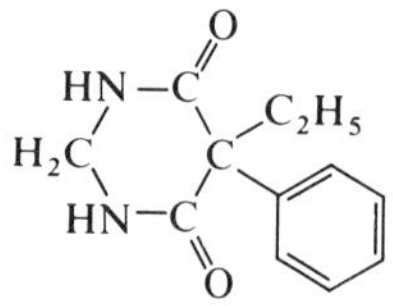 (7.13)

methylphenobarbitone **(7.12)** is converted to the active metabolite phenobarbitone whilst primidone **(7.13)** is oxidized to phenobarbitone.

The non-steroidal anti-inflammatory drug sulindac **(7.14)** is converted *in vivo* to the active form **(7.15)**.

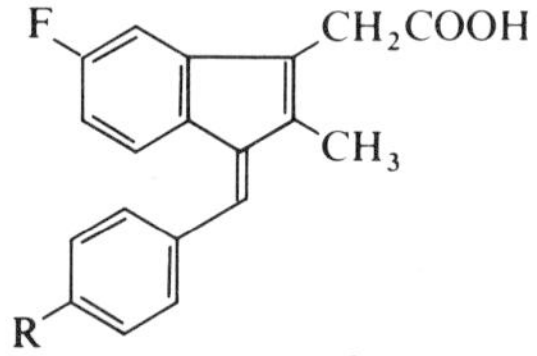

(7.14) R $= -\overset{O}{\underset{\uparrow}{S}}CH_3$
(7.15) R $= -SCH_3$

Several drugs giving active metabolites were initially considered to be pro-drugs but were subsequently shown to possess activity themselves.

Phenylbutazone (butazolidine, **(7.16)**) is converted by the body into the two hydroxylated forms, oxyphenbutazone **(7.17)** and **(7.18)**. The drug is used in therapy mainly as an anti-inflammatory agent and this activity resides in form **(7.17)**. However another use of the drug is as a uricosuric agent, in the treatment of gout, and this action is attributable to the form **(7.18)**. The observation that

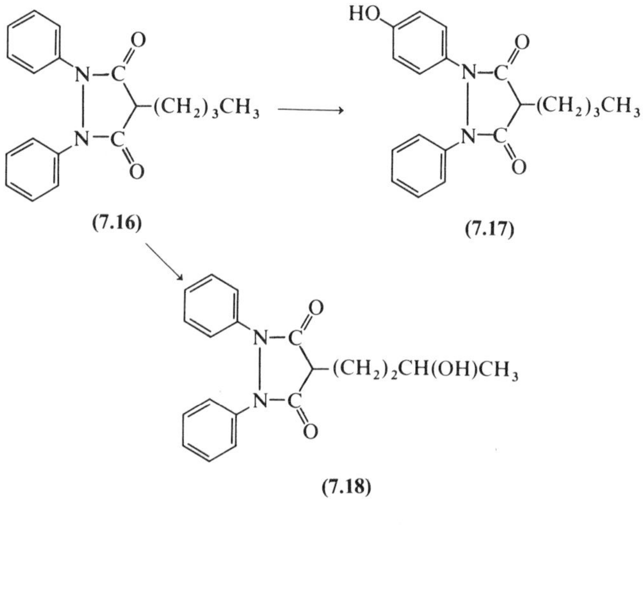

(7.16) (7.17)

(7.18)

substitution in the side-chain of phenylbutazone results in enhanced uricosuric action has led to the discovery of several other agents which have this action, in particular sulphinpyrazone (7.19).

Phenacetin (7.20), an analgesic and antipyretic agent, is mainly metabolized in the body to an active metabolite, N-acetyl-p-aminophenol (paracetamol (7.21)), as well as to an inactive metabolite, the glucuronide of 2-hydroxy phenacetin (7.22),

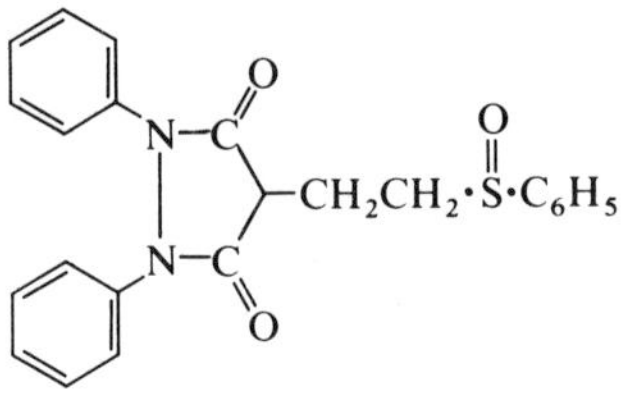

(7.19) 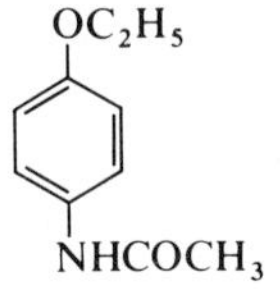   (7.20) 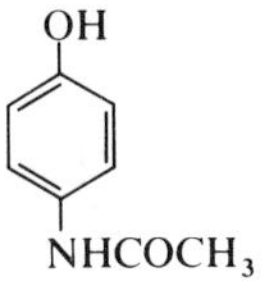   (7.21) 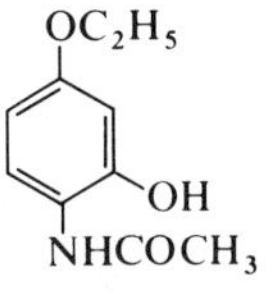   (7.22)

in small amounts. Paracetamol has replaced phenacetin in therapy since it is usually free from toxic effects, associated with phenacetin, e.g. methaemoglobin formation. However, extensive hepatic necrosis may occur when overdoses are ingested since the normal biotransformation pathway (conjugation with glutathione) is then saturated and a highly reactive metabolite is formed which binds irreversibly to hepatic tissue. More recent work has shown that phenacetin itself possesses antipyretic activity and that this activity is not dependent on metabolism to paracetamol.

The tranquillizer, diazepam (7.23), is converted in the body by demethylation and hydroxylation to three active metabolites N-demethyldiazepam (7.24), N-methyloxazepam (7.25) and oxazepam (7.26). The three metabolites are at least as

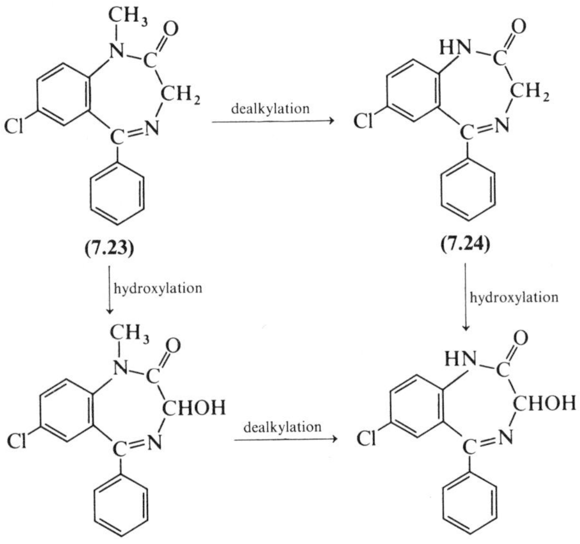

(7.23)

(7.24)

(7.25)

Oxazepam
(7.26)

active as diazepam in animal tests and have the advantage that they have reduced toxicity. Oxazepam is available commercially and is used for the same purpose as diazepam.

7.2 DESIGN OF PRO-DRUGS TO IMPROVE THE PHYSICAL AND BIOLOGICAL PROPERTIES OF A DRUG

The physical and biological properties of a drug such as taste, colour, irritability in the gastrointestinal tract and poor absorption in the intestine may be improved by selective chemical modification of the parent drug to an inactive pro-drug form. After administration or absorption of the pro-drug, the active drug is released either by catalysed hydrolysis by liver or intestinal enzymes or simply by hydrolysis:

$$\text{Active drug} \xrightarrow[\text{modification}]{\text{chemical}} \underset{\text{(inactive)}}{\text{Pro-drug}} \xrightarrow[\text{HOH}]{\text{Enzymes}} \text{Active drug.} \tag{7.1}$$

7.2.1 Enzymes concerned in activation of pro-drugs

The inactive zymogen precursors of α-chymotrypsin, trypsin and elastase are produced in the pancreas and enter the duodenum where they are converted by proteolytic enzymes to the active enzyme. These enzymes degrade proteins and polypeptides by hydrolysis of peptide linkages.

A peptide bond on the carboxyl side of tryptophan, tyrosine and phenylalanine residues is more rapidly hydrolysed by α-chymotrypsin than when it is situated adjacent to hydrophobic residues (leucine, methionine) or elsewhere in the peptide structure. Ester and amide derivatives of tryptophan, tyrosine and phenylalanine are also good substrates of the enzyme, as are non-specific substrates with a good leaving group, e.g. p-nitrophenylacetate. In a similar manner, trypsin rapidly hydrolyses peptide bonds, ester and amide derivatives of the basic L-amino acids, arginine and lysine, whilst elastase shows specificity towards derivatives of amino acids with uncharged, non-aromatic side-chains (glycine, alanine, valine, leucine, isoleucine and serine).

Carboxylesterases, mainly present in the liver, kidney, duodenum and brain, rapidly hydrolyse esters and, to a much slower extent, some amides. They are much more efficient at hydrolysing non-specific labile esters than α-chymotrypsin, the relative rate being 10^4–10^5 greater. Pancreatic lipase, present in the digestive tract, also hydrolyses esters provided that they are not completely soluble in water. It would appear that the enzyme requires a minimum degree of molecular aggregation before it can exert its activity.

7.2.2 Modification leading to increased absorption of a drug

Many penicillins are not absorbed efficiently when administered orally and their lipophilic esters have been used to improve absorption. Simple aliphatic esters of penicillins are not active *in vivo* and activated esters are necessary for release of the active penicillin from the inactive pro-drug ester. Ampicillin **(7.27)**, a wide spectrum antibiotic, is readily absorbed orally as the inactive pro-drugs, pivampicillin **(7.28)**, bacampicillin **(7.29)** and talampicillin **(7.30)** which are then converted by enzymic hydrolysis to ampicillin. The preferred pro-drug is pivampicillin since minimal hydrolysis occurs in the intestine before absorption. Pivampicillin, the

(7.27) ampicillin, R = H

(7.28) pivampicillin, R = $-CH_2-O-\overset{\overset{\displaystyle O}{\|}}{C}-C(CH_3)_3$

(7.29) bacampicillin, R = $-CH(CH_3)-O-\overset{\overset{\displaystyle O}{\|}}{C}-O-C_2H_5$

(7.30) talampicillin, R =

pivaloyloxymethyl ester, contains an acyloxymethyl function which is rapidly hydrolysed by enzymes to the hydroxymethyl ester. This ester, being a hemiacetal of formaldehyde, spontaneously cleaves with release of ampicillin and formaldehyde. In a similar manner, bacampicillin and talampicillin are cleaved and decompose to give ampicillin together with acetaldehyde and 2-carboxybenzaldehyde respectively.

The non-lability of simple esters of penicillin *in vivo* may be due to formation of a stable acyl-enzyme due to steric hindrance by the penicillin nucleus with release of the alcohol fragment, i.e. methanol for methyl ester (*see* p. 122). The acyloxymethyl esters form an acyl-enzyme which is less sterically hindered and more readily deacylated, since the penicillin nucleus is released in the alcohol fragment.

Acyloxymethyl esters of cephalosporins have also been prepared and found to have enhanced oral absorption characteristics when compared with the parent compounds.

Phosphate esters of steroidal alcohols and other alcoholic drugs have been used for a number of purposes. These esters are water-soluble derivatives of the drug and are stable at pH 7 as the di-anionic form. *In vivo*, the widely distributed phosphatase enzymes convert the pro-drug to the active form. The poorly water-soluble anti-inflammatory steroidal alcohol, dexamethasone, when injected as the water-soluble phosphate **(7.31)** rapidly ($t_{\frac{1}{2}} = 10$ min) liberates the active steroid *in vivo*.

Oxyphenbutazone **(7.17)**, as the water-soluble phosphate ester **(7.32)**, is rapidly hydrolysed *in vivo* and gives higher blood levels of oxyphenbutazone on oral or intramuscular administration than the parent drug dose.

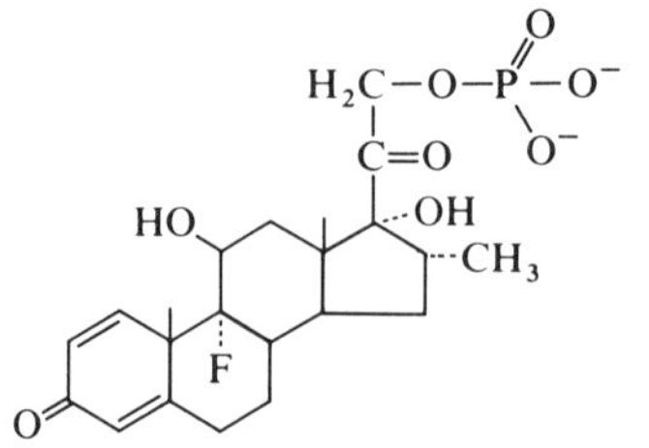

202   INTRODUCTION TO THE PRINCIPLES OF DRUG DESIGN

(7.31)

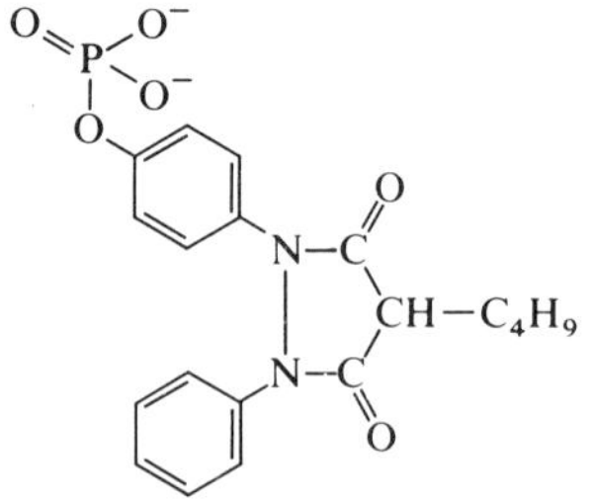

(7.32)

The antibiotic erythromycin is destroyed by gastric acid and, as an alternative to enteric-coated tablets, it is administered orally as a more stable ester. The inactive erythromycin estolate (laurylsulphate salt of the propionyl ester), when administered as a suspension, is rapidly absorbed and the propionyl ester converted by body esterases to the active erythromycin. The propionyl ester gives higher blood levels after oral administration on an equi-dose basis than the acetate or butyrate esters. The ethyl succinate ester is also used.

Theophylline used in the treatment of asthma is administered frequently due to its rapid elimination from the body. Larger doses to sustain the effect cannot be given due to its narrow therapeutic index. 7,7'-Succinylditheophylline is an insoluble pro-drug which has a slow dissolution rate but in solution is rapidly hydrolysed to theophylline in the body and is a useful controlled release dosage form of theophylline.

Highly polar drugs do not pass the blood–brain barrier. Better penetration of the nerve gas antagonist, pralidoxine (see p. 111), into the CNS has been achieved using (7.33) as a non-polar pro-drug which can cross the barrier and is then rapidly oxidized to the active form.

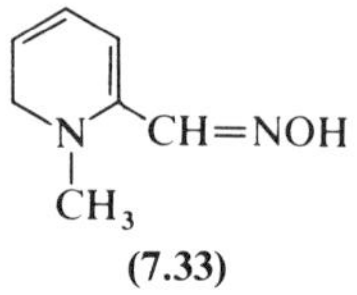

(7.33)

The bioavailability of the β-adrenergic receptor blocking drug, propranolol, is low when administered orally and is subject to wide inter-patient variations. The hemisuccinate ester (7.34) is a pro-drug which gives considerably increased and less variable oral absorption in dogs than propranolol, probably as a result of reduced

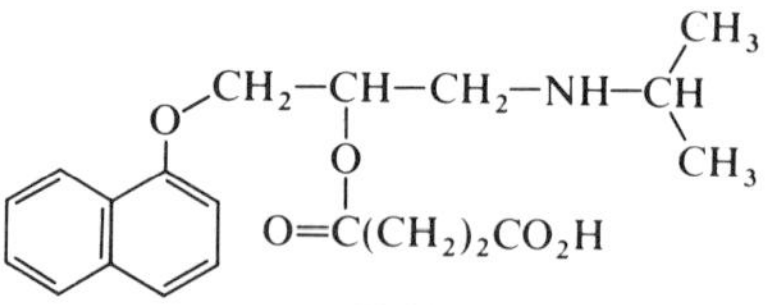

(7.34)

O-glucuronidation of the blocked hydroxyl group during first pass metabolism (*see* p. 27) in the liver.

7.2.2.1 *Current research*

Current research in animal experiments has shown that the oral absorption of certain basic drugs may be increased by the preparation of 'soft' quaternary salts.

The 'soft' quaternary salt is formed by reaction between an α-chloromethyl ester **(7.35)** and the amino group of the drug (Equation 7.2). The quaternary salt

$$R_1\text{--}\overset{\overset{\displaystyle O}{\|}}{C}\diagdown_{Cl} + R_2CHO \longrightarrow R_1\text{--}COO\text{--}\overset{\overset{\displaystyle R_2}{|}}{C}H\text{--}Cl \longrightarrow Drug\text{--}\overset{\overset{\displaystyle R_2}{\overset{|}{N}}}{\underset{Cl^-}{\overset{+}{|}}}\text{--}\overset{\overset{\displaystyle R_2}{|}}{C}H\text{--}O\text{--}\overset{\overset{\displaystyle O}{\|}}{C}\text{--}R_1 \qquad (7.2)$$

$$\underset{\text{(7.35)}}{} $$

$$+$$

$$Drug\text{--}\overset{|}{\underset{|}{N}}{:}$$

formed is termed a 'soft' quaternary salt since, unlike normal quaternary salts, e.g. $R\text{--}\overset{+}{N}(CH_3)_3$, it can release the active basic drug on hydrolysis (Equation 7.3).

$$Drug\text{--}\overset{\overset{\displaystyle R_2}{|}}{\underset{\underset{Cl^-}{|}}{N^{\pm}}}\text{--}\overset{|}{C}H\text{--}O\text{--}\overset{\overset{\displaystyle O}{\|}}{C}\text{--}R_1 \xrightarrow{H_2O} Drug\text{--}\overset{+}{\underset{\underset{Cl^-}{|}}{N}}H + R_1COO^- + R_2CHO + H^+ \qquad (7.3)$$

'Soft' quaternary salts have useful physical properties compared with the basic drug or its salts. Water solubility may be increased compared with other salts, such as the hydrochloride, but more important there may be an increased absorption of the drug from the intestine. Increased absorption is probably due to the fact that the 'soft' quaternary salt has surfactant properties and is capable of forming micelles and un-ionized ion pairs with bile acids etc., which are able to penetrate the intestinal epithelium more effectively. The pro-drug, after absorption, is rapidly hydrolysed with release of the active parent drug.

Pilocarpine is rapidly drained from the eye and its miotic effect is of short duration. The 'soft' quaternary salt hexadecanoylmethyl pilocarpine, containing a lipophilic side-chain, is better absorbed in rabbits and at 1/10th the concentration of pilocarpine gives a more prolonged effect. The action of **(7.36)** has been shown to be due to release of pilocarpine on hydrolytic cleavage of the ester, followed by the release of formaldehyde.

(7.36)

The antimalarial drug (7.37) has a low water solubility and is poorly absorbed after oral administration. Attempts to increase solubility by preparing salts did not increase absorption, due to the low pK_a of the two nitrogen atoms in the molecule. Introduction of a more basic group into the molecule by preparation of the dimethylaminoacetate ester (7.38) increased solubility but did not give high blood levels of the drug. The 'soft' quaternary derivative (7.39) of the dimethyl-aminoacetate ester, however, had good solubility properties and led to dramatic increases in blood levels of the drug in dogs.

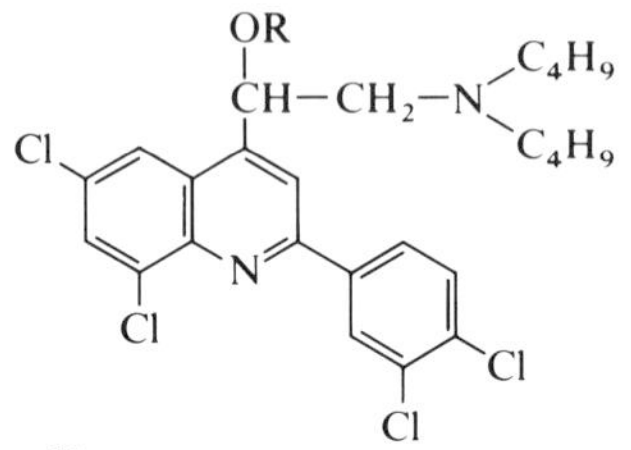

(7.37)   R = H
(7.38)   R = —CO—CH₂—N(CH₃)₂
(7.39)   R = —CO—CH₂—Ṅ(CH₃)₂—CH₂—O—CO—C₆H₅

7.2.3   Modification leading to elimination of unwanted physical properties of a drug

Ethyl mercaptan, C_2H_5SH, is a foul-smelling liquid which was originally used in the treatment of leprosy. It is now administered by rubbing into the skin as the colourless, inactive diisophthalyl thio ester (ditophal) and this is metabolized by the body to the active parent drug.

Although not currently used clinically, much ingenuity has been used to overcome the unpalatable nature of the hypnotic chloral hydrate. Before the introduction of trichlofos, the phosphate ester of the active metabolite trichloro-ethanol, chloral hydrate was modified to other pro-drugs which were more palatable. Examples are chlorhexadol (7.40) and petrichloral (7.41) which, as hemiacetals of chloral hydrate, are readily hydrolysed and release chloral hydrate after ingestion.

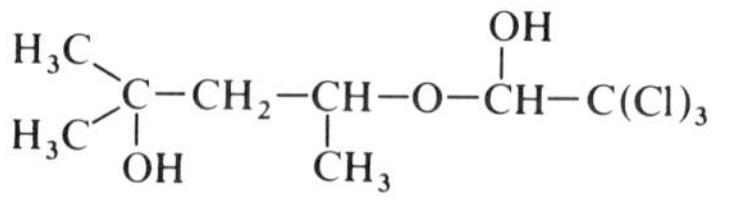

Chlorhexadol
(7.40)

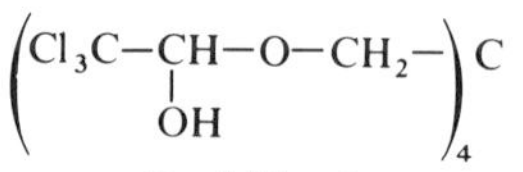

Petrichloral
(7.41)

The antibiotic chloramphenicol (7.42) is little used currently by oral admini-stration, except in the treatment of typhoid fever and salmonella infections, due to the drug's life-threatening toxic effects. It has an extremely bitter taste and is entirely unsuitable for administration as a suspension to children. Very young children generally require liquid medication since they are usually not amenable to swallowing capsules or coated tablets. Chloramphenicol for such purposes is now usually formulated as the inactive tasteless palmitate **(7.43a)** or cinnamate **(7.43b)**

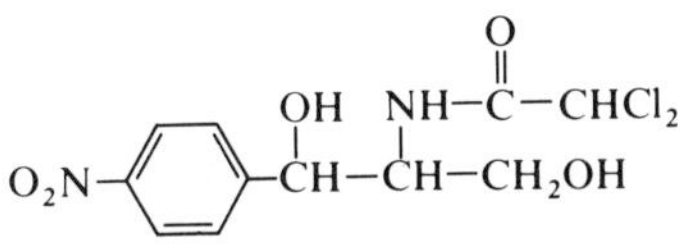

(7.42)

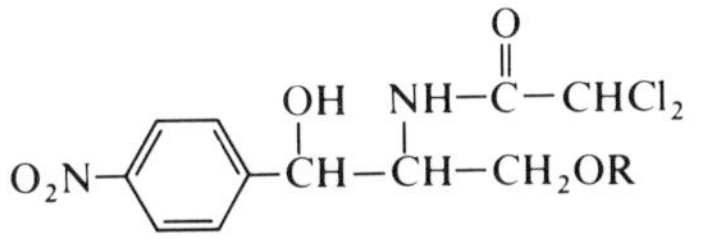

(7.43) (a) R = $CH_3(CH_2)_{14}CO-$
(b) R = $C_6H_5CH{=}CH-CO-$

esters. The active parent drug is released from these compounds by esterases present in the small intestine. The bitter taste of the antibiotics clindamycin and erythromycin are similarly masked in the palmitate ester and hemisuccinate ester pro-drugs respectively.

7.2.4 Modification leading to restriction of a drug to a specific site in the body

The modification of a drug to a pro-drug may lead to enhanced efficacy for the drug by differential distribution of the pro-drug in body tissues before the release of the active form. More extensive distribution of ampicillin occurs in the body tissues when the methoxymethyl ester of hetacillin (a 6-side-chain derivative of ampicillin) is administered, than is obtained with ampicillin itself. Alternatively, decreased tissue distribution of a drug may occur – as was observed when adriamycin as its DNA-complex was administered as a pro-drug. Decreased tissue distribution restricts the action of a drug to a specific target site in the body and so decreases the toxic side-effects of the drug, resulting from its reaction at other sites. Improved selective localization of drugs has been achieved with anticancer drugs, which can suppress growth in normal as well as neoplastic tissue, by using non-toxic pro-drugs which release the active drug within the cancer cell as a result of either the enhanced enzyme activity or the decreased pH associated with the cancer cell.

7.2.4.1 *Enhanced enzyme activity*

Oestrogens have proved useful in the treatment of malignant neoplasms of the prostate gland but have an associated feminizing side-effect. The pro-drug stilboestrol phosphate **(7.44)** was specifically designed to overcome this side-effect on the premise that the active drug (stilboestrol), released by acid phosphatases present in high concentration in the cancerous prostate tissue, would remain localized in the target tissue. Unfortunately, acid phosphatase activity is more widespread than therapeutically desired and the pro-drug offers no great clinical

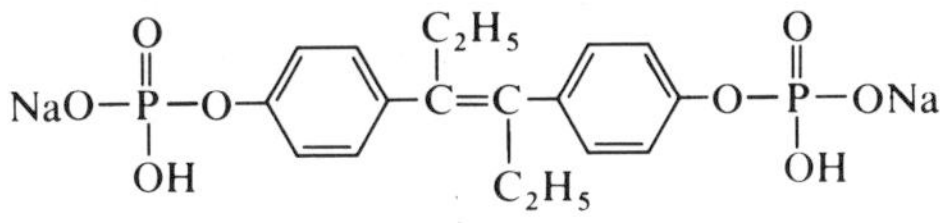

(7.44)

advantage over normal oestrogen therapy. Pro-drugs of colchicine, which are substrates for prostatic acid phosphatase, release the active drug within the cancerous tissue.

The pro-drug cyclophosphamide (7.45) is used for the treatment of certain forms of cancer and as an immunosuppressant after organ transplant. It does not possess alkylating properties and consequently is not a tissue vesicant since the electron-withdrawing properties of the adjacent phosphono-function decreases the nucleophilic properties of the β-chloroethylamino-nitrogen atom and prevents formation of the reactive alkylating ethyleniminium ion (see p. 172). The pro-drug is metabolized via liver hydroxylation to the active alkylating species, (7.46) and normustine, by the series of reactions depicted in Equation 7.4.

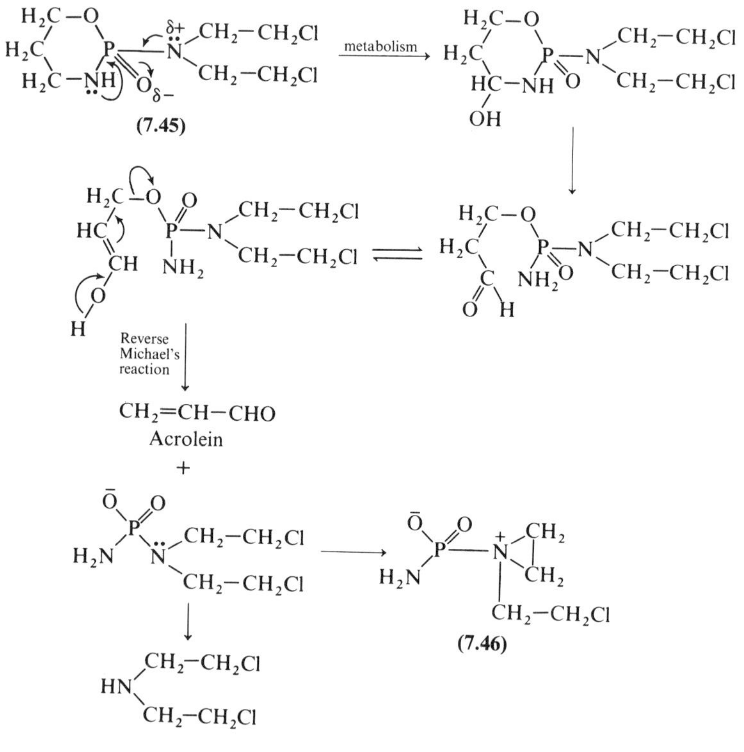

(7.4)

The action of this alkylating species would be expected to be restricted to the target tissue but unfortunately in practice the action of the drug is more widespread and it shows toxicity to normal tissue, one of the apparent effects being alopecia.

A series of other non-toxic nitrogen mustard pro-drugs have been designed to regenerate the parent alkylating agent in neoplastic tissues, by taking advantage of the difference in the level of enzymatic amidase between normal and neoplastic cells. N,N-diallyl-3(1-aziridino)propionamide (DAAP) is active against certain forms of leukaemia but does not cause leucopenia, a common toxic side-effect observed with other bifunctional alkylating agents. This observation suggests that DAAP is selective in its action against dividing (neoplastic) cells where a high amidase level occurs.

7.2.4.2   Differential pH

Neoplastic cells have a slightly lower relative pH than normal cells, in some circumstances, due to their high rate of production of lactic acid resulting from enhancement of glycolysis metabolism. Pro-drugs which are acid-labile with release of the anticancer drug are potentially selective in their action on neoplastic cells due to this pH difference. For example, it has been shown that mice implanted with L-1210 carcinoma when dosed with 5-dimethyltriazeno-imidazole-4-carboxamide (dacarbazine (7.47)) had their lifespan increased by 57% over controls. Structure (7.47) is acid-labile and is considered to release the anticancer drug 5-diazoimidazole-4-carboxamide (7.48) within the neoplastic cell.

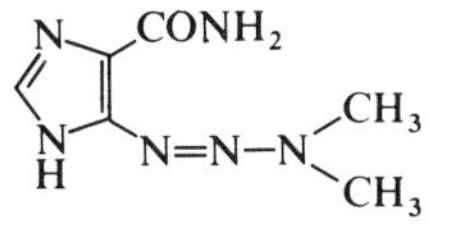

(7.47) 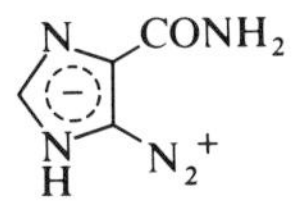   (7.48) 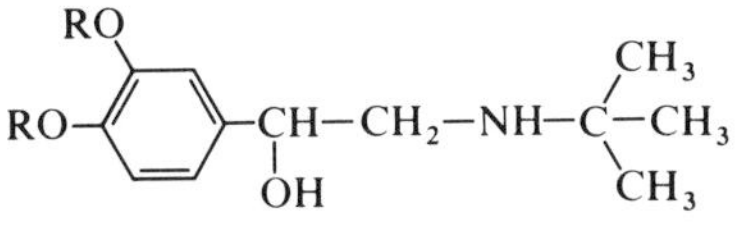   (7.49)   R = p-toluoyl
                               (7.50)   R = H

7.2.5   Modification leading to increased duration of action

The pro-drug, bitolterol (7.49), which is the di-p-toluate ester of N-t-butyl noradrenaline (7.50) has been shown in dogs to provide a longer duration of bronchodilator activity than the parent drug. Furthermore, the pro-drug is preferentially distributed in lung tissues rather than plasma or heart so that the bronchodilator effect, following subsequent biotransformation of the pro-drug, is not associated with undesirable cardiovascular effects.

The phenothiazine group of drugs, acting as tranquillizers, have been converted to long acting forms by conversion to pro-drugs which are administered by intramuscular injection. Not only is the frequency of administration reduced but the problem associated with patient compliance which sometimes arises is also eliminated. Flupenthixol (7.51) when administered as the decanoate ester (7.52) in an oily vehicle is released intact from the depot and subsequently hydrolysed to the parent drug, possibly after penetration of the blood–brain barrier. Maximum

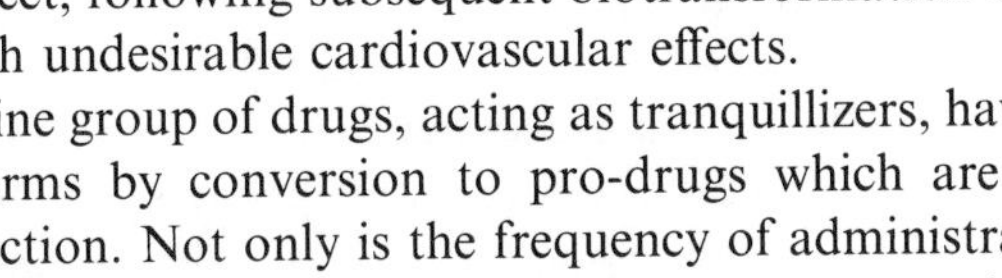

(7.51)   R = H

(7.52)   R = —C—(CH$_2$)$_8$CH$_3$

blood levels are observed within 11–17 days after injection and the plateau serum levels averaged 2–3 weeks in duration. Similarly, perphenazine has been used as the enanthate ester (7.53) and pipothiazine (7.54) as the undecanoate (7.55) and palmitate (7.56) esters.

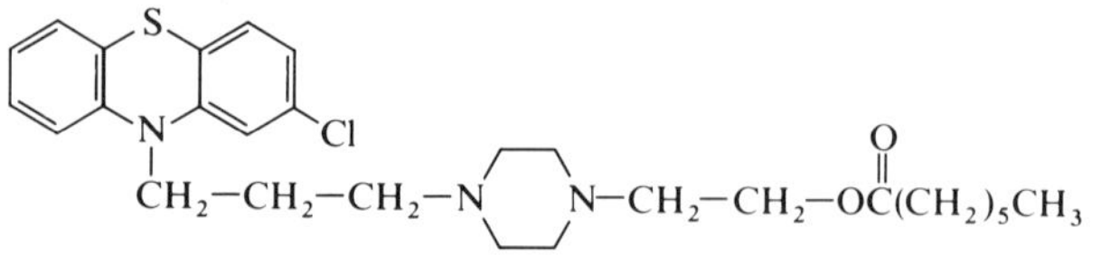

(7.53)

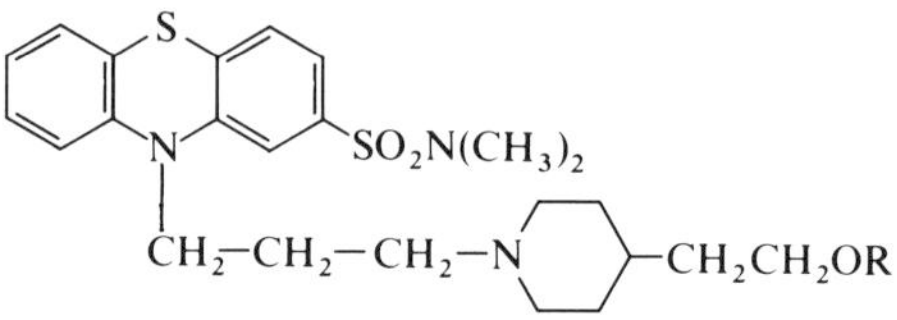

(7.54) R = H

$$(7.55)\ R = -\overset{O}{\underset{\|}{C}}(CH_2)_9CH_3$$

$$(7.56)\ R = -\overset{O}{\underset{\|}{C}}(CH_2)_{14}CH_3$$

7.3 DESIGN OF MORE EFFICIENT DRUGS FROM A KNOWLEDGE OF DRUG METABOLISM

There is a wealth of knowledge available concerning the range of metabolic processes occurring, in the body, to which drugs may be subjected – thereby converting them to biologically inactive products. In certain instances this knowledge may suggest to the medicinal chemist suitable chemical manipulation of an *active* parent drug to give an *active* drug which may, from a particular therapeutic aspect, have a better performance than the parent drug. For example, chemical manipulation might be designed to either shorten or increase the duration of action of a parent drug by modifying it in a predictable manner in order to affect its rate of metabolism and consequently the duration of its plasma level above the threshold responsible for the pharmacological effect (*see* Fig. 7.1). This more rational approach to drug design can, of course, only be applied to existing drugs or basic types associated with a known action but it means that once a desired biological activity is detected in a parent molecule the pathway of the development to a therapeutically acceptable product is more direct and sure than previously.

7.3.1 Modification leading to shorter action

Introduction into a drug molecule of a grouping which is vulnerable to the metabolic processes occurring in the body will give a drug with a shorter duration of action than the parent drug. This is assuming of course that modification leaves

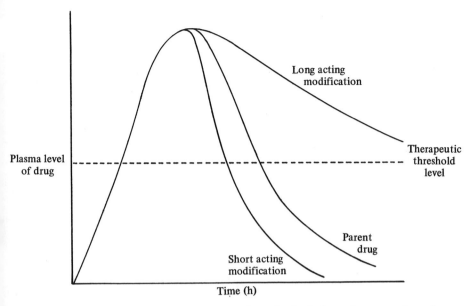

Fig. 7.1   Effect of duration of therapeutic effect of a single dose of a parent drug after chemical manipulation to increase or decrease the rate of metabolism.

unaltered the activity, absorption and distribution characteristics of the parent compound. Very few examples are known where a shorter acting derivative is more therapeutically desirable than the parent compound except where the drug is to be used on a limited number of occasions as for example in a surgical operation. Usually, chronic therapy is more suitable with drug administration kept to the minimum by the use of long acting drugs.

A muscle relaxant is used as an adjuvant to anaesthesia in surgical operations to obtain greater muscle relaxation. Where a short period of anaesthesia is required, a long acting neuromuscular blocking agent such as decamethonium **(7.57)** would produce unnecessary muscular pain after the patient has gained consciousness. In such situations shorter acting muscle relaxants are used and one of these is suxamethonium chloride **(7.58)** which contains two vulnerable ester groups

$$CH_2CH_2CH_2CH_2CH_2\overset{+}{N}(CH_3)_3$$
$$|$$
$$CH_2CH_2CH_2CH_2CH_2\overset{+}{N}(CH_3)_3$$

(7.57)

$$CH_2 \cdot \overset{O}{\overset{\|}{C}}O \cdot CH_2CH_2\overset{+}{N}(CH_3)_3$$
$$|$$
$$CH_2\overset{O}{\overset{\|}{C}}O \cdot CH_2CH_2\overset{+}{N}(CH_3)_3$$

(7.58)

between the two cationic nitrogen atoms. Hydrolysis of suxamethonium chloride by plasma esterases to the inert products, succinic acid and choline accounts for this short duration of action.

The barbiturate diethylbarbitone **(7.59)** is a long acting hypnotic sometimes used as an anticonvulsant in the treatment of epilepsy. Modification of the 5-substituents of this type of drug with the introduction of branched, cyclic or unsaturated chains generally produces a drug with a briefer duration of action than observed for the corresponding drug containing linear saturated chains with the same number of carbon atoms. This is due to the introduction of vulnerable unsaturated linkages and branching points where metabolism can occur to produce inert metabolites. Drugs such as butobarbitone (**7.59a**) and allobarbitone (**7.59b**) have an intermediate duration of action (3–6 h), whereas others such as cyclobarbitone (**7.59c**) and secobarbitone (**7.59d**) have a short duration of action (3 h) and are used for insomnia, the advantage being that the patient awakens in the morning and the effects of the drug have worn off.

(**7.59**)　barbitone;　$R^1 = R^2 = -C_2H_5$
(**7.59a**)　butobarbitone; $R^1 = -C_2H_5$, $R^2 = -CH_2 \cdot CH_2 \cdot CH_2 \cdot CH_3$
(**7.59b**)　allobarbitone; $R^1 = R^2 = -CH_2-CH=CH_2$

(**7.59c**)　cyclobarbitone; $R^1 = -C_2H_5$, $R^2 = $

(**7.59d**)　secobarbitone;　$R^1 = -CH_2-CH=CH_2$, $R^2 = -CH(CH_3)C_3H_7$

Replacement of the oxygen at C-2 by sulphur shortens the onset and duration of action and these drugs are used as general anaesthetics. The thiobarbiturates are more lipophilic in the un-ionized form that the barbiturates and rapidly penetrate the central nervous system to exert their effect. However, their short duration of action is not due to rapid metabolism but rapid clearance from the plasma by storage in the fatty deposits of the body tissues.

7.3.2 Modification leading to longer action

A parent drug may be converted to a drug with a longer duration of action in one of two ways. The group in the parent drug which is metabolized to give an inert product is either (*a*) protected from metabolic attack by placing other groupings in close proximity so that it is more sterically hindered or, (*b*) replaced by a group which is less vulnerable to metabolic attack, provided that such a change is not associated with a loss in activity.

7.3.2.1　*Steric hindrance of a vulnerable group*

A vulnerable group in a parent drug can be sterically hindered to a metabolic process by introduction of alkyl groups in its vicinity. The success of this procedure is seen by the increase in biological life of the series of alcohols, $(CH_3)_3COH > (CH_3)_2CHOH > CH_3CH_2OH$, where the vulnerable alcohol group is attached to a carbon atom which is successively substituted by alkyl groups.

The prostaglandin, PGF$_{2\alpha}$ **(7.60)**, is metabolized by oxidation of the C-15 hydroxyl group to give the inert ketone. The C-16 dimethyl analogue **(7.61)** has a much longer biological half-life in man, presumably due to protection of the vulnerable group by the adjacent methyl groups.

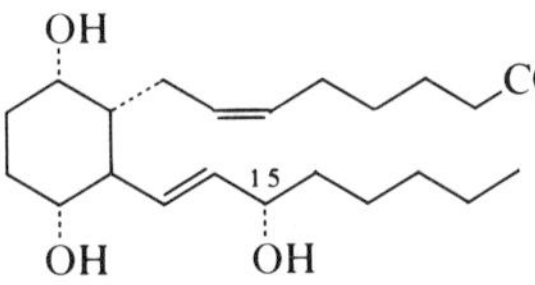

PGF$_{2\alpha}$
(7.60)

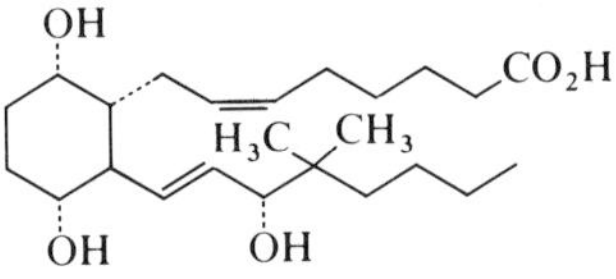

(7.61)

Lignocaine **(7.62)**, a local anaesthetic, has also been used in the treatment of cardiac arrhythmia. It is administered by injection since it is ineffective orally. This is because after absorption through the intestinal wall it is carried to the liver where it is metabolized (first-pass metabolism, *see* p. 27 to the metabolite **(7.63)** which, although active, is rapidly hydrolysed to inactive metabolites by microsomal amidases. An analogue of lignocaine, tocainide **(7.64)**, is an effective oral

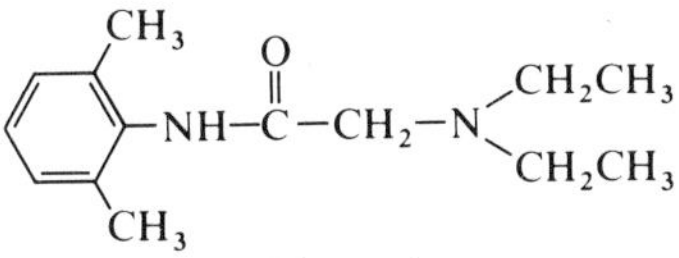

Lignocaine
(7.62)

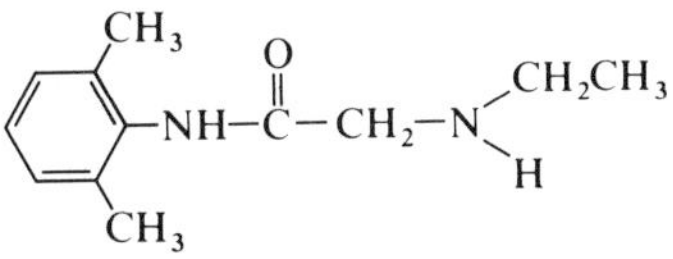

(7.63)

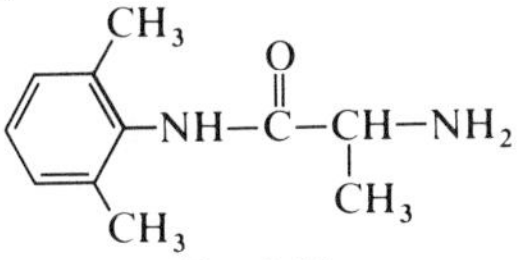

Tocainide
(7.64)

anti-arrhythmic agent since it is only slowly metabolized in the liver, possibly due to the fact that amido-compounds containing primary amino groups are poor substrates of the enzyme.

7.3.2.2   *Replacement of a vulnerable group*

Replacement of a vulnerable ester group by a less vulnerable amide group may lead to loss of activity, as noted with the more stable amide analogue of acetylcholine which has very little acetylcholine-like activity. However, isosteric replacement of the vulnerable ester group in the local anaesthetic procaine **(7.65)** by the more stable amide group to give procainamide **(7.66)** is associated with a decrease in local anaesthetic activity but an enhanced activity in the treatment of the condition of cardiac arrhythmia. The transient action of procaine towards this condition is the result of rapid hydrolysis of the ester function by blood esterases, an effect which is decreased in procainamide and the related drug lignocaine where the amide function is further protected by flanking methyl substituents.

$$H_2N-\underset{}{\overset{}{\bigcirc}}-COOCH_2CH_2N\overset{C_2H_5}{\underset{C_2H_5}{\diagdown}}$$

(7.65)

$$H_2N-\underset{}{\overset{}{\bigcirc}}-CONHCH_2CH_2N\overset{C_2H_5}{\underset{C_2H_5}{\diagdown}}$$

(7.66)

2,2-Diethyl-1,3-propanediol (7.67) and related compounds possess anticonvulsant and muscle-relaxing properties but are not useful drugs since they are rapidly metabolized and their action is of short duration. Replacement of the vulnerable hydroxyl groups by conversion to esters or carbamates prolongs their action, the carbamates being the most effective. The carbamate drug found to be most useful as a mild tranquillizer is meprobamate (7.68).

$$\underset{CH_2OH}{\overset{CH_2OH}{C_2H_5-C-C_2H_5}}$$

(7.67)

$$\underset{\underset{O}{\overset{}{\parallel}}{H_2C-O-C-NH_2}}{\overset{\overset{O}{\overset{}{\parallel}}}{\underset{C_3H_7-C-CH_3}{H_2C-O-C-NH_2}}}$$

(7.68)

$$H_3C-\underset{}{\overset{}{\bigcirc}}-SO_2NHCONHC_4H_9$$

(7.69)

$$Cl-\underset{}{\overset{}{\bigcirc}}-SO_2NHCONHC_3H_7$$

(7.70)

Tolbutamide (7.69) is a sulphonyl urea used as an antidiabetic drug for elderly people where insulin output is low. It has a short duration of action due to oxidation of the vulnerable nuclear-substituted methyl group. Replacement of the methyl group by a chlorine atom, with shortening of the alkyl chain, extends the biological half-life of the modified drug, chlorpropamide (7.70) six-fold.

FURTHER READING

1. Stella V. J., Mikkelson T. J. and Pipkin J. D. (1980) Prodrugs: the control of drug delivery via bioreversible chemical modification. In Juliano R. L. (ed.) *Drug Delivery Systems.* Oxford University Press, pp. 112–76.
2. Sinkula A. A. (1978) Methods to achieve sustained drug delivery. The chemical approach. In Robinson J. R. (ed.) *Sustained and Controlled Release Drug Delivery Systems.* New York and Basel, Marcel Dekker Inc., pp. 411–555.
3. Sinkula A. A. and Yalkowsky S. H. (1975) Rationale for design of biologically reversible drug derivatives: prodrugs. *J. Pharm. Sci.,* 64, 181–210.
4. Amidon G. L., Pearlman R. S. and Leesman G. D. (1977) Design of prodrugs through consideration of enzyme–substrate specificities. In Roche E. B. (ed.) *Design of Biopharmaceutical Properties Through Prodrugs and Analogues.* Washington, American Pharmaceutical Association, pp. 281–315.
5. Ariens E. J. (1971) Modulation of pharmacokinetics by molecular manipulation. In Ariens E. J. (ed.) *Drug Design,* Vol. III. New York, Academic Press, pp. 1–127.

Chapter 8

Quantitative structure–activity relationships and drug design

Quantitative structure–activity relationships and drug design

8.1 INTRODUCTION

Medicinal chemists have tried to quantify relationships between chemical structure and biological activity since before the turn of the century. However, it was not until the early 1960s, through the joint efforts of Corwen Hansch and his computer, that a workable methodology was developed and the subject that was to become known as quantitative structure–activity relationships (QSAR), was born. Since then, hundreds of research papers, articles and reviews on QSAR have emerged, with unfamiliar symbols and parameters, and with results which are expressed in a format different from that of traditional medicinal chemistry. It is the object of this chapter to explain these methods of expression, what they are meant to convey, and how the technique may be used in drug design.

The traditional method of searching for new medicinal compounds has sometimes been described as chemical roulette. A chemical structure, known to have a particular biological activity, is chosen, and attempts are made to improve it by modifications based on chemical intuition and isosteric considerations, (*see* Section 5.2) until a highly active compound with minimal side-effects is produced. A plan of the probable receptor site is built up as the number of compounds synthesized and tested increases, and the selection of further new compounds becomes progressively more rational. Beckett's work on analgesics is a classical example of this procedure. By carefully choosing his compounds, he was able to chart a map of the analgesic receptor site, which is reproduced in Fig. 8.1. It can be seen that there is a hollow which will accommodate a protruding group, a flat area which will fit a similar flat surface, and a negatively charged site. Methadone ((8.1) X = H) will fit this receptor. It has a phenyl group which can lie on the flat surface, and an alkyl chain which will occupy the hollow. Using this approach, one is able to anticipate the shapes of biologically active molecules, and speculate on the types and positions of groups which will bring about the optimal stereochemistry required for activity (*see also* Section 3.2.3).

The quantitative structure–activity approach uses parameters which have been assigned to the various chemical groups that can be used to modify the structure of a drug. The parameter is a measure of the potential contribution of its group to a particular property of the parent drug. In the present situation a steric parameter, which assesses the bulkiness of the group occupying the hollow on the drug receptor, would be appropriate. In a typical procedure, a series of related compounds are examined, and the relevant parameters of their substituent groups compared with the biological activities of the compounds and then, by mathematical procedures, the structure of the most promising derivatives are predicted.

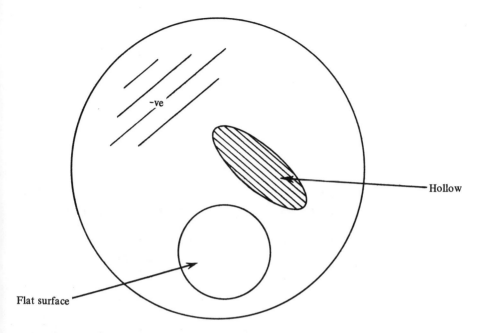

Fig. 8.1   Analgesic receptor site (as proposed by Beckett A. H. (1956). Analgesics and their antagonists: some steric and chemical considerations. Part 1. The dissociation constants of some tertiary amines and synthetic analgesics; the conformation of methadone compounds. *J. Pharm. Pharmacol.* **8**, 848–59).

Parameters governing several different properties can be employed, but the three most commonly used are steric and electronic parameters and parameters related to solubility.

8.2   ELECTRONIC PARAMETERS

The negatively charged site on the analgesic receptor suggests that an electron-deficient group on a potential analgesic molecule, positioned so that it will come into contact with the negative site, will help the molecule to bind to the receptor. The electron-deficient centre in methadone is provided by the protonated amine group. If the electron-density on the amine group is decreased, its electrostatic attraction for the receptor will become stronger. This can be achieved by attaching an electron-withdrawing group, such as chlorine (**(8.1)** $X = Cl$) to the amine

$$
\begin{array}{c}
CH_3 \quad CH_3 \\
| \qquad | \\
CH{-}N \\
| \qquad | \\
CH_2 \quad CH_2X \\
C \\
COOC_2H_5
\end{array}
$$

(8.1)

group, while an electron-donating group, such as methoxy ((**8.1**) X = OCH$_3$) will have the opposite effect. Considerations of this sort approach drug design in only a qualitative manner. It is more effective to quantify these qualities; electronic parameters perform this function by giving a value which is a measure of the degree of electron-donating or electron-withdrawing power. The best known electronic parameter is the Hammett substituent constant.

8.2.1   Hammett constants

In 1940, Hammett introduced his substituent constants to predict equilibrium constants and rate constants for chemical reactions. He reasoned that an electron-withdrawing group, attached to the aromatic ring of benzoic acid would increase the acid strength of the carboxyl group, and the greater the electron-withdrawing power, the greater the increase in strength. He was therefore able to assign substituent constants (σ) to groups according to their influence on the acid strength of benzoic acid. Hammett's substituent constant is defined by

$$\sigma_x = \log (K_x/K_0). \tag{8.1}$$

K_0 represents the dissociation constant of benzoic acid ((**8.2**) X = H), and K_x that

COOH

(8.2)

of benzoic acid substituted by the group X. More conveniently, σ can be expressed in terms of Equation 8.2. Thus, considering benzoic acid

$$\sigma_x = pK_a{}^0 - pK_a{}^x, \tag{8.2}$$

which has a pK_a value of 4·19, and p-toluic acid ((**8.2**) X = p-CH$_3$) which has a pK_a value of 4·36, the change in acid strength brought about by the methyl group ($\sigma_{p\text{-CH}_3}$) is equal to 4·19 − 4·36 = −0·17. A small selection of Hammett substituent constants is given in Table 8.1, from which it can be seen that electron-withdrawing groups have positive values, electron-donating groups have negative values, and hydrogen has a value of zero.

Scrutiny of Table 8.1 now shows that the analgesic activities of methadone analogues should increase in the order X = OCH$_3$ < CH$_3$ < H < Cl < NO$_2$. Unfortunately the situation is not so simple, because there are other factors which influence analgesic activity, in particular the migration of the drug from the site of administration to the site of action. Also, Hammett substituent constants apply specifically to groups attached to an aromatic system, while the part of the parent compound being modified may be aliphatic, as in the present example. Biological results which fit the concept precisely were generated by Fukata and Metcalf, who measured the toxic concentrations of nuclear substituted phenyldiethyl phosphates

(8.3) on houseflies. A plot of their results against σ, shown in Fig. 8.2, gives a good straight line, indicating that biological activity is mainly dependent on the electron density on the aromatic ring, and provides a means of predicting activities of potential new compounds before time is spent synthesizing them.

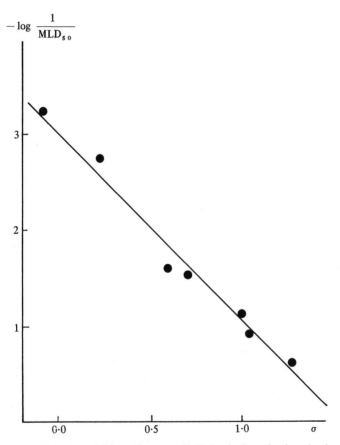

Fig. 8.2   Insecticidal activities of some diethyl-substituted phenyl phosphates. (Results taken from Fukata T. R. and Metcalf R. L. (1956) Structure and insecticidal activity of some diethyl-substituted phenyl phosphates. *J. Agr. Food Chem.* **4**, 930–5; Metcalf R. L. and Fukata T. R. (1962) Meta-sulfurpentafluorophenyldiethyl phosphate and meta-sulfapentafluorophenyl-*N*-methyl carbamate as insecticides and anticholinesterases. *J. Econ. Entomol.* **55**, 340–1).

Fukata and Metcalf's results can be expressed in the form of Equation 8.3, which is the equation for the best straight line through the points in Fig. 8.2.

$$\log(1/\mathrm{MLD}_{50}) = 1 \cdot 963\sigma - 3 \cdot 030. \qquad (8.3)$$

MLD_{50} is the minimum lethal dose for 50% of the flies treated. The equation was calculated using a mathematical process called regression (least squares) analysis. The calculation is not difficult, but is rather protracted. It is, therefore, only since the introduction of computers and electronic calculating machines that these so-called regression equations have been used extensively.

A regression equation is a convenient way of quantitatively expressing a correlation, but on its own it does not give as much information as a graph, because the graph indicates how many results were considered, how scattered they were around the best-fitting line, and how representative of the results the line is. Additional data should therefore be given, the basic minimum being shown in Equation 8.4. where it is laid out in the conventional manner. k_1 is the intercept,

$$\log(1/C) = k_1 + k_2\sigma,$$

n	s	r
(number of results)	(standard deviation about the regression line)	(correlation coefficient)

(8.4)

and k_2 the coefficient for σ. The correlation coefficient is a number which varies from zero to 1. The higher the number, the better the correlation. What constitutes a satisfactory correlation coefficient depends on the number of results, the greater the number of results, the lower the acceptable correlation coefficient. In quantitative structure–activity relationships, a figure in excess of $0 \cdot 9$ is aimed for. A useful feature of the correlation coefficient is that it is the square root of the explained variation, for example, a relationship having a correlation coefficient of $0 \cdot 990$ explains $0 \cdot 990^2 \times 100 = 98\%$ of the variation between results.

Additional statistical information, in particular the F value for the equation, is sometimes quoted. The F value is a numerical indicator of whether or not the relationship expressed by the equation is coincidental, the higher the value, the less likely the relationship is due to chance. The format for expressing F distribution and other data is shown in Equation 8.26, and the interpretation explained in Section 8.5.2.

The reason for using the logarithm of biological response in Fig. 8.2 and Equation 8.3 has thermodynamic origins. The free energy of a transition involving a given molecule is assumed to be the sum of the free energies of its substituent groups. Thus for example, the excess free energy of ionization of p-toluic acid (**(8.2)** X = p-CH$_3$) over that of benzoic acid is equal to the contribution of the p-methyl group. Equation 8.1 uses $\log(K_x/K_0)$ instead of free energy because equilibrium constants are logarithmically related to free energy (ΔG) through the van't Hoff equation (8.5) in which R is the gas constant and T is temperature. Log (K_x/K_0) and σ are therefore also additive. Because of this direct relationship, Hammett's and equivalent equations are said to be linear free energy relationships (LFER). It is therefore logical that the logarithms of biological parameters should be used in quantitative structure–activity relationships.

$$\Delta G = -2 \cdot 303 RT \log K. \tag{8.5}$$

Hammett substituent constants can only be used for nuclear aromatic substituents and their effects upon side-chain groups in the meta or para position to them. There are no ortho Hammett substituent constants. Numerous other electronic substituent constants have been introduced since Hammett's original work, many of which have been used in quantitative structure–activity relationships, but only two of them have been used to any great extent. These are the inductive substituent constant and the Taft substituent constant. For information on other constants, the reader is referred to the more comprehensive treatises listed at the end of the chapter.

8.2.2   Inductive substituent constants

Hammett substituent constants are a measure of both inductive and mesomeric effects. The p-substituent constant (σ_p) has a greater resonance component than the equivalent meta constant (σ_m), and the inductive contribution can be calculated from Equation 8.6. σ_I is the inductive substituent constant, and can be used in

$$\sigma_I = \tfrac{1}{2}(3\sigma_p - \sigma_m). \tag{8.6}$$

aliphatic compounds in which the influencing and influenced groups do not form part of a conjugated system. Inductive substituent constants have also been obtained from the dissociation constants of 4-substituted bicyclo(2,2,2)octane carboxylic acids (**8.4**), and α-substituted acetic acids. A small selection of inductive

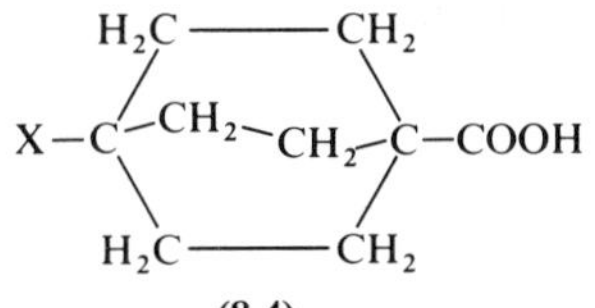

(8.4)

substituent constants is given in Table 8.1. More comprehensive lists can be found in the references cited below the table and at the end of the chapter.

8.2.3   Taft's substituent constants

Taft's substituent constants (σ^*) are a measure of the polar effects of substituents in aliphatic compounds when the group in question does not form part of a conjugated system. They are based on the hydrolysis of esters and are calculated from Equation 8.7, where k represents the rate constants for the hydrolysis of the

Table 8.1   Electronic substituent constants

Group	Hammett constants[a]		Inductive constants[b]	Taft constants[c]
	σ_m	σ_p	σ_I	σ^*
—H	0·00	0·00	0·00	0·49
—CH_3	−0·07	−0·17	−0·05	0·00
—C_2H_5	−0·07	−0·15	−0·05	−0·10
—Cl	0·37	0·23	0·47	—
—Br	0·39	0·27	0·45	—
—I	0·35	0·30	0·39	—
—NO_2	0·71	0·78	—	—
—OH	0·12	−0·37	0·25	—
—OCH_3	0·12	−0·27	0·25	—
—C_6H_5	0·06	−0·01	0·10	0·60

[a] Hammet L. P. (1940) *Physical Organic Chemistry.* New York and London, McGraw-Hill, p. 186.
[b] Charton M. (1964) Definition of 'inductive' substituent constants. *J. Org. Chem.* **29**, 1222–7.
[c] Taft R. W. (1956) Separation of polar, steric and resonance effects. In Newman M. S. (ed.), *Steric Effects in Organic Chemistry.* New York, John Wiley, pp. 559–675.

More comprehensive lists of electronic substituent constants can be found in:
Tute M. S. (1971) Principles and practice of Hansch analysis: A guide to structure–activity correlation for the medicinal chemist. In Harper N. J. and Simmonds A. B. (ed.), *Advances in Drug Research*, Vol. 6. London, Academic Press, pp. 1–77.
Hansch C. and Leo A. (1979) *Substituent Constants for Correlation Analysis in Chemistry and Biology.* New York, John Wiley.

substituted compound, and k_0 those of the methyl derivative. The bracketed term with the subscript *B* represents basic hydrolysis and the other, with the subscript *A*,

$$\sigma^* = (1/2{\cdot}48)\,[\log{(k/k_0)_B} - \log{(k/k_0)_A}]. \tag{8.7}$$

acid hydrolysis. The factor 2·48 brings the constants on to the same scale as the Hammett constants. The equation depends on the fact that although both basic and acid hydrolysis are sensitive to steric effects, the effect is the same. Only basic hydrolysis is influenced by polar effects, so that by subtracting the acid term from the basic term, only the polar effect remains. A limited list of Taft substituent constants is given in Table 8.1, larger compilations can be found in the literature.

Taft substituent constants are different from the others in that methyl, rather than hydrogen, is the standard group, for which the constant is zero. However, they can be compared with other constants by writing the methyl group in the form, CH_2—H, and identifying it as the group for H. Another substituent constant, representing a group X can then be compared by using the Taft constant for CH_2—X. Under these circumstances, Taft and inductive substituent constants are approximately related by:

$$\sigma^* = 2{\cdot}51\sigma_I. \tag{8.8}$$

8.3   STERIC SUBSTITUENT CONSTANTS

Steric effects can be expressed in a similar way to electronic effects. A steric substituent constant is a measure of the bulkiness of the group it represents, and its effect on the closeness of contact between the drug and the receptor site.

8.3.1   Taft's steric substituent constants

This constant (E_s) is a corollary of Equation 8.7. It depends on the fact that acid hydrolysis is determined almost completely by steric factors, and is defined by Equation 8.9. Kutter and Hansch used E_s values to examine the effects of

$$E_s = \log{(k/k_0)_A}. \tag{8.9}$$

substituents X on the antihistaminic activities (the biological response, R_b) of some analogues of diphenhydramine **(8.5)**, and derived Equations 8.10 and 8.11.

	n	s	r	
$\log R_b = 0.440 E_s - 2.204,$	30	0.307	0.886.	(8.10)
$\log R_b = 2.814\sigma - 0.223,$	30	0.519	0.629.	(8.11)

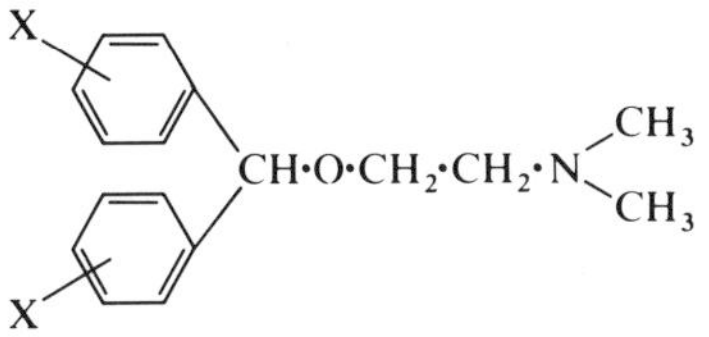

(8.5)

The standard deviations and correlation coefficients clearly show that the important factor is stereochemical, since the observed results are nearly twice as scattered about the line represented by Equation 8.11, in comparison with Equation 8.10, and Equation 8.10 explains 78% of the variation, while the correlation coefficient of Equation 8.11 is unacceptably low. It can be argued that Equation 8.11 does explain 40% of the variation, and that a precise correlation between $\log R_b$ and a combination of the two substituent constants is probable. The three variables can be correlated by multiple regression analysis, and the result is expressed in Equation 8.12. The arithmetic is similar to, but more complex than,

	n	s	r	
$\log R_b = 0.492 E_s - 0.585\sigma - 2.445,$	30	0.301	0.889.	(8.12)

linear regression and can be handled by most computers. Equation 8.12 cannot be expressed on graph paper, but can be represented by a three-dimensional model. When the number of variables exceeds 3, the results cannot be expressed in the form of either graph or model, since all dimensions will have been exhausted. A regression equation is, therefore, the only method of expression which can be used in such situations. Equation 8.12 confirms that the effect is predominantly steric, since introduction of σ has produced only an insignificant improvement in either correlation coefficient or standard deviation.

E_s values are given in Table 8.2. The list is limited by the experimental difficulties in obtaining the physico-chemical data upon which E_s values are based.

Table 8.2   Taft steric parameters[a]

Substituent	E_s	Substituent	E_s
—CH$_3$	0·00	C$_2$H$_5$	−0·07
CH$_3$COCH$_2$—	−0·19	BrCH$_2$	−0·27
C$_6$H$_5$CH$_2$—	−0·38	n-C$_4$H$_9$	−0·39
i-C$_4$H$_9$	−0·93	t-C$_4$H$_9$	−1·54
c-C$_6$H$_{11}$	−0·79		

[a] Taft R. W. (1956) Separation of polar, steric and resonance effects. In Newman M. S. (ed.) *Steric Effects in Organic Chemistry*. New York, John Wiley, pp. 559–675.

More comprehensive lists of Taft steric parameters can be found in:
Tute M. S. (1971) Principles and practice of Hansch analysis: A guide to structure–activity correlation for the medicinal chemist. In Harper N. J. and Simmonds A. B. (ed.), *Advances in Drug Research*, Vol. 6. London, Academic Press, pp. 1–77.
Hansch C. and Leo A. (1979) *Substituent Constants for Correlation Analysis in Chemistry and Biology*. New York, John Wiley.

8.3.2   van der Waals' dimensions

van der Waals' volume (V_w) and radius (r_v) represent the actual dimensions of the group. Since chemical groups are rarely symmetrical, the van der Waals' radius depends on the axis along which it is measured, and three types are defined, $r_{v(min)}$, the minimum radius, $r_{v(max)}$, the maximum radius, and $r_v\|$, which is the distance the group protrudes from the bulk of the parent molecule. van der Waals' radii can be correlated with biological results in the same ways as E_s, to which they are linearly related. $r_{v(min)}$ is usually preferred because groups are expected to take up positions which will minimize the degree of steric interaction. Sometimes the mean of the three radii ($r_{v(av)}$) is used.

8.3.3   Molecular connectivities

Molecular connectivities, designated $^m\chi$, can be employed as steric parameters. The superscript m denotes the order of the parameter. Zero order connectivity ($^0\chi$) is the simplest and is defined by Equation 8.13, where

$$^0\chi = \Sigma(\delta_i)^{-\frac{1}{2}}.$$ (8.13)

δ_i is a number assigned to each non-hydrogen atom, reflecting the number of non-hydrogen atoms bonded to it. Thus for *n*-butane (**8.6**),

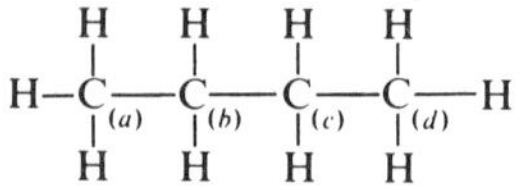

(8.6)

$\delta_{C_a} = 1$ (because C_a is attached to C_b only),

$\delta_{C_b} = 2$ (because C_b is attached to C_a and C_c),

$$\therefore {}^{0}\chi = (1/\sqrt{\delta_{C_a}}) + (1/\sqrt{\delta_{C_b}}) + (1/\sqrt{\delta_{C_c}}) + (1/\sqrt{\delta_{C_d}})$$
$$= (1/1) + (1/\sqrt{2}) + (1/\sqrt{2}) + (1/1) = 3.414.$$

The first order connectivity ($^{1}\chi$) is derived for each bond by calculating the product of the numbers associated with the two atoms of the bond. The reciprocal of the square root of this number is the bond value. Bond values are summed to give the first order connectivity for the molecule, so that the value for n-butane is,

$$^{1}\chi = (1/\sqrt{2}) + (1/\sqrt{4}) + (1/\sqrt{2}) = 1.914.$$

8.3.4 The parachor

The parachor [P] is molar volume V which has been corrected for forces of intermolecular attraction by multiplying by the fourth root of surface tension γ. It is expressed mathematically by Equation 8.14; M is molecular weight and D is

$$[P] = V\gamma^{\frac{1}{4}} = M\gamma^{\frac{1}{4}}/D. \tag{8.14}$$

density. The parachor has an advantage as a steric parameter in that it is easy to calculate, either from atomic contributions or from the component chemical bonds.

8.3.5 Charton's steric constants

The principal problem with van der Waals' radii and Taft's E_s values is the limited number of groups to which these constants have been allocated. Charton introduced a corrected van der Waals' radius U, in which the minimum van der Waals' radius of the substituent group ($r_{v(min)}$) is corrected for the corresponding radius for hydrogen (r_{vH}), as defined by Equation 8.15. They were shown to be a

$$U = r_{v(min)} - r_{vH} = r_{v(min)} - 1.20. \tag{8.15}$$

good measure of steric effect by correlation with E_s values, and also found to be rectilinearly related to the rates of esterification of substituted carboxylic acids with methanol and ethanol. Since there were ample data for these reactions, Charton was able to extend his list of constants to 62, by substituting rate constants into the regression equations linking esterification rates to U. The large number of constants available makes this a useful source of steric parameters for QSAR studies.

8.3.6 Minimal steric difference (MSD)

This parameter assesses the difference between molecules in terms of the parts which do not overlap when one chemical formula is placed on top of the other. If for example, piperidine (8.7) is compared with pyrrolidine (8.8), the methylene group, surrounded by the dotted circle, will determine the MSD, since this is the

only portion which does not overlap. The rules of the calculation are as follows,
 (i) hydrogen atoms are ignored,
 (ii) elements in the second period of the periodic table have a weighting of 1,
 (iii) elements in the third period have a weighting of 1·5 and
 (iv) elements in higher periods have a weighting of 2.
Thus the MSD between piperidine and pyrrolidine is 1, and that between
pyrrolidine and indole (8.9) is 4.

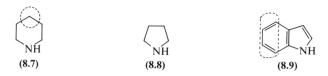

(8.7)   (8.8)   (8.9)

8.3.7 Sterimol parameters

A criticism of the steric parameters described so far is that they represent only one
aspect of the shape of the group. Thus for example, parachor represents the total
volume of the group, and r_v the width along one plane. Sterimol parameters were
developed to overcome this weakness. Each chemical group is allocated 5 sterimol
parameters: L, which is the distance the group protrudes from the parent molecule,
and B_1–B_4, which give the widths of the group in four directions, 90° to each other
and perpendicular to the L axis. Cross sectional dimensions increase from B_1 to
B_4. The procedure is shown diagramatically in Fig. 8.3.

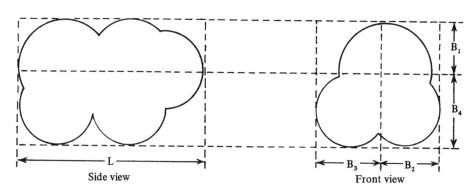

Side view   Front view

Fig. 8.3   Sterimol parameters.

8.4 PARTITION COEFFICIENTS

Partition coefficients P are equilibrium constants, and are therefore logarithmically
related to free energy. It follows that it should be possible to split log P into
parameters, characteristic of the chemical groups which make up the parent
molecule.

8.4.1 Hansch substituent constants

Most of the work in quantitative structure–activity relationships has been based on the system 1-octanol–water, and the substituent constants quoted in a dimensionless form (π), defined by Equation 8.16. π is the Hansch substituent constant. The

$$\pi = \log (P_x/P_H). \tag{8.16}$$

subscript H represents the unsubstituted compound and the subscript x represents the derivative in which hydrogen has been replaced by the group x.

Values can be used to calculate 1-octanol–water partition coefficients in the same way as Hammett constants can be used to estimate dissociation constants. Thus, the partition coefficient of butan-2-one between 1-octanol and water is 2·01 ($\log P_x = 0·32$), therefore the partition coefficient for hexan-2-one in the same system should be antilog $(0·32 + 0·52 \times 2) =$ antilog $1·36 = 22·9$, $(\pi_{CH_2} = 0·52)$. Values may also be correlated directly with biological activities, as will be discussed later.

Collander showed that partition coefficients in one solvent system (P_1) are related to those in another (P_2) by:

$$\log P_1 = k_1 \log P_2 + k_2. \tag{8.17}$$

where k_1 and k_2 are constants. Partition coefficients for an extensive range of compounds can be found in the literature, together with values of k_1 and k_2, to convert from one solvent system to another, using Equation 8.17.

Hansch constants for groups attached to aromatic nuclei fall roughly into three categories, depending on the nature of the group already in the ring, and these are,

  (i) strong electron-donating groups,
  (ii) strong electron-withdrawing groups and
  (iii) groups lying between these two extremes.

The differences involved can be seen from Table 8.3, which shows a selection of Hansch substituent constants. It has been recommended that for structure–activity relationships involving substitution on an aromatic ring, π constants based on phenoxyacetic acid should be used for systems in the third group, and constants based on phenol should be used for those in the first group.

As an alternative to π values, log partition coefficients can be correlated with biological activies. When π values are not available, they can be determined experimentally, or when the solubility is considerably higher in one solvent than in the other, can be estimated as the ratio of the solubilities in the individual solvents.

8.4.2 Fragmentation constants

Under some circumstances the π approach is inadequate, for example the values for $-CH_3$ and $-CH_2$ are the same in the Hansch scheme. Equation 8.18 provides an alternative method of calculating 1-octanol–water partition coefficients, and is

$$\log P = \Sigma af. \tag{8.18}$$

Table 8.3   Hansch substituent constants

(1) *Groups Attached to Non-conjugated Systems*

Group	π	Group	π
—OH (primary)	$-1 \cdot 16$	—OH (secondary)	$-1 \cdot 39$
—OH (tertiary)	$-1 \cdot 43$	—OCH$_3$	$-0 \cdot 47$
—Cl	$0 \cdot 39$	—Br	$0 \cdot 60$
—I	$1 \cdot 00$	—NH$_2$	$-1 \cdot 19$
—COCH$_3$	$-0 \cdot 71$	—NO$_2$	$-0 \cdot 85$
—CH$_3$, —CH$_2$, —CH	$0 \cdot 52$		

(2) *Groups Conjugated to Aromatic Systems*

Entering Group	\u2014OCH$_2$COOH	\u2014CH$_2$COOH	Occupying group \u2014COOH	\u2014CH$_2$OH	\u2014OH	\u2014NO$_2$
—H	0·00	0·00	0·00	0·00	0·00	0·00
3-Cl	0·76	0·68	0·83	0·84	1·04	0·61
4-Cl	0·70	0·70	0·87	0·86	0·93	0·54
3-CH$_3$	0·51	0·49	0·52	0·50	0·56	0·57
4-CH$_3$	0·52	0·45	0·42	0·48	0·48	0·52
3-OH	−0·49	−0·52	−0·38	−0·61	−0·66	0·15
4-OH	−0·61	—	−0·30	−0·85	−0·87	0·11
3-OCH$_3$	0·12	0·04	0·14	—	0·12	0·31
4-OCH$_3$	−0·04	0·01	0·08	0·00	−0·12	0·18
3-NO$_2$	0·11	−0·01	−0·05	0·11	0·54	−0·36
4-NO$_2$	0·24	−0·04	0·02	0·16	0·50	−0·39

More comprehensive lists of Hansch substituent constants can be found in:
Tute M. S. (1971) Principles and practice of Hansch analysis: A guide to structure–activity correlation for the medicinal chemist. In Harper N. J. and Simmonds A. B. (ed.), *Advances in Drug Research*, Vol. 6. London, Academic Press, pp. 1–77.
Hansch C. and Leo A. (1979) *Substituent Constants for Correlation Analysis in Chemistry and Biology.* New York, John Wiley.

theoretically better; it assumes additivity, but attempts to take account of constitutive effects by introducing correction factors. f represents the hydrophobic fragmentation constants of the various groups in the molecule, and a the number of times the group occurs.

Fragmentation constants have been derived from the 1-octanol–water partition coefficients of a large number of compounds for which reliable values are available. A small selection of f values is given in Table 8.4. Using these, the value of log P for n-propanol, $CH_3(CH_2)_2OH$, is $(3 \times 0 \cdot 20) + (7 \times 0 \cdot 23) - (2 \times 0 \cdot 12) - 1 \cdot 64 = 0 \cdot 33$, which agrees well with the experimental value of $0 \cdot 34$. The result, using Hansch constants from Table 8.3, is $(0 \cdot 52 \times 3) - 1 \cdot 12 = 0 \cdot 44$. This is a simple example, numerous corrections have been built in to allow for proximity effects, folding effects, aromaticity, etc.

8.4.3   Chromatographic R_m values

When the solubility of a solute is considerably greater in one phase than in the other, partition coefficients become difficult to determine experimentally. Parameters related to partition coefficient have therefore had to be used, in particular

Table 8.4   Fragmentation constants[a]

Fragment	f	Fragment	f
$\overset{\displaystyle |}{\underset{\displaystyle |}{-\text{C}-}}$	0·20	—COOH	$-1\cdot11$
—H	0·23	—NH$_2$	$-1\cdot54$
—OH	$-1\cdot64$	—O—	$-1\cdot82$

For hydrocarbon chains, $0\cdot12(n-1)$ is subtracted, where n is the number of bonds between carbons and between carbon and hetero atoms excepting hydrogen.

[a] Rekker R. F. (1977) *The Hydrophobic Fragment Constant.* Oxford, Elsevier. pp. 39–106.

A comprehensive account of fragmentation constants can be found in Hansch C. and Leo A. (1979) *Substituent Constants for Correlation Analysis in Chemistry and Biology.* New York, John Wiley.

the R_f value of chromatography, which is related to partition coefficient P through:

$$R_m = \log[1/R_f + 1]. \tag{8.19}$$

$$\log P = R_m + \text{a constant.} \tag{8.20}$$

Special chromatographic methods have had to be developed for highly lipophilic materials, which give rise to R_f values outside the normally acceptable range. Reversed-phase paper chromatography is a useful technique in this respect. Another method involves development on a thin layer impregnated with liquid paraffin, with acetone–water mixtures as moving phase, and extrapolating the R_f values to zero acetone concentration. R_m values have been used as a substitute for partition coefficients in QSAR investigations.

8.5   BIOLOGICAL RELATIONSHIPS

8.5.1   Ferguson effect

Ferguson was probably the first person to connect free energy with biological activity. He abstracted toxicity data from the literature, and noted that in homologous series of normal aliphatic alcohols, the logarithm of toxic concentration varied with carbon number in the same way as properties which were linearly related to free energy. He suggested that concentration in a body fluid is not a critical factor controlling the biological activity of a drug, and that it is the concentration within the receptor cell which is critical. If the cell contents are in equilibrium with the surrounding body fluid, the partial free energies, or thermodynamic activities, in the two phases will be equal. Ferguson expressed this activity as C_e/C_s for solutions, where C_e is the effective concentration and C_s the solubility. Also, since gas concentrations are measured in terms of their partial pressures, the activities for gases and vapours are given by p_e/p_s, where p_e is the effective vapour pressure and p_s the saturated vapour pressure.

The theory worked well with general anaesthetics. The compounds examined by Ferguson had widely different chemical structures, for example N_2O, $CHCl_3$, $(C_2H_5)_2O$, and potencies, the narcotic concentrations being in the range 0·5–100%. However, p_e/p_s remained reasonably constant. It also worked well with the *in vitro* antimicrobial activities of phenols. However, with homologous series, the thermodynamic activity was frequently found to increase with carbon number. This behaviour shows up as an increase in biological activity as the series is ascended, followed by a sudden abrupt fall, i.e. a cut-off point. An attractive explanation is that at the point at which biological activity falls, the biologically effective concentration is greater than the solubility of the homologue. A supersaturated solution would therefore be necessary to achieve an effect.

8.5.2 Hansch analysis

Hansch explained the cut-off point noted in certain homologous series, by suggesting that the equilibrium conditions required by Ferguson's theory were not established. The systems with which Ferguson's approach was successful (general anaesthetics, phenols) were ones in which equilibrium is quickly established. Two stages were postulated in drug action.

(a) A 'random walk' from the point of administration to the site of action. This will involve passage over a series of membranes, and is therefore related to partition coefficient. It is expressed mathematically as $f(P)$, a function of the partition coefficient.

(b) Attachment to the receptor site, expressed mathematically as k_x, which depends on
(i) the shape of the molecule, and hence on the stereochemistry of its substituent groups,
(ii) the electron density on the attachment groups.
The methods of quantifying the attachment to the receptor site have already been discussed in the form of electronic and steric substituent constants.

Biological activity will also be dependent on concentration C, so that the complete relationship is

$$R_b = f(P)k_x C. \tag{8.21}$$

$f(P)$ represents a mathematical function of partition coefficient.

The random walk involves passage across hydrophilic barriers and lipophilic barriers. Substances with low aqueous solubilities will be impeded (or, if the solubility is sufficiently low, prevented) from crossing hydrophilic barriers and there is a similar connection between low lipid solubilities and ease of crossing lipid barriers. Somewhere between the two extremes, there will be an optimum balance between hydrophilic and lipophilic properties, so that a plot of hydrophilic–lipophilic nature against the likelihood of the molecule completing the random walk would be expected to take the form shown in Fig. 8.4.

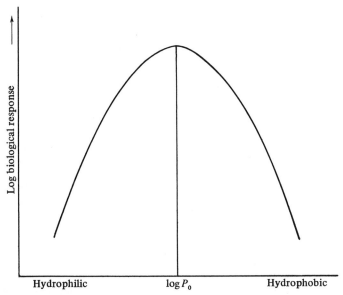

Fig. 8.4   Parabolic dependency of biological response on octanol–water partition coefficient.

Hydrophilic–lipophilic nature can be expressed in terms of a lipid–water partition coefficient, so that $\log P$, where P is the 1-octanol–water partition coefficient, can be used as the abcissa scale. The plot approximates to a parabola, for which the general equation is

$$y = a + bx + cx^2, \qquad (8.22)$$

and therefore the random walk can be expressed as

$$\log R_b = k_1 + k_2 \log P + k_3 (\log P)^2, \qquad (8.23)$$

or alternatively for a group of related compounds as

$$\log R_b = k_1 + k_2 \pi + k_3 \pi^2, \qquad (8.24)$$

where k_1, k_2 and k_3 represent the relevant coefficients. The choice of 1-octanol as non-aqueous solvent is completely arbitrary. Its use is justified by Equation 8.17, as would be the choice of any other solvent which is not appreciably miscible with water. The complete biological process can therefore be fitted into equations of the form

$$\log R_b = k_1 + k_2 \log P + k_3 (\log P)^2 + k_4 \sigma + k_5 E_s. \qquad (8.25)$$

The second and third terms on the right hand side represent the random walk, and the fourth and fifth terms, the electronic and steric factors governing the attachment to the receptor site. Any of the other electronic and steric parameters could be substituted for σ and E_s. Hydrophobic effects may also contribute to receptor binding as well as to transport.

The factors which control biological activity can be identified by fitting the experimental data into regression equations. Suppose 17 compounds were submitted to a pharamacological test, and that Equations 8.26–8.30 were obtained when the biological responses were correlated with various combinations of Hammett constants, Taft steric parameters and 1-octanol–water partition coefficients. The numbers in brackets in the equations, immediately preceding $\log P$, σ and E_s are the standard errors of the coefficients, and should be ignored until their significance is explained in Section 8.5.2(d).

$$
\begin{array}{llll}
 & n & s & r \\
\end{array}
$$

$$
\log R_b = 5{\cdot}816 + 2{\cdot}342(0{\cdot}105)\log P + 0{\cdot}731 \qquad 17 \quad 0{\cdot}126 \quad 0{\cdot}957 \qquad (8.26)
$$
$$
(0{\cdot}0413)(\log P)^2 + 0{\cdot}0361(0{\cdot}0190)\sigma
$$
$$
+ 0{\cdot}195(0{\cdot}1762)E_s.
$$
$$
F_{4,12} = 10{\cdot}9;\ F_{4,12}\alpha,\ 0{\cdot}05 = 3{\cdot}18;
$$
$$
F_{4,12}\alpha,\ 0{\cdot}001 = 9{\cdot}07.
$$

$$
\log R_b = 6{\cdot}303 + 3{\cdot}416(0{\cdot}0961)\log P + 0{\cdot}942 \qquad 17 \quad 0{\cdot}141 \quad 0{\cdot}938 \qquad (8.27)
$$
$$
(0{\cdot}0114)(\log P)^2.
$$

$$
\log R_b = 2{\cdot}416 + 4{\cdot}981(0{\cdot}994)\log P. \qquad\qquad 17 \quad 0{\cdot}314 \quad 0{\cdot}895 \qquad (8.28)
$$

$$
\log R_b = 2{\cdot}002 + 0{\cdot}0714(0{\cdot}0697)\sigma. \qquad\qquad 17 \quad 0{\cdot}280 \quad 0{\cdot}246 \qquad (8.29)
$$

$$
\log R_b = 5{\cdot}972 + 0{\cdot}0146(0{\cdot}0209)E_s. \qquad\qquad 17 \quad 0{\cdot}303 \quad 0{\cdot}209 \qquad (8.30)
$$

Much information can be derived from these equations, as explained below.

(a) Correlation coefficient   The correlation coefficient of Equation 8.26, because it is close to 1·00, indicates that the relationship represents the experimental results reasonably well, and explains $0{\cdot}957^2 \times 100 = 91{\cdot}6\%$ of the variation. However, if the steric and electronic parameters are omitted, to give Equation 8.27, the new equation still has a good correlation coefficient. It is doubtful whether the correlation coefficient of Equation 8.26 is significantly better, since Equation 8.26 contains two extra variables. If there were 17 variables for example, r would equal 1·000, irrespective of the data. The strongest evidence comes from the correlation coefficients of Equations 8.29 and 8.30, which are very low, indicating that neither σ nor E_s contributes to biological activity. Furthermore, the significantly lower correlation coefficient of Equation 8.28 in comparison with that of Equation 8.27 suggests that the relationship between $\log R_b$ and $\log P$ is binomial.

(b) Coefficients   The coefficients to the variables give support to the evidence given by the correlation coefficients. The coefficients of σ and E_s in Equation 8.29 and 8.30 are small, and in comparison with the intercepts and coefficients of $\log P$ and $(\log P)^2$, suggest that Equations 8.29 and 8.30 represent plots in which the regression lines would be almost parallel with the σ and E_s axes. The larger

coefficients in $\log P$ in Equations 8.26 and 8.27 support the conclusions given by the correlation coefficients, that biological activity is dependent on the hydrophilic–lipophilic nature of the compounds under test.

The lower coefficients in $(\log P)^2$ might give the impression that the squared term is not important, for example, the coefficient of $(\log P)^2$ in Equation 8.26 is only 0·731, in comparison with 2·342 with $\log P$. However, it must be remembered that $(\log P)^2$ is usually bigger than $\log P$. Thus if P is of the order of 1000, $(\log P)^2 = 3 \log P$, and one would anticipate a correspondingly larger coefficient for $\log P$, as is the case in Equations 8.26 and 8.27. A similar pitfall occurs when parameters of considerably different magnitude are compared, for example Equation 8.31, in which V is molar volume (molecular weight/density) in cm^3, suggests that molecular size is not a controlling factor. However, molar volumes are of the order of 10^2 cm^3, while σ has a value less than 1·00. In this light the coefficients are comparable.

$$\log R_b = 1\cdot313 + 2\cdot456\sigma + 0\cdot02456V. \tag{8.31}$$

(c) Standard deviation   The standard deviations support the conclusions given above.

(d) Standard error of the coefficient   The figures in brackets following the coefficients represent the standard error of the coefficient, which means that if the experiment is repeated the coefficient should lie between these limits, for example, the coefficient for σ in Equation 8.26 should be $0\cdot0361 \pm 0\cdot0190$, Obviously the higher the standard error, the less reliable is the coefficient, and the less is the likelihood that the variable it represents is related to the biological response.

The confidence in the term can be assessed by dividing the coefficient by the standard error. Thus for the second term on the right hand side of Equation 8.26, the ratio is $2\cdot342/0\cdot105 = 22\cdot3$, which, because it is a high number, suggests that the term is important. When there is doubt whether the ratio can be considered sufficiently high, it may be compared with the limiting Student's t value. Most statistical text books give tables of these. Some limiting t values are given in Table 8.5, and it can be seen that they depend on the probability level and on the number of degrees of freedom. The probability level is invariably 0·05 for QSAR. The number of degrees of freedom (ϕ) is $(n-m)$, where n is the number of sets of data (17 in the example) and m is the number of variables (5 in Equation 8.26). ϕ is therefore 12, which from Table 8.5 gives a t value of 2·179 for a probability of 0·05.

Table 8.5   Student t values

Degrees of freedom ϕ	Probability	
	0·05	0·01
12	2·179	3·055
13	2·160	3·012
14	2·145	2·977
15	2·132	2·947

This is less than 22·3, indicating that the term in log P is significant. The same test rejects the σ and E_s terms in Equation 8.26.

(e) F values For convenience, F distribution results are only given for Equation 8.26. The two numbers in the subscript (4 and 12) following the letter F are $m-$ and $n-m$, as defined in the previous paragraph, and the 10·9 following is the experimental F value which fits the data. The F value indicates the probability that the equation is a true relationship between the results, or merely coincidence. If the experimental figure exceeds the limiting value, the relationship is a true one, within the given probability level. Limiting F values can be obtained from statistical tables, from which Table 8.6 has been abstracted. The numbers running along the top represent the first number in the subscript following F, and those running down the left hand side, the second number in the subscript. Thus for Equation 8.26. $v_1 = 4$ and $v_2 = 12$ in Table 8.6, giving $F = 3·26$. Table 8.6 is

Table 8.6   0·05 Probability points of the *F*-distribution

$v_1 =$	1	2	3	4	5
$v_2 = $ 1	161·4	199·5	215·7	224·6	230·2
2	18·5	19·0	19·2	19·2	19·3
12	4·75	3·89	3·49	3·26	3·11
13	4·67	3·81	3·41	3·18	3·03
14	4·60	3·74	3·34	3·11	2·96

based on a probability of 0·05 (α,0·05 $= 3·26$), therefore there is less than a 1 in 20 chance that the relationship is a coincidence, and better than a 19 in 20 chance that the results are truly related in the manner given. $F = 10·9$ is obviously much greater than 3·26, and it would be of interest to know precisely how good it is. Consultation of a table for 0·001 points of the F distribution gives $F_{4,12}\alpha,0·001 = 9·63$, so that the probability of Equation 8.26 representing a chance relationship is less than 1 in 1000.

The mechanism of calculating the statistical parameters of regression, used above, are considered to be outside the scope of this book, which seeks to explain the interpretation, rather than preparation of QSAR data. The necessary arithmetic can be built into the computer program.

(f) Optimum partition coefficient   An advantage of the parabolic relationship between log R_b and log P is that the biological activity goes through a maximum corresponding to an optimum value of P, which is easily calculated, as shown in the following example.

The concentrations (HD_{50}) producing hypnosis in 50% of mice by a series of barbiturates **(8.10)** was found to be related to the octanol–water partition coefficient (P) by:

$$\log 1/HD_{50} = 2·501 + 0·864 \log P - 0·219(\log P)^2. \tag{8.32}$$

The change in log $1/HD_{50}$ with log P will be zero when the biological effect is at a maximum, therefore differentiation of log $1/HD_{50}$ with respect to log P, and placing the result equal to zero will give the optimum partition coefficient (P_0), i.e.

$$\frac{d(\log 1/HD_{50})}{d(\log P)} = 0 \cdot 864 - 0 \cdot 438 \log P = 0, \qquad (8.33)$$

therefore,

$$\log P_0 = 0 \cdot 864/0 \cdot 438 = 1 \cdot 97.$$

The optimum octanol–water partition coefficient therefore, is antilog $1 \cdot 97 = 93$.

Hansch and Fujita suggested that the Ferguson effect was represented by the left hand side of the parabola, where the plot was approximately rectilinear, and that the fall off in biological activity as the homologous series was ascended, was a consequence of the change in slope in the region of the maximum.

(g) Comparison of slopes and intercepts   If two sets of compounds are submitted to the same biological test, and yield rectilinear equations having similar slopes, the indication is that they have similar modes of action. Similarly, if two biological tests are applied to the same set of compounds, and are found to yield rectilinear equations with similar slopes, the tests are probably measuring the same response. The compounds giving the greater intercept in the first case are the more potent, and the test giving the greater intercept in the second is the more sensitive. Intercepts can only be compared when the equations have similar slopes.

8.5.3   Free–Wilson analysis

This is an alternative procedure to Hansch analysis, in that substituent constants based on biological activities are used, rather than physical properties. As one of their examples, Free and Wilson used the antimicrobial activities of some 6-deoxy tetracyclines (8.11) against *Staphylococcus aureus*. The compounds they examined

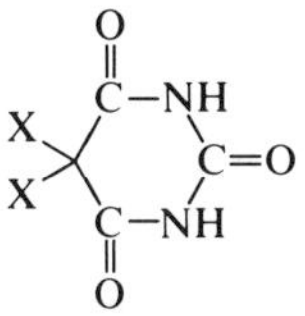

(8.10) 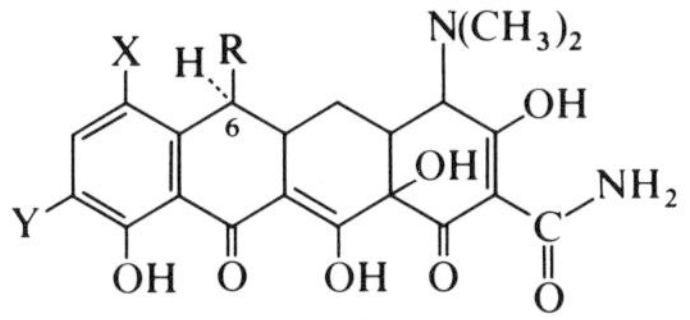   (8.11)

are summarized in Table 8.7, together with their antimicrobial activities. Biological activities can be expressed in terms of the constituent groups in the molecules, for example, Equation 8.34 can be used to describe the antimicrobial activity of the first compound in Table 8.7.

$$\mu + a[H] + b[NO_2] + c[NO_2] = 60. \qquad (8.34)$$

μ is the overall average antimicrobial activity for the whole series, and a, b and c the contributions of the groups —R, —X and —Y respectively. The identity of the

Table 8.7   Antimicrobial activities of 6-deoxytetracyclines against *Staphylococcus aureus*[a,b]

Compound	R H	R CH3	Supposed partial biological activity	X Br	X Cl	X NO2	Y NO2	Y NH2	Y CH3CONH	Experimental biological activity
I	√	—	5·9	—	—	√	√	—	—	60
II	√	—	2·2	—	√	—	√	—	—	21
III	√	—	1·4	√	√	—	—	—	—	15
IV	√	—	50·4	√	√	—	—	√	—	525
V	√	—	32·5	—	—	√	—	√	—	320
VI	—	√	29·2	—	—	—	√	√	—	275
VII	—	√	13·2	—	—	—	√	√	—	160
VIII	—	√	5·2	—	—	—	—	√	—	15
IX	—	√	14·6	√	—	—	—	√	√	140
X	—	√	6·0	√	—	—	—	—	√	75

[a] Spencer J. L., Hlavka J. J., Petisi J., Krazinski H. M. and Boothe J. R. (1963) 6-Deoxytetracyclines. V. 7,9-Disubstituted products. *J. Med. Chem.* **6,** 405–7.
[b] Free S. M. and Wilson J. W. (1964) A mathematical contribution to structure–activity studies. *J. Med. Chem.* **7,** 395–9.

terms prefixed by the letters a, b and c can best be explained if it is imagined that the contributions to the total antimicrobial activities made by the groups in position R can be determined experimentally, and are given in column 4 of Table 8.7. $a[H]$ will then be defined by Free–Wilson analysis as the mean of the figures in column 4 involving R = H, minus the mean of all the figures in column 4, i.e.

$$a[H] = \frac{(5\cdot9+2\cdot2+1\cdot4+50\cdot4+32\cdot5+29\cdot2)}{6} - \frac{160\cdot6}{10} = 4\cdot2. \qquad (8.35)$$

Similarly,

$$a[CH_3] = -6\cdot3.$$

Obviously it is not possible to determine partial biological activities of this sort, but the calculation given above serves to show that

$$6a[H]+4a[CH_3]=6\times4\cdot2-4\times6\cdot3=0, \quad \text{or} \quad 4a[CH_3] = 6a[H], \qquad (8.36)$$

and this relationship applies no matter what numbers are displayed in column 4 of Table 8.7. Similarly,

$$4b[Br]+2b[Cl]+4b[NO_2] = 0 \qquad (8.37)$$

and

$$3c[NO_2]+5c[NH_2]+2c[CH_3CONH] = 0. \qquad (8.38)$$

Table 8.7 yields 10 equations analogous to Equation 8.34, with 9 unknowns, μ, and the contributions of R = —H or —CH$_3$, X = —NO$_2$ or —Br or —Cl and Y = —NO$_2$ or —NH$_2$ or CH$_3$CONH—. μ can be equated to the mean experimental response, and three of the remainder can be eliminated through Equations 8.36–8.38, leaving five unknowns. Calculation of the best values to fit the 10 equations can be carried out using a computer, and gives the substituent constants shown in Table 8.8, from which the antimicrobial properties of new compounds can be predicted. Thus for example, if R = —CH$_3$, X = —Cl and Y = —NH$_2$, the predicted antimicrobial activity will be,

$$1606/10 - 112 + 84 + 123 = 256.$$

1606 is the total experimental biological activity.

Table 8.8 Calculated substituent constants for antimicrobial activities or 6-deoxytetracyclines against *Staphylococcus aureus*[a]

R		X		Y	
$a[H]$	75	$b[Cl]$	84	$c[NH_2]$	123
$a[CH_3]$	−112	$b[Br]$	−16	$c[CH_3CONH]$	18
		$b[NO_2]$	−26	$c[NO_2]$	−218

[a] Free S. M. and Wilson J. W. (1964) A mathematical contribution to structure–activity studies. *J. Med. Chem.* 7, 395–9.

The major weakness of this approach is that it can be used only for relationships which are rectilinear. The technique has been extended to parabolic relationships by introducing terms representing interactions between substituent groups, and by using equations involving both Hansch and Free–Wilson parameters. In recent investigations, activity has been replaced by log activity, which is related to free energy, and therefore additive. Another innovation is that the activity of the unsubstituted compound (in which the substituent is hydrogen) is used as standard, thereby eliminating the need for restricting equations.

8.6   SOME LIMITATIONS AND PITFALLS OF QSAR

The concept of quantitative structure–activity relationships has been continuously under fire since it was introduced, but most of the shots have been directed against the ways in which the technique has been used, rather than against the overall idea. QSAR is dependent on the accuracy of the biological results which, by their nature, are susceptible to considerable experimental error. There is therefore a built-in scatter which cannot be explained mathematically. The true relationships can be hidden within this scatter (or alternatively, false correlations can evolve) and their failure to fit as closely as is desirable is blamed on biological variation. Accurate biological data are essential for this technique.

The success of QSAR predictions is highly dependent on the number of results from which they are derived, the greater the number, the more reliable the correlation. Five biological results for every variable on the right hand side of the correlation equation are generally regarded as a minimum acceptable level, and the more this figure is exceeded, the better. Correlations derived from the first results emanating from a structure–activity exercise can change considerably when more results come to hand. Coefficients can change, and physico-chemical parameters which were originally considered significant can cease to be important. Many of the earlier publications on QSAR were based on too few results.

It has been suggested that the results generated in QSAR are by their nature co-related, and that random biological responses can be correlated with physico-chemical parameters. Bias of this sort can be demonstrated, but the chance of coincidental relationships with correlation coefficients greater than 0·9 is highly improbable. Distributions consisting of two clusters of results, as exemplified by Fig. 8.5, can yield good linear correlation coefficients, and yet have no predictive value.

In much of the early QSAR work, biological data were correlated successively to each, and combinations of a range of physical parameters, on a trial and error basis. A theory of biological action was then evolved, fitting the parameters which gave the best correlation. Whilst this approach can be justified in separating the influences of steric, electronic and distribution effects, its use in comparing parameters depending on the same basic property usually stretches the technique too far. Thus dipole moments have been successfully correlated with biological results which could not be related to Hammett σ constants. In such situations it

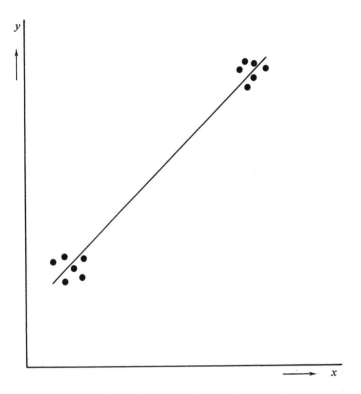

Fig. 8.5   Distribution consisting of two clusters.

would be tempting to derive a theory in which dipole moment is a unique factor governing biological activity. However, Hammett constants and dipole moments are rectilinearly related to each other. Differentiation between the two properties was therefore not permissible. Similarly, several workers have found that one electronic parameter has fitted their data, and others did not. Forty-one different electronic parameters have been listed, and all can be expressed as linear parameters of an inductive substituent constant $\mathscr{F}$ and a resonance substituent constant $\mathscr{R}$. Even σ and π have been shown to be related. Strictly speaking therefore, expressions of the form shown in Equation 8.39 should be employed in seeking quantitative structure–activity relationships, but the procedure is impracticable, even if only for the single consideration that a prohibitively large number of results would be required to make the expression meaningful.

$$\log 1/C = k_1\pi^2 + k_2\pi + k_3\sigma + k_4E_s + k_5\pi\sigma + k_6\pi E_s + k_7\sigma E_s + k_8\pi\sigma E_s + k_9. \quad (8.39)$$

Interrelationships between parameters must be eliminated before a correlation is accepted. For example, before an expression of the form of Equation 8.40 can be considered valid, linear regressions should be carried out between each pair of

$$\log 1/C = k_1\pi + k_2\mathscr{R} + k_3\mathscr{F} + k_4E_s \quad (8.40)$$

parameters. This is best expressed in the form of a correlation matrix, for example for Equation 8.40, the squared correlation matrix given below could apply.

	π	$\mathscr{R}$	$\mathscr{F}$	E_s
π	1·00	0·84	0·08	0·03
$\mathscr{R}$		1·00	0·39	0·17
$\mathscr{F}$			1.00	0·20
E_s				1·00

The figures in the matrix represent the squares of the correlation coefficients of the various linear correlation equations. Thus, the regression equation of the form $\pi = k_2\mathscr{R}$ has a correlation coefficient of $\sqrt{0·84}$. There is no objection to using unsquared coefficients in the matrix, but the squared form is more convenient because the reader can see the extent of the variation immediately. Inspection of the matrix indicates that π and $\mathscr{R}$ are co-linear, and that either π or $\mathscr{R}$ is not required.

A correlation matrix is specific to the chemical groups and physical parameters chosen for its construction, and some combinations of results give rise to greater co-linearity than others. An obvious example would be a correlation matrix for an homologous series of compounds, which would be expected to show significant co-linearity between distribution coefficient and steric parameters. Compounds used in a QSAR exercise can be selected by a process of trial and error, involving construction of numerous correlation matrices, but the procedure is time consuming and inefficient. Cluster analysis is a mathematical procedure for allocating substituents to cluster sets. The substitutents within a given set are co-linear, but co-linearity between sets is minimal. The result of a cluster analysis is given in Table 8.9. It tells us that in planning a QSAR exercise, one should not choose more than one substituent from each set. It is obvious, for example, that molar volume (a steric parameter) in set 3 will increase from left to right, as also will log octanol–water distribution coefficients. Similarly, co-linearity between σ and steric constants for set 1 would be anticipated. The substituents in Table 8.9 were chosen to illustrate the procedure by using sets whose behaviour can be predicted. Less

Table 8.9   A model cluster set table

Cluster set	Substituents
1	—F, —Cl, —Br, —I
2	—NO$_2$, —NO, —CN
3	—H, —CH$_3$, —C$_2$H$_5$, —C$_3$H$_7$
4	—OH, —NH$_2$
5	—CH$_2$OH, —C$_2$H$_4$COOH, —C$_3$H$_6$COOH
6	—NHCONH$_2$, —NHCOCH$_3$
7	—CONH$_2$, —CONHC$_2$H$_5$, —COOH
8	—OCH$_3$, —OC$_2$H$_5$, —OC$_3$H$_7$

Further cluster sets can be found in:
Hansch C. and Leo A. (1979) *Substituent Constants for Correlation Analysis in Chemistry and Biology*. New York, John Wiley.

obvious interrelationships, and larger collections of substituents demand involved mathematical procedures. More comprehensive cluster set tables can be found in the literature.

Readers of communications involving QSAR should guard against the temptation to overestimate the precision of comparisons between experimental and predicted results. It is traditional to compare log values of experimental and predicted results, a practice which gives greater credibility to relationships than they really merit. As an example, experimental and predicted results of 1·98 and 2·28 could be cited as evidence of a good correlation. Although this conclusion may well be justified within the context of the particular situation, conversion to the real values, 95 and 191 (antilog 1·98 and antilog 2·28), brings the reader down to bare reality.

8.7 SUMMARY

Quantitative structure–activity relationships can be said to have brought drug design into the computer age. It has introduced a quantitative element into a subject which had hitherto been entirely qualitative. The medicinal chemists of old used their instinct and experience to predict conformational changes which should bring about increased biological activity, but had little idea of the magnitude of those changes. QSAR requires less instinct and experience, and also estimates the extent of the biological activity. Hansch and Free–Wilson analysis are lead-optimizing techniques. This means that it is necessary to begin with a 'lead' compound, having the basic pharmacological properties; analogues are prepared and tested, and the resultant data used to plan new compounds which will have enhanced biological activity. The technique demands that compounds be selected in a highly rational manner, with a systematic and stepwise progression throughout. Because of this stringent approach, much of the early structure–activity data in the literature is not adaptable to QSAR. These techniques are also self-limiting; as more results become available, the picture becomes clearer, but the number of possible new compounds becomes more restricted.

Powerful new mathematical techniques in which the computer is made to recognize molecular structures, are being extended to drug design, and could move the concept of QSAR from lead-optimizing to lead-generating.

FURTHER READING

1. Buisman J. A. K. (1977) *Biological Activity and Chemical Structure*. Amsterdam, Elsevier.
2. Hansch C. and Leo A. (1979) *Substituent Constants for Correlation Analysis in Chemistry and Biology*. New York, Wiley.
3. James K. C. (1974) Linear Free Energy Relationships and Biological Action. In: Ellis G. P. and West G. B. (ed.) *Progress in Medicinal Chemistry*, Vol. 10. Amsterdam, North-Holland Publishing, pp. 205–43.
4. Kier L. B. and Hall L. H. (1976) *Molecular Connectivity in Chemistry and Drug Research*. London, Academic Press.
5. Tute M. S. (1971) Principles and practice of Hansch analysis: a guide to structure–activity correlation for the medicinal chemist. In: Harper N. J. and Simmonds A. B. (ed.) *Advances in Drug Research*, Vol. 6. London, Academic Press, pp. 1–77.
6. Wells P. R. (1968) *Linear Free Energy Relationships*. London, Academic Press.

Chapter 9

Design of antimicrobial chemotherapeutic agents

Design of antimicrobial chemotherapeutic agents

9.1 INTRODUCTION

The design of a new chemotherapeutic agent, suitable for clinical use in the treatment of human infections, must take into account two aspects above all others. First, the drug must possess high antimicrobial activity and secondly it must be non-toxic to human tissues. Paul Ehrlich's early concept of a selectively toxic 'magic bullet' is thus just as true in the modern world as when it was first propounded. A host of antimicrobial agents has been examined and many shown to be effective inhibitors of micro-organisms *in vitro*; unfortunately, several of these have been found to be harmful to human tissues and consequently have no useful role to play in chemotherapy. This chapter will thus concentrate on several of those chemotherapeutic agents that have proved their worth when employed internally (usually orally or parenterally). Antimicrobial compounds that are used for their disinfectant, antiseptic or preservative qualities will not be dealt with here.

Two important properties of any chemotherapeutic agent were mentioned briefly above. Any drug must ideally have a broad spectrum of activity, with a rapid bactericidal action. Some bacteria produce enzymes that can inactivate or modify antibiotics, and insusceptibility of a drug to such degradation or modification could result in its playing an important part in therapy. Likewise, some bacteria possess an outer membrane that acts as a permeability barrier to the entry of some, but not all, antibiotics. Drugs that can readily penetrate this barrier might again be expected to be of possible clinical importance. These two aspects are considered in greater detail later (Sections 9.4.1 and 9.4.2).

In addition to being non-toxic, an antibiotic should not cause any hypersensitive reactions (such as those induced in a minority of patients by the penicillins and, to a lesser extent, the cephalosporins). It should, however, be readily absorbed to give high blood and tissue levels and it should be stable to gastric acid. Binding to serum proteins should be of a low order. In urinary infections, high urine levels are desirable but some antibiotics are excreted so rapidly that, on occasion, it may be necessary to delay the rate of excretion. These and other pharmacological properties are considered further where appropriate.

Finally, the design of any chemotherapeutic agent must involve a consideration of its chemical and physical properties, since these will be of paramount importance to the pharmacist responsible for formulating a suitable product. Such properties include its aqueous solubility, and its stability in solution at different pHs and temperatures. These aspects are considered to be outside the scope of the present chapter.

9.2 PRODUCTION OF CHEMOTHERAPEUTIC AGENTS

The demonstration in the early 1920s that lysozyme possessed antibacterial activity, the accidental discovery of 'penicillin' by Fleming in the late 1920s and the finding that the azo dye, prontosil, owed its antibacterial properties to the release *in vivo* of sulphanilamide, all stimulated research towards the development of chemotherapeutic agents.

Fleming, in 1929, published the results of his chance finding that a *Penicillium* mould caused lysis of staphylococcal colonies on an agar plate. He also showed that the filtrate of a culture of the mould, growing in a liquid medium, possessed significant activity against Gram-positive bacteria and Gram-negative cocci, although most other types of Gram-negative organisms were resistant. In retrospect, it was indeed fortunate that the original plates of staphylococci did not contain organisms that produced an inactivating enzyme (β-lactamase: Section 9.4.1) otherwise the mould would not have shown any activity and could well have been discarded! It is, of course, highly unlikely with today's knowledge and techniques that benzylpenicillin (the product obtained from the *Penicillium* mould) would have been lost to mankind, but rather that its introduction into medicine would have been delayed.

It is now known that benzylpenicillin is thermolabile. At the time of Fleming's finding, however, great difficulty was experienced in extracting the antibiotic from the culture medium, as this property was not appreciated. Later studies by Florey, Chain and their colleagues at Oxford University, and in the United States, used a cold solvent extraction method that succeeded in extracting and purifying the elusive active principle. Extensive research on composition of culture media and on induction of mutants of the mould resulted in conditions that gave enhanced antibiotic yields.

These facts are all relevant to the subsequent development of antibiotics, since the commercial production of benzylpenicillin stimulated world-wide efforts into examining soil samples with a view to obtaining other antibiotics. Studies at Rutgers (by Waksman and his colleagues) and elsewhere were responsible for the development of streptomycin, the tetracyclines and chloramphenicol. These and many other antibiotics – some of them clinically useful – were obtained from *Streptomyces* species, which comprise the most prolific source of antibiotics. In the 1950s, a *Cephalosporium* mould isolated off the coast of Sardinia was found to produce significant antibiotic activity and was sent to Oxford University where, as a result of the efforts of Abraham and his colleagues, the birth of the cephalosporins resulted.

Important though these early findings are, they do not in themselves present any coherent pattern in the deliberate design of an antibiotic. This development had to await further discoveries in antibiotic production and an improved knowledge of mechanism of action, bacterial resistance and pharmacokinetics. Towards the end of the 1950s Chain, in collaboration with scientists at Beecham Research Laboratories, observed the production of 6-aminopenicillanic acid (6-APA **(9.1)**) in media in which *Penicillium chrysogenum* was growing when phenylacetic acid

($C_6H_5 \cdot CH_2 \cdot COOH$; phenylethanoic acid) was omitted. Phenylacetic acid is the precursor of the side-chain of benzylpenicillin ((9.2) R = $C_6H_5CH_2CO$) and 6-APA is the nucleus to which a side-chain is attached. This finding has had far-reaching developments since it has become the starting point in the deliberate

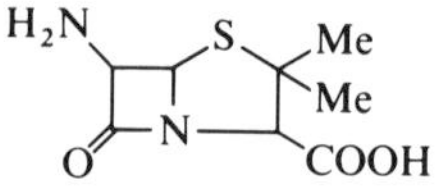

6-APA
(9.1)

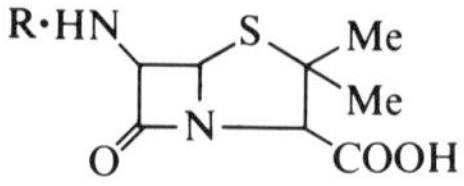

'General structure'
of penicillins
(In benzylpenicillin, R is
$C_6H_5 \cdot CH_2 \cdot CO$—)
(9.2)

design and synthesis of a family of penicilllins having different or improved properties from existing members. This aspect is considered in more detail in Section 9.5.1. It must be added that an early procedure in designing penicillins was to add various compounds to the fermentation broth to see whether different penicillins could be produced.

6-APA is a naturally occurring antibiotic. In contrast, the nucleus (7-aminocephalosporanic acid, 7-ACA (9.3)) of the cephalosporin group does not

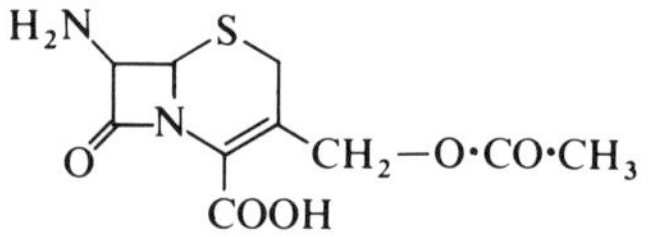

7-ACA
(9.3)

occur naturally. Studies at Oxford revealed that *C. acremonium* produced more than one antibiotic: 'cephalosporin P' (active against Gram-positive bacteria, but subsequently shown not to be a cephalosporin) and 'cephalosporin N' (with activity against Gram-negative bacteria and later found to be a penicillin). Further studies disclosed that 'cephalosporin N' was actually contaminated with a true cephalosporin, cephalosporin C (9.4) which showed a high degree of stability to

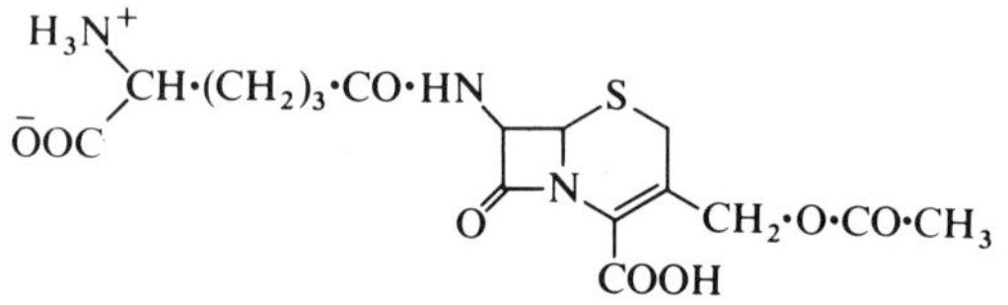

Cephalosporin C
(9.4)

staphylococcal β-lactamase. Cephalosporin C is converted to 7-ACA by appropriate chemical means. Like 6-APA, 7-ACA can be considered as being the starting point in the development of newer antibiotics. The cephalosporins are discussed in Section 9.5.2.

The production of semisynthetic β-lactam antibiotics has formed part of an exciting era in chemotherapy. In the meantime, other semisynthetic antibiotics, e.g. some members of the tetracyclines, have been described and some antibiotics, notably chloramphenicol, have been totally synthesized chemically. Contrary to earlier predictions, new naturally occurring β-lactam antibiotics continue to be found, notably: important β-lactamase inhibitors (Section 9.5.4) such as clavulanic acid and olivanic acids; thienamycin, one of the broadest spectrum antibiotics yet reported; nocardicins; and monobactams. These are considered later in Section 9.5.

9.3   MECHANISM OF ACTION OF CHEMOTHERAPEUTIC AGENTS

The great majority of studies of the mechanism of action of chemotherapeutic agents have involved investigations of individual compounds or of drugs within a particular group. A considerable amount of information is now available (Table 9.1) and will be summarized in this section, since in the space available only a bare

Table 9.1   Mechanism of action of antibacterial agents

Effect	Example(s)	Comments
Inhibition of cell wall synthesis	D-cycloserine	Competitive inhibition of alanine racemase and synthetase
	β-lactams	Inhibition of transpeptidases Binding to PBP1: cephaloridine, cefoxitin PBP2: mecillinam PBP3: cefotaxime, cephalexin
Effect on the cytoplasmic membrane	Polymixins	Affect outer membrane of Gram-negative bacteria also
	Ionophores	Specific cation conductors
	Polyenic antibiotics	Bind to membrane sterols in fungi (bacteria unaffected)
Inhibition of protein synthesis	Streptomycin	Inhibits initiation stage
	Tetracyclines	Inhibits binding of aminoacyl-tRNA to 30S ribosomal unit
	Chloramphenicol	Inhibits peptidyl transferase
	Erythromycin Puromycin	Inhibits translocation
Inhibition of RNA synthesis	Actinomycin D	Binds to double stranded DNA
	Rifampicin	Inhibits RNA polymerase
Inhibition of DNA synthesis	Mitomycin C[a]	Covalent linking to DNA
	Nalidixic acid	Effect on DNA gyrase
	Novobiocin	Effect on DNA gyrase
Inhibition of tetra-hydrofolate synthesis	Sulphonamides	Competitive inhibitors of dihydropteroate synthetase (see text also)
	Trimethoprim	Inhibits dihydrofolate reductase

[a] Highly toxic agent formerly used in the treatment of malignant conditions.

outline can be presented. Where possible, ways in which this knowledge can be used to further the design of new antibiotics will be discussed.

9.3.1   Inhibitors of cell wall synthesis

The bacterial cell wall is a complex structure (*see also* Section 9.4.2 and Fig. 9.1). Differences occur between walls of Gram-positive and Gram-negative bacteria,

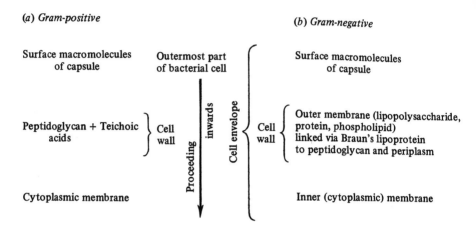

Fig. 9.1   Outer layers of (*a*) Gram-positive (*b*) Gram-negative bacteria.

but they all contain a basal peptidoglycan (murein, mucopeptide). This consists of amino sugars such as *N*-acetylglucosamine (GlcNAc) and *N*-acetylmuramic acid (MurNAc) to which are attached amino acids, some in the unnatural D-configuration. In brief, peptidoglycan synthesis involves the stepwise addition of amino acids to MurNAc, the linking to GlcNAc to form a linear polymer and finally a cross-linking (transpeptidation, via a transpeptidase) of the linear polymers to form a rigid structure, in which the degree of cross-linking varies. A simplified example of cross-linked peptidoglycan is given in Fig 9.2(*a*). D-cycloserine (**9.5**), a structural analogue of D-alanine (**9.6**) inhibits two enzymes (a racemase and a synthetase) involved in the synthesis of a D-alanyl-D-alanine dipeptide. β-lactam antibiotics inhibit the cross-linking (transpeptidation) reaction (*see* Fig. 9.2(*b*)).

Considerable progress has been made recently in understanding the action of β-lactam antibiotics at the molecular level. Bacterial cell membranes (inner membranes) contain several proteins, known as penicillin binding proteins (PBPs) with which β-lactam antibiotics may combine. Most of these antibiotics bind to only one or two PBPs and, very importantly, the morphological effects induced by various β-lactams is determined by the PBP to which they bind predominantly (examples are provided in Table 9.1). PBPs 1A, 1B, 2 and 3 appear to be the most important, since binding to PBPs 4, 5 and 6 has no adverse effect on the cells. Thus,

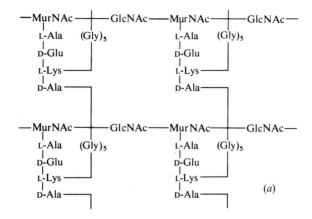

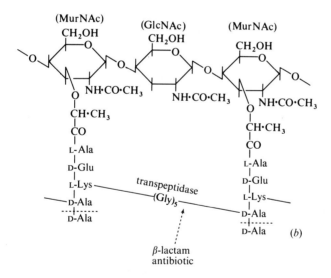

Fig. 9.2   Cross-linked peptidoglycan (*a*) and role of transpeptidase (*b*) in *Staphylococcus aureus*. MurNAc, N-acetylmuramic acid; GlcNAc, N-acetylglucosamine; AGLA...respectively L-alanine, D-glutamine, L-lysine, D-alanine; (Gly)₅...5 molecules of glycine.

a future possibility might well be to design a combination of two β-lactam antibiotics which have different PBP specificity in order to achieve a synergistic

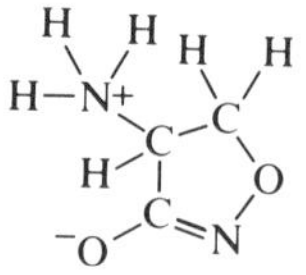

D-Cycloserine
(9.5)

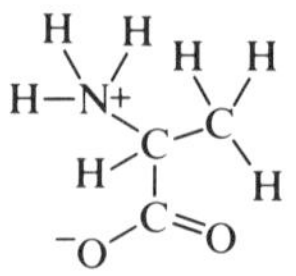

D-Alanine
(9.6)

result. β-lactams that bind to PBP1 induce rapid cell lysis, whereas those binding predominantly to PBP3 induce filamentation.

9.3.2   Membrane-active agents

The term 'membrane-active agent' is generally taken to mean an agent that affects the cytoplasmic membrane in micro-organisms. Gram-negative bacteria, however, also possess an outer membrane (Section 9.4.2) which may act as a penetration barrier to some drugs. The polymyxins, for example, cause the leakage of intracellular constituents by damaging the cytoplasmic membrane of Gram-negative bacteria, but they also disrupt the outer membrane lipopolysaccharide. They are highly toxic to mammalian cells.

Polyenic antibiotics combine with sterols in the cytoplasmic membrane of yeasts, fungi and mammalian cells. However, nystatin and amphotericin B have some selective action against fungi because they exhibit a greater binding to ergosterol than to cholesterol (Section 9.7.1).

Ionophoric drugs facilitate the passage of specific inorganic cations across the cytoplasmic membrane of Gram-positive bacteria, e.g. valinomycin and monactin are K^+-conducting ionophores. Unfortunately, they show a lack of specific toxicity, as they exert the same effect on mammalian membranes also.

9.3.3   Inhibitors of protein synthesis

Bacterial ribosomes have different characteristics (sedimentation coefficient of 70, i.e. are 70S, with 50S and 30S subunits) from those of mammalian ribosomes (80S, with 60S and 40S subunits). Most antibacterial antibiotics that are clinically important inhibitors of protein synthesis have a preferential effect on 70S ribosomes. For example, chloramphenicol affects 70S ribosomes, but not 80S. In contrast, the tetracyclines inhibit protein synthesis on isolated 70S and 80S ribosomes. The reason for their selective inhibition of bacterial protein synthesis *in vivo* resides in the energy-dependent active transport mechanism, present in bacterial but not mammalian cells, that transports these antibacterial agents into bacteria.

The tetracyclines bind to the 30S subunit, as does streptomycin. In contrast, erythromycin binds entirely to the 50S subunit.

Bacterial protein synthesis, i.e. peptide chain extension, is carried out on 70S ribosomes. In brief, an amino acid, activated and attached to its transfer RNA (tRNA) binds to the acceptor site of the ribosome. The peptide in the donor site is transferred, as a result of peptidyl transferase, to the new amino acid at the acceptor site. Subsequently, translocation of the extended peptide from the acceptor site to the donor site takes place with loss of the preceding tRNA and movement of the ribosome relative to messenger RNA (mRNA) which specifies the next amino acid.

The action of some antibiotics is shown in Table 9.1.

One antibiotic, puromycin (9.7), has a similar structure to the terminal aminoacyl adenosine grouping (9.8) of tRNA (*see also* Section 5.2.2.2). Puromycin

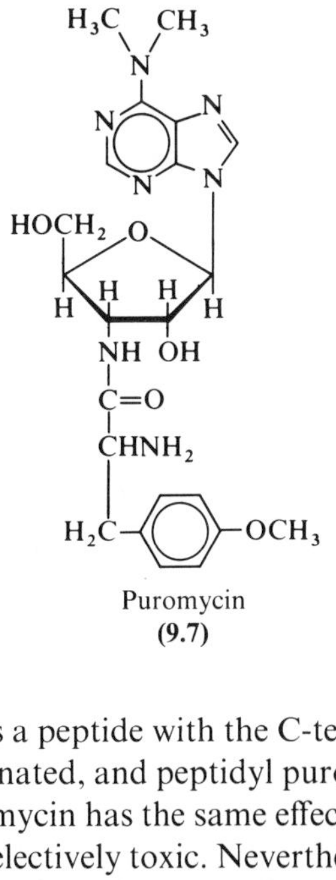

Puromycin
(9.7)

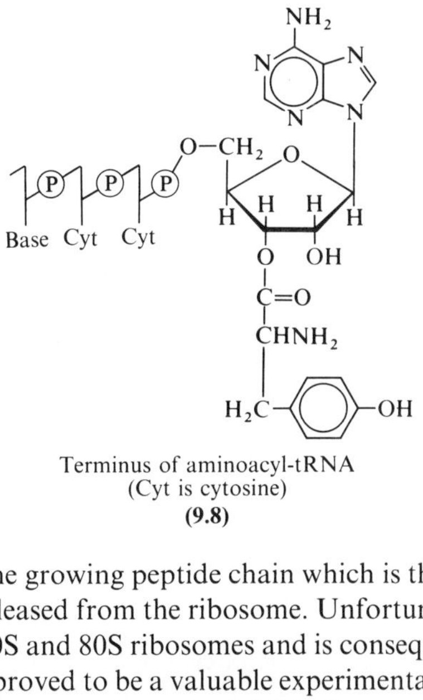

Terminus of aminoacyl-tRNA
(Cyt is cytosine)
(9.8)

forms a peptide with the C-terminus of the growing peptide chain which is thereby terminated, and peptidyl puromycin is released from the ribosome. Unfortunately, puromycin has the same effect on both 70S and 80S ribosomes and is consequently not selectively toxic. Nevertheless, it has proved to be a valuable experimental tool, since other inhibitors of protein synthesis may or may not inhibit the puromycin reaction, depending on whether they act on the 50S ribosomal subunit or the 30S subunit, respectively.

9.3.4 Inhibitors of nucleic acid syntheses

Inhibitors of nucleic acid syntheses fall into two main categories: (*a*) those that inhibit the synthesis of purine and pyrimidine nucleotides, e.g. azaserine, a glutamine analogue, although this is not selectively toxic as it is also harmful to mammalian cells; (*b*) those that inhibit synthesis at the polymerization level. This involves the appropriate polymerase, with nucleic acid as a template, and is the stage where condensation of nucleoside triphosphates into a polynucleotide chain, with joining by 3′,5′-phosphodiester linkages, takes place.

Some drugs are intercalating agents (e.g. acridines: *see* Section 3.5.1) and inhibit DNA synthesis and DNA-dependent RNA synthesis in whole cells and in cell-free systems. Another intercalating agent, actinomycin D, has a selective action on RNA synthesis. Mitomycin C cross-links to DNA but, like actinomycin D, is also toxic to mammalian cells (*see* also Section 3.5.3).

An important antimicrobial agent, nalidixic acid (9.9) has a selective action on

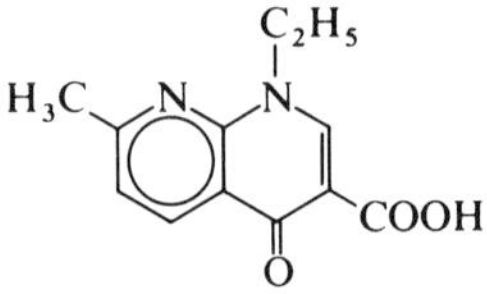

Nalidixic acid
(9.9)

DNA synthesis by acting on the enzyme DNA gyrase, which is found in prokaryotic but not eukaryotic cells. Rifampicin (9.10), a useful antitubercular

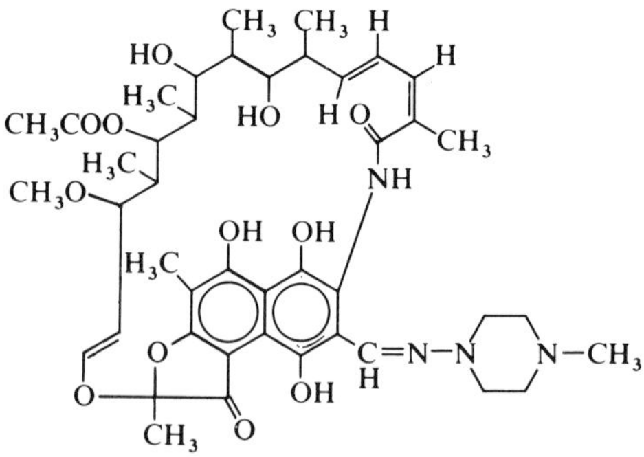

Rifampicin
(9.10)

antibiotic and a member of the rifamycin group, does not interact with DNA but binds to and inhibits DNA-dependent RNA polymerase with a consequent specific action on RNA synthesis. RNA polymerase from rifampicin-resistant bacteria is not inhibited by the drug. Rifampicin does not bind to or inhibit mammalian RNA polymerase.

Other drugs inhibit nucleic acid synthesis by being incorporated into the DNA template. These are considered more fully in Section 9.8.

9.3.5 Antibacterial folate inhibitors

Sulphonamides (9.11) act by competitively inhibiting dihydropteroate synthetase, an enzyme involved in the production from *p*-aminobenzoate (PAB (9.12)) of dihydropteroate (9.13) during dihydrofolate (9.14) biosynthesis. This inhibitory effect is reversed by excess PAB. It has also been found that these drugs can replace

PAB as a substrate, so that they become incorporated in a false dihydropteroate or dihydrofolate (*see also* Sections 4.3.1.1 and 4.3.1.2).

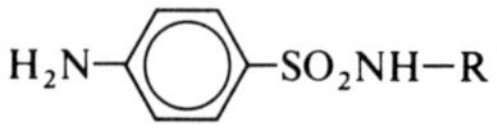

General structure of
sulphonamides
(9.11)

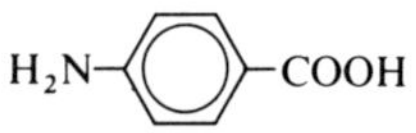

p-Aminobenzoic acid
(9.12)

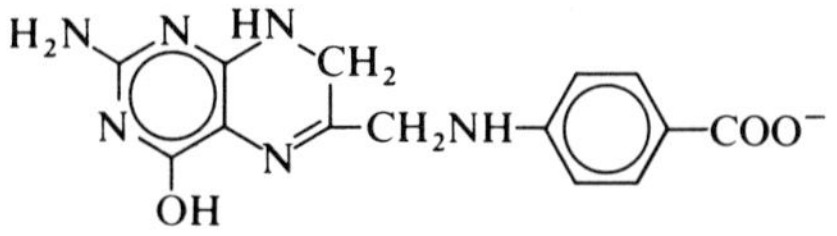

Dihydropteroate
(9.13)

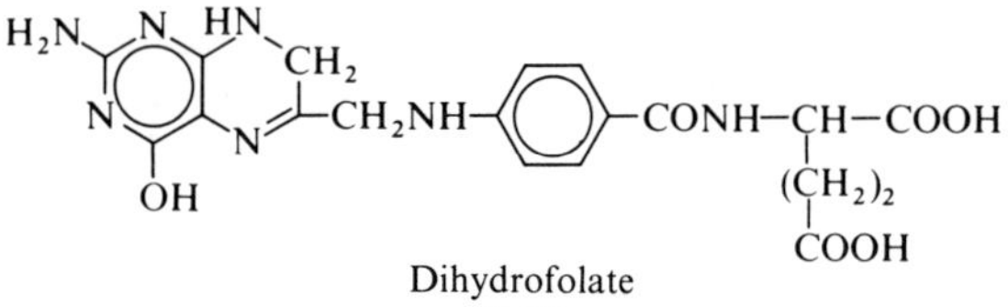

Dihydrofolate
(9.14)

Diaminopyrimidines structurally dissimilar from folic acid have been known for some time to be antagonists of folic acid. The best known example, trimethoprim **(9.15)** is a potent inhibitor of dihydrofolate reductase (DHFR, the enzyme responsible for converting dihydrofolate **(9.14)** to tetrahydrofolate **(9.16)**) in

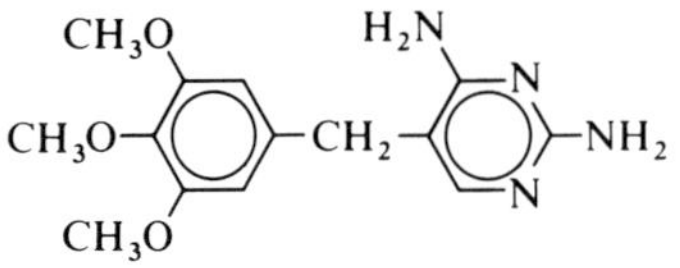

Trimethoprim
(9.15)

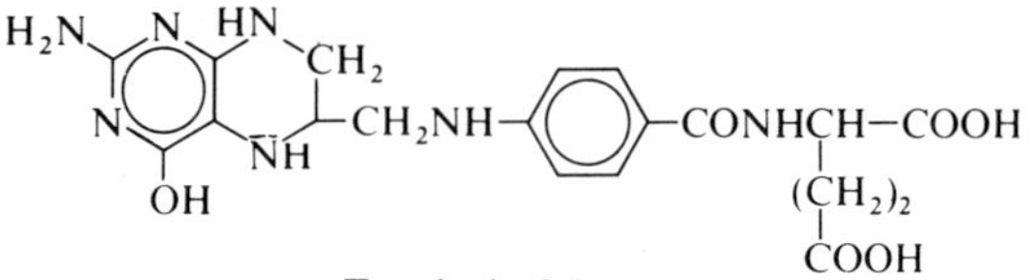

Tetrahydrofolate
(9.16)

Escherichia coli but not in man. Other antifolate inhibitors of DHFR are described later in Table 9.5 (*see* p. 274), from which it can be seen that tetroxoprim **(9.17)** also possesses significant antibacterial activity, whereas pyrimethamine is an antimalarial agent (*see* also Section 4.3.2.2) and methotrexate is used in cancer chemotherapy (*see* also Section 4.3.2.1).

Since sulphonamides and trimethoprim appear to inhibit sequential stages in

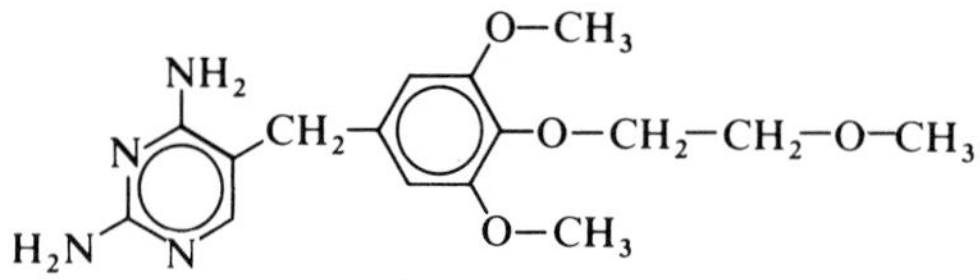

Tetroxoprim
(9.17)

tetrahydrofolate synthesis, it was a logical step to use a combination of an appropriate sulphonamide (sulphamethoxazole **(9.18)**)) with trimethroprim as an

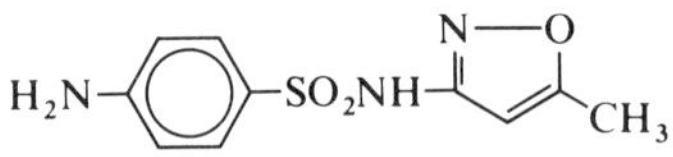

$$H_2N-\bigcirc-SO_2NH-\underset{\underset{CH_3}{\overset{N\!-\!O}{\diagdown}}}{\diagup}$$

Sulphamethoxazole
(9.18)

antibacterial mixture. Such a combination undoubtedly shows synergism *in vitro* but not necessarily *in vivo*. This aspect is discussed more fully in Section 9.6.5.

9.3.6   Conclusions and comments

There is no doubt that the mechanism of action of antibiotics is now being understood at the molecular level. This is most desirable, since such drugs have proved to be very important laboratory tools in elucidating cellular reactions and furthermore studies of this nature must increasingly lead to the development of selectively toxic chemotherapeutic agents, although progress in this area to date has been somewhat disappointing.

9.4   BACTERIAL RESISTANCE TO CHEMOTHERAPEUTIC AGENTS

The resistance of bacteria to chemotherapeutic agents has long posed a problem and will continue to do so for the foreseeable future. Much is now known about the mechanisms of bacterial resistance, and this section will provide a summary of the available information, because the design of new antibiotics is, to a considerable extent, linked to methods of combatting this problem.

Bacterial resistance can arise in several different ways (Table 9.2), e.g. by

Table 9.2   Mechanisms of bacterial resistance to antibiotics

Mechanism of resistance	Example(s)
Enzymatic inactivation	Some β-lactam antibiotics
	Chloramphenicol
Enzymatic modification	Some aminoglycoside antibiotics
Permeability barrier	Some β-lactam antibiotics
	Tetracyclines
	High molecular weight antibiotics
Tolerance	β-lactam antibiotics
Decreased affinity of target enzyme	β-lactam antibiotics
	Trimethoprim[a]
	Sulphonamides[b]
Alteration in binding site	Streptomycin[c]
	Erythromycin[d]

[a] Altered dihydrofolate reductase.
[b] Altered dihydropteroate synthetase.
[c] Altered 30S ribosomal subunit.
[d] Altered 50S ribosomal subunit.

mutation and indirect selection, by adaptation, by the presence of antibiotic-destroying or -modifying enzymes, by an outer membrane permeability barrier (predominantly in Gram-negative bacilli), by changes in the target site or target enzyme and by tolerance to β-lactam antibiotics (as a result of autolytic-deficient bacterial strains). It is not possible to discuss all of these in this chapter and consequently attention will be focussed on the role of bacterial enzymes and on impermeability mechanisms. These are particularly relevant to the design of various groups of antibacterial agents as depicted in Sections 9.5 and 9.6. It must also be noted (see later in this Section) that some bacteria possess the ability to transfer resistance.

9.4.1   Enzyme-mediated resistance

Resistance of bacteria to β-lactam antibiotics may be associated with enzymes termed β-lactamases. Some bacteria are capable of producing enzymes that modify streptomycin or other aminoglycoside antibiotics. A description, therefore, of the various types of enzymes is important in understanding the development and design of antibiotics.

9.4.1.1 β-lactamases

β-lactamases occur widely in nature. They are produced by various Gram-positive and Gram-negative bacteria. In Gram-positive organisms such as staphylococci and *Bacillus* species, β-lactamase is an inducible enzyme, with low concentrations of various β-lactam antibiotics acting as appropriate inducers, and is released extracellularly. In contrast, β-lactamases of Gram-negative bacteria are usually constitutive, but are induced by high concentrations of appropriate inducing agents in organisms such as *Pseudomonas aeruginosa* and *Enterobacter cloacae*. The β-lactamases of Gram-negative bacteria are intracellular, being located in the periplasm situated between the inner and outer membranes, and are less potent enzymes than those produced by Gram-positive bacteria. They may be chromosomally- or plasmid-mediated (Section 9.4.3).

The effects of β-lactamases generally on susceptible penicillins and cephalosporins are shown in Figs. 9.3 and 9.4, respectively. Susceptible penicillins are converted to the corresponding penicilloic acid (9.19) which is inactive; this results from an opening of the β-lactam ring (see Fig. 9.3). The situation with susceptible

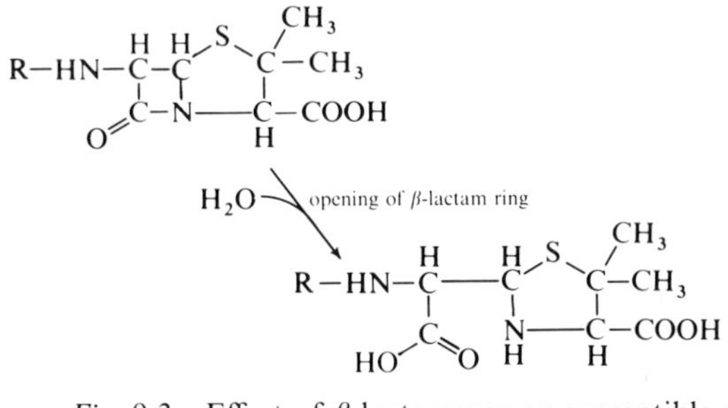

Fig. 9.3   Effect of β-lactamases on susceptible penicillins.

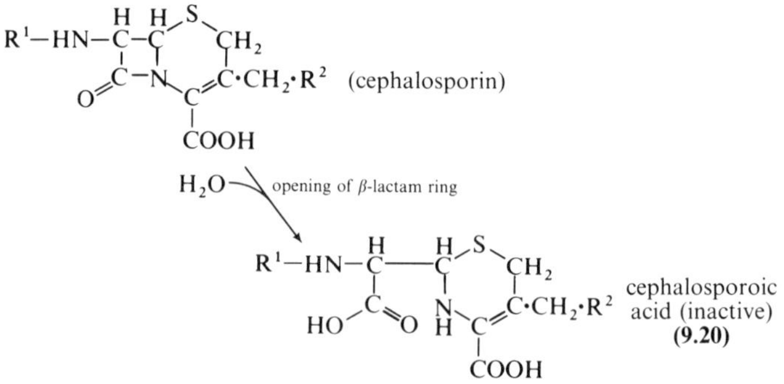

With expulsion of R^2 (except in Cephalexin, where $R^2 = H$) and fragmentation of structure

Fig. 9.4 Effect of β-lactamases on susceptible cephalosporins.

cephalosporins is more complex. Opening of the β-lactam ring again occurs **(9.20)** and this is accompanied by expulsion of the group at R^2 (except in cephalexin, where R^2 is H). The molecule finally breaks up into fragments (*see* Fig. 9.4).

Extensive studies have shown that several different types of β-lactamases exist among Gram-negative bacteria. These have been classified into several different groups on the basis of their substrate profile (the rate at which different β-lactam substrates are inactivated) and whether their activity is inhibited by *p*-chloromercuribenzoate (PCMB) and cloxacillin. A simplified summary of the different types is presented in Table 9.3. Four types of enzymes are of major clinical

Table 9.3 Types of β-lactamases of Gram-negative bacteria

Class of enzyme	*Mediation*[a]	*Predominant activity*	*Inhibition*[c] *by*	
			PCMB[b]	*Cloxacillin*
I	C	Cephalosporinase	–	+
II	C	Penicillinase	–	+ or –
III	R-factor	Cephalosporinase & Penicillinase	–	+
IV	C	Cephalosporinase & Penicillinase	+	–
V	R-factor	Cephalosporinase	–	–

[a] Chromosomally (C) or R-factor mediated.
[b] PCMB....*p*-chloromercuribenzoate.
[c] +, Sensitivity of enzyme to inhibitor; –, no inhibition of enzyme (cloxacillin may, in fact be a substrate for the Type V enzyme).

significance, *viz.* staphylococcal (Gram-positive) and K1 (Type IV), P99 (Type I) and TEM (Type III). Cephalosporins are generally more resistant to staphylococcal β-lactamases than are penicillins, but P99 β-lactamase (from *Enterobacter* species) is a powerful cephalosporinase type enzyme active against many cephalosporins. The K1 enzyme (from *Klebsiella aerogenes*) and the TEM type (found in many R^+ *E. coli* strains and in gonococci) attack a wide range of substrates. Amino acid sequences in the different β-lactamases are now being actively studied.

9.4.1.2 *Aminoglycoside-modifying enzymes*

β-lactam antibiotics are destroyed by β-lactamases. In contrast, aminoglycoside antibiotics are not totally inactivated by plasmid-coded enzymes but rather modified in the outer regions of the resistant cell and are thus not transported to the target site (ribosome). Only a small proportion of the external aminoglycoside need be modified for resistance to be expressed.

Aminoglycoside-modifying enzymes are of three types:

(i) acetyltransferases (AAC), which transfer an acetyl group from acetylcoenzyme A to susceptible —NH$_2$ groups in the antibiotic;

(ii) adenylyltransferases (AAD), which transfer adenosine monophosphate (AMP) from adenosine triphosphate (ATP) to susceptible —OH groups in the antibiotic;

(iii) phosphotransferases (APH), which phosphorylate susceptible —OH groups, ATP acting as the source of phosphate.

Kanamycin **(9.21)** can be modified in at least six different ways. Thus, the development of aminoglycosides such as amikacin (Section 9.6.1 **(9.22)**), with considerably greater resistance to many of these enzymes, is a significant improvement to the currently available range of antibiotics.

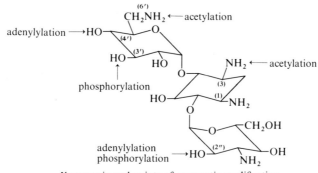

Kanamycin and points of enzymatic modification
(9.21)

Amikacin and points of enzymatic modification
(9.22)

9.4.1.3   *Chloramphenicol-inactivating enzymes*

Some bacteria, notably some R^+ Gram-negative and *Staphylococcus* containing transducible plasmids (Section 9.4.3) can produce an enzyme, chloramphenicol acetyltransferase that acetylates the hydroxyl groups in the side-chain of chloramphenicol (9.23) to produce initially 3-acetoxychloramphenicol (9.24) and finally 1,3-diacetoxychloramphenicol (9.25) which is inactive. In *S. aureus*, the acetyltransferase is an inducible enzyme, whereas in Gram-negative bacteria the enzyme

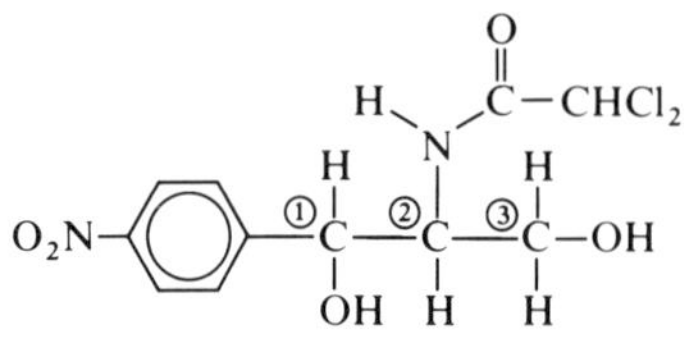

Chloramphenicol
(9.23)

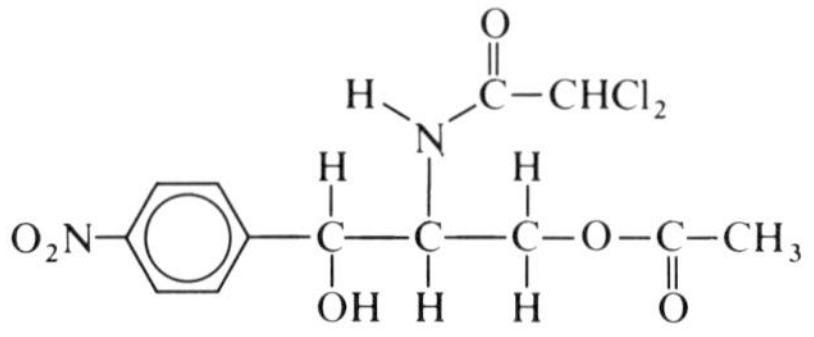

3-acetoxychloramphenicol
(9.24)

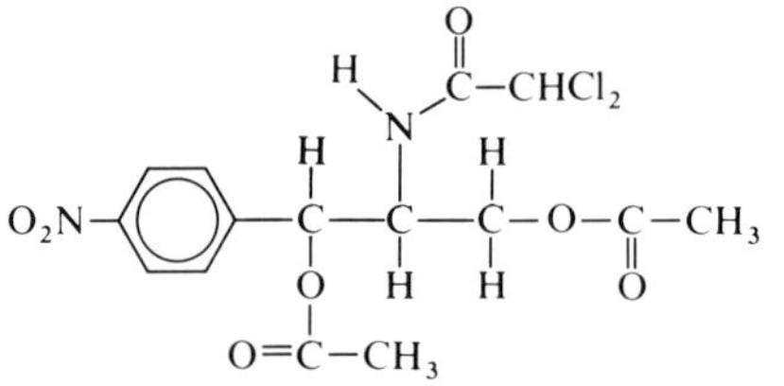

1,3-diacetoxychloramphenicol
(9.25)

is constitutively synthesized. The recent design of new chloramphenicol derivatives (in which the terminal hydroxyl is replaced by fluorine) could be a major advance, since these do not function as substrates for chloramphenicol acetyltransferase.

9.4.2   Outer membrane barrier

Another way in which bacteria show resistance to antibiotics is by an intrinsic type of resistance associated, in Gram-negative bacteria especially, with the outer membrane of the cell. The cell envelope of such organisms is considerably more chemically complex than the envelopes of Gram-positive bacteria, which consist predominantly of peptidoglycan (murein, mucopeptide) and teichoic acids (Fig. 9.1*a*).

Fig. 9.1*b* presents a simplified version of the cell envelope of Gram-negative cells. The outer membrane acts as a barrier to the entry of many high molecular weight hydrophobic molecules, whereas low molecular weight (less than about 550–650 daltons) hydrophilic antibiotics can pass through hydrophilic channels, known as porins, which consist of outer membrane protein molecules. Removal of much of the outer membrane lipopolysaccharide by exposure of cells to ethylenediamine tetraacetate (EDTA), a chelating agent (*see* p. 140) with a strong affinity for envelope Mg^{2+}, renders the organisms sensitive to several types of hydrophobic antibiotics. This is believed to result from a re-orientation of the phospholipid molecules, with the head-groups on the outside, thereby forming a classical type of membrane structure.

Many of the β-lactam antibiotics, especially cephalosporins, readily enter Gram-negative cells via hydrophilic channels. Of interest, in this context, have been the findings that porin-deficient *Salmonella typhimurium* cells are resistant to cephaloridine and that the porins of *Ps. aeruginosa* are much larger than those of other Gram-negative bacteria (*see above*) and have an exclusion limit of about 9000 daltons. It would, therefore, be logical to predict that *Ps. aeruginosa* is *more* sensitive to antibiotics than other Gram-negative bacteria, which is the exact opposite of known fact. The reason for its increased resistance has yet to be elucidated, but one possibility is that the outer membrane of pseudomonads contains fewer porins or that some of the porins are closed.

Resistance to the tetracyclines in R^+ bacteria (*see below*: Section 9.4.3) appears to be linked to the presence of additional outer membrane and inner (cytoplasmic) membrane proteins that prevent uptake of the antibiotics and passage to their target sites (ribosomes). Tetracyclines have been developed that are active against such resistant bacteria (*see* Section 9.6.2).

9.4.3 Transferable resistance

Genetic information can be transferred from one bacterial cell to another by three ways: transduction (phage-mediated), transformation (absorption of extracted DNA by 'competent' cells) and conjugation. The last is the most important in the spread of bacterial resistance and thus will be the only one considered here.

In the late 1950s, it was observed during a dysentery outbreak in Japan that a *Shigella* strain was resistant to four chemically unrelated antibiotics. It was unlikely that resistance in this strain arose by spontaneous mutation. Other multiple-resistant strains of Gram-negative bacteria were also isolated and it was proposed that blocks of resistance genes were being transferred between bacteria of the same or different species. For this transference (conjugation) to occur, cell-to-cell contact is necessary and this is achieved via a cytoplasmic bridge (pilus) between mating bacteria. It is now known that some (R^+) Gram-negative bacteria carry small, autonomously replicating extrachromosomal elements known as plasmids which are double stranded DNA molecules. These consist of a resistance transfer factor (RFT) (which is responsible for pilus synthesis) to which may be attached one or more fragments of resistance determinants (genes) which confer drug resistance. Thus, during conjugation between R^+ and R^- cells, the plasmids (and hence resistance determinants) pass via the pilus from donor to recipient cells and there specify the production of, for example, drug-inactivating or -modifying enzymes.

9.4.4 Conclusions and comments

Bacterial resistance to antibiotics is often achieved by the constitutive possession or inducibility of drug-inactivating or -modifying enzymes. This problem can, at least to some extent, be overcome by designing new drugs (e.g. by chemical alteration of an existing molecule) that (*a*) are insusceptible to this enzyme attack or (*b*) will inactivate the enzyme concerned thereby protecting enzyme-labile antibiotics that, in the absence of the enzyme, would be highly active antibacterially. Some degree of success has been achieved in both aspects, as discussed in Section 9.5.

Another problem concerns the lack of penetration of many drugs into Gram-negative bacteria. On the basis of current knowledge, it would seem logical that any design of new agents should at least consider the need for hydrophilic, low molecular weight compounds that can penetrate the outer membrane of these cells via aqueous channels (porins). In this context, the development of amino acid analogues with antibacterial activity is worthy of consideration. These penetrate poorly into bacteria but when attached to small peptides are transported into cells via relatively non-specific permeases. One such example is alaphosphin (L-alanyl-L-1-aminoethylphosphonic acid, alafosfalin, (9.26)) which is rapidly accumulated by, and concentrated within, bacteria where it is converted to L-1-aminoethylphosphonic acid (9.27) which acts as an inhibitor of peptidoglycan

$$\underset{\substack{| \\ H_2N-CH-CO-NH-CH-\underset{|}{\overset{\parallel}{P}}-OH \\ OH}}{\overset{CH_3 CH_3 \ \ O}{}}$$

Alaphosphin
(L-alanyl-L-1-aminoethylphosphonic acid)
(9.26)

$$\underset{\substack{| \\ H_2N-CH-\underset{|}{\overset{\parallel}{P}}-OH \\ OH}}{\overset{CH_3 \ \ O}{}}$$

L-1-aminoethylphosphonic
acid
(9.27)

synthesis (Section 9.3.1). Alaphosphin belongs to a group of compounds, the phosphonopeptides, which are peptide mimetics with C-terminal residues that simulate natural amino acids. Their mechanism of action results from transport into the bacterial cell followed by release of the alanine mimetic. These agents are an important concept in designing new antibacterially active compounds.

Despite extensive research, the design of clinically effective antimetabolites has generally been disappointing.

9.5 DESIGN OF β-LACTAM ANTIBIOTICS

It was pointed out in Section 9.2 that 6-APA **(9.1)** and 7-ACA **(9.3)** formed the starting point in the development of new penicillins and cephalosporins, respectively. This Section will continue this consideration and will also explain current thinking in the design of new β-lactam antibiotics (or of combinations of β-lactams) that can effectively counter the unwanted effects of β-lactamases (Section 9.4.1.1) and bacterial impermeability (Section 9.4.2). In addition, pharmacokinetic aspects will be considered where relevant.

9.5.1 Penicillins

The original penicillins, benzylpenicillin (penicillin G, **(9.2)**) and phenoxymethyl-penicillin (penicillin V, **(9.28)**) suffered clinically in the context that both were narrow spectrum, β-lactamase-labile antibiotics. The former is also acid unstable and is thus normally administered by injection, whereas penicillin V is acid stable and is thus given orally. The first semisynthetic penicillin produced from 6-APA of any consequence was methicillin **(9.29)** which, although inactive against Gram-negative bacteria, possesses significant activity against β-lactamase staphylococcal

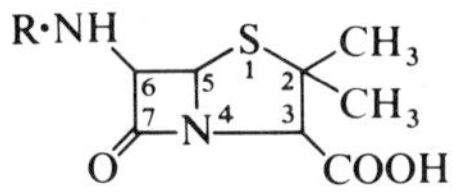

(9.28)   Phenoxymethylpenicillin $C_6H_5OCH_2CO-$ **(9.29)**   Methicillin

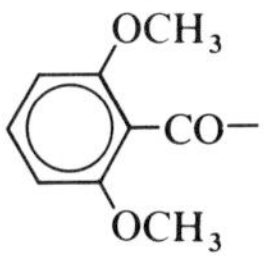

producers. Its intrinsic potency is, however, less that that of benzylpenicillin against non-β-lactamase staphylococci, and acid instability precludes the oral usage of methicillin. Methicillin was soon followed by ampicillin **(9.30)**, and this was another significant advance, because ampicillin was the first semisynthetic penicillin to possess marked activity against Gram-negative organisms (although *Ps. aeruginosa* is resistant). Ampicillin is stable to acid and is administered orally or by injection, but is susceptible to the β-lactamases produced by *S. aureus* and most Gram-negative bacteria.

There then followed many other important new semisynthetic penicillins, such as cloxacillin **(9.31)** (the first oral, β-lactamase-stable penicillin, but again without

(9.30)   Ampicillin   **(9.31)**   Cloxacillin

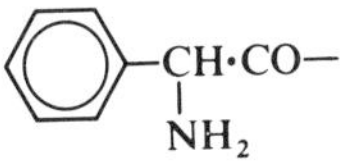

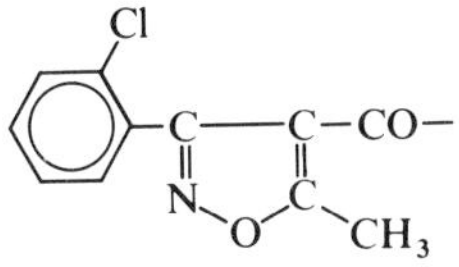

significant action on Gram-negative cells); its derivative flucloxacillin **(9.32)** claimed to give higher blood levels; carbenicillin **(9.33)** the first penicillin with activity against *Ps. aeruginosa*; amoxycillin **(9.34)** with a similar spectrum to

(9.32)   Flucloxacillin   **(9.33)**   Carbenicillin

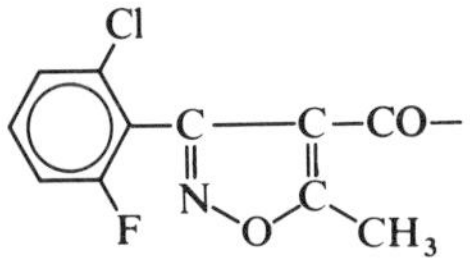

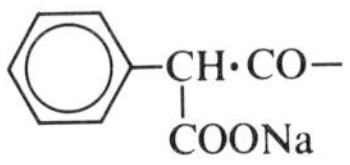

(9.34)   Amoxycillin

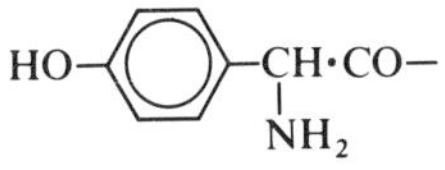

ampicillin, but which is much better absorbed; and several others.

The design of all the semisynthetic penicillins has had one common goal: to achieve, by the introduction of a different R group **(9.2)**, a new antibiotic with an improved spectrum of activity and/or enhanced stability to β-lactamases. This deliberate design concept, therefore, has achieved some notable successes.

The above examples all illustrate development of new penicillins by substitution at the 6-position in the molecule. Position 3 is also uniquely important, since the introduction of various groups here has led to the design of new esters ('pro-drugs': *see* Chapter 7) which hydrolyse *in vivo* to give the active antibiotic. Esters (pivampicillin, talampicillin and bacampicillin: *see* **(9.35)**, **(9.36)** and **(9.37)**,

(9.35) Pivampicillin

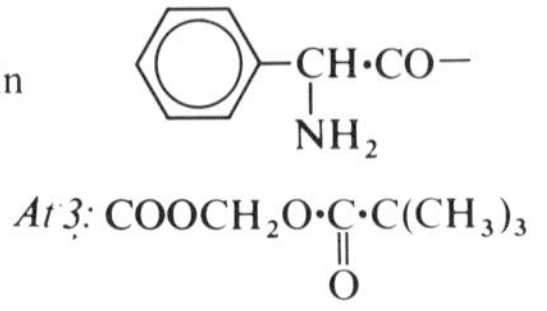
CH·CO—
NH2
At 3: COOCH2O·C·C(CH3)3
O

(9.36) Talampicillin

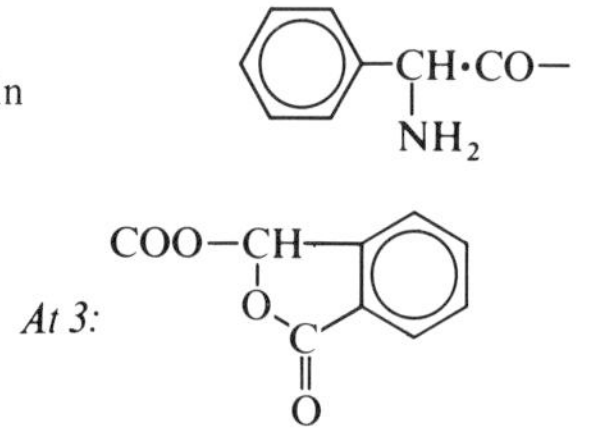
CH·CO—
NH2
At 3:
COO—CH
O
C
O

(9.37) Bacampicillin

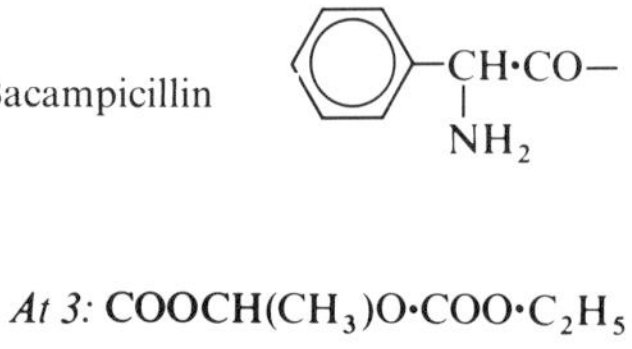
CH·CO—
NH2
At 3: COOCH(CH3)O·COO·C2H5

respectively) at position 3 of the ampicillin molecule break down *in vivo* to produce higher blood levels of ampicillin than would be obtained if ampicillin itself had been given at an equivalent concentration. Carbenicillin is not absorbed when given orally but esters (carfecillin **(9.38)**, carindacillin **(9.39)**) in the side-chain at

(9.38) Carfecillin

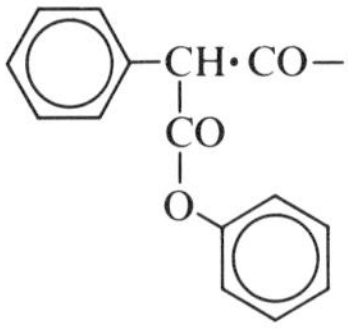
CH·CO—
CO
O

(9.39) Indenyl carbenicillin (Carindacillin)

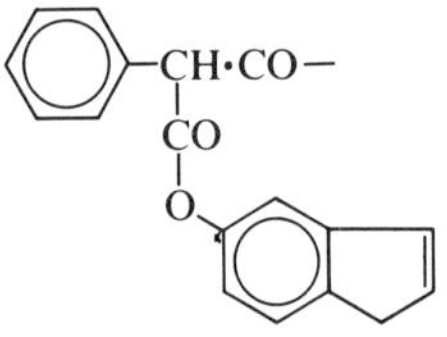
CH·CO—
CO
O

position 6, when given orally will hydrolyse *in vivo* to give a similar blood level to that obtained with an equivalent dose of carbenicillin given intramuscularly. Thus, 'pro-drugs' form a useful development in β-lactam design. Substituted ampicillins, such as piperacillin **(9.40)**, azlocillin **(9.41)** and mezlocillin **(9.42)**, appear to combine the spectra and degree of activity of ampicillin and carbenicillin.

Mecillinam **(9.43)** a 6β-amidinopenicillin, has limited activity against Gram-positive bacteria but is active against Gram-negative organisms. It binds preferentially to PBP2.

Thus, alterations in the molecule (and especially at positions 6 and 3) can produce penicillins with changes in microbiological and/or pharmacological properties.

Substitution at other sites has also been examined in the quest for improved design: removal of the sulphur atom of the thiazolidine ring usually leads to a reduction of activity, although the oxapenicillin (clavam), clavulanic acid (Section 9.5.4.2) is an important β-lactamase inhibitor. Additionally, the carbapenems

(9.40) Piperacillin

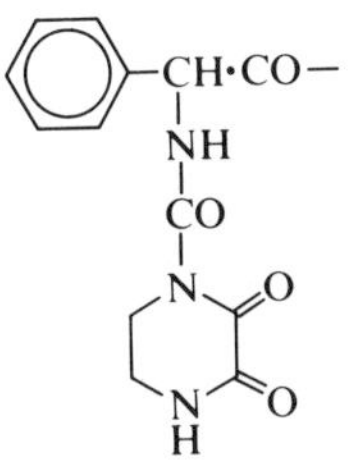

(9.41) Azlocillin

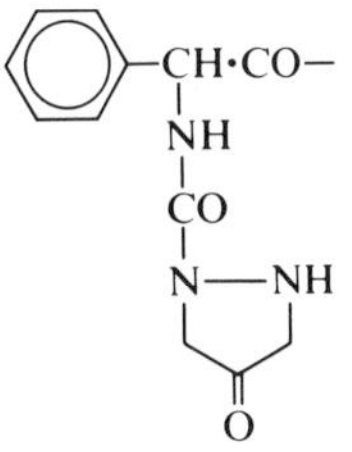

(9.42) Mezlocillin

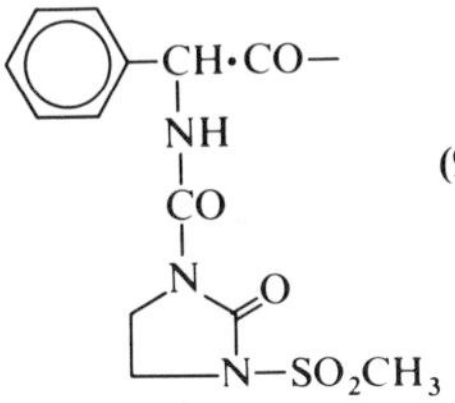

(9.43) Mecillinam
(a 6β-amidino-
penicillanic acid)

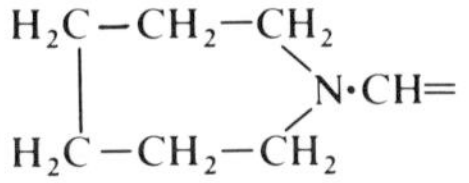

(Section 9.5.5.2), in which sulphur is isosterically replaced by a methylene group but which have a double bond in the 5-membered ring, may possess significant activity. Substitution at the C-5 position reduces antibacterial activity, and substitution at the C-2 locus produces penicillins with activity against Gram-positive but not Gram-negative bacteria.

9.5.2 Cephalosporins

Current research on cephalosporins and cephamycins (methoxycephalosporins) is proceeding at a bewildering pace. The cephalosporins may be considered as semisynthetic derivatives of 7-ACA. Several of the early (first generation) cephalosporins differed more in their pharmacokinetic than in their antibacterial properties. Subsequent developments have been to improve:
  (i) antibacterial activity, especially in the context of increasing resistance to β-lactamases produced by Gram-negative bacteria, although it must be added that decreased enzyme lability is sometimes paralleled by a reduction in antibacterial potency;
  (ii) pharmacokinetic properties by making appropriate substitutions in the molecule, especially at positions 3 and 7.
  A classification of the cephalosporins, in which due attention is paid to both β-lactamase response and pharmacological properties, is given in Table 9.4.

9.5.2.1 Structure–activity relationships

The cephalosporins (Δ^3-cephalosporins) and penicillins are structurally related in that the β-lactam ring is fused to different rings. The position of the double bond in

Table 9.4 Classification of cephalosporin antibiotics[a]

Oral administration		Parenteral administration	
β-lactamase sensitive[c]	β-lactamase resistant	β-lactamase sensitive[c]	β-lactamase resistant
Cephalexin	None	Cephalothin[b]	Cefuroxime
Cephradine		Cephapirin[b]	Cefamandole
Cefaclor		Cephacetrile[b]	Cefotaxime
		Cephaloridine	Cefoxitin
		Cefazolin	
		Cefazedone	

[a] Based on O'Callaghan (1979).
[b] Metabolically unstable, i.e. conversion of cephalosporins with a 3-acetoxymethyl group to the less active 3-hydroxymethyl derivative.
[c] Cephalosporins are generally much less sensitive than penicillins to inactivation by staphylococcal β-lactamase. On the other hand, the 'β-lactamase-sensitive' cephalosporins in the table may be hydrolysed by β-lactamases from some, but not all, Gram-negative species. The 'β-lactamase-resistant' cephalosporins are considerably more stable to these enzymes, although cefamandole is less resistant than the others in this group.

Δ^3-cephalosporins is very important, since Δ^2-cephalosporins **(9.44)**, irrespective of the composition of the side-chains, are not significantly antibacterial. In contrast, Δ^2-penicillins are highly active against Gram-positive and Gram-negative bacteria (Sections 9.5.4.2 and 9.5.5.2).

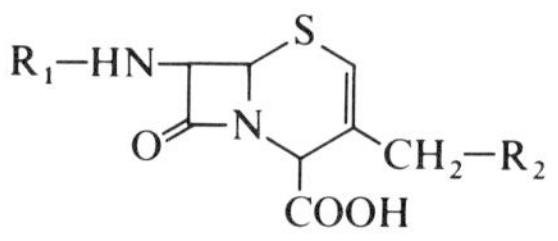

Δ^2-Cephalosporins
(9.44)

The 7α-methyl cephalosporin derivatives have a greatly reduced antibacterial activity, whereas the introduction of a 7α-methoxy group gives compounds with high antibacterial activity, and possessing considerable stability to most β-lactamases. There is, however, a rapid decrease in activity as the size of the ether group is increased.

Oxacephems (oxcephamycins; *see* Section 9.5.5.1) have been produced by synthetic means and may have high antibacterial activity, including β-lactamase stability.

An example of the interplay of various factors in antibacterial activity is demonstrated by the following findings. 7α-methoxy substitution of cefuroxime, cefamandole and cephapirin gives reduced activity against *E. coli* because of a smaller affinity for penicillin binding proteins and not because of reduced permeability. In contrast, similar substitution of cefoxitin enhances activity because of greater penetration through the outer membrane barrier rather than an increased affinity for penicillin binding proteins.

The 3-acetoxymethyl compounds cephalothin (9.45), cephacetrile (9.46) and cephapirin (9.47) have different 7-acyl groups, which are monosubstituted

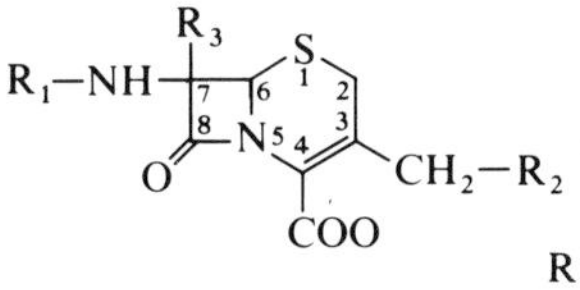

R_1—NH

R_3 is —OCH_3 in cefoxitin and — H in all other antibiotics

		R_1	R_2
(9.45)	Cephalothin	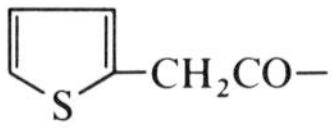 —CH_2CO—	—$OCOCH_3$
(9.46)	Cephacetrile	$N\equiv C\cdot CH_2\cdot CO$—	—$OCOCH_3$
(9.47)	Cephapirin	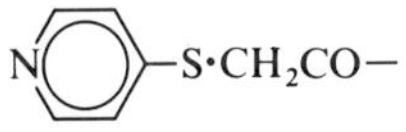 —$S\cdot CH_2CO$—	—$OCOCH_3$

acetamido groups, and have similar antibacterial activity. They are active against Gram-positive bacteria and against β-lactamase-negative Gram-negative organisms.

9.5.2.2 Pharmacokinetic properties

The 3-acetoxymethyl compounds are converted *in vivo* by esterases to the antibacterially less active 3-hydroxymethyl derivatives and are excreted partly as such. The rapid excretion means that such cephalosporins have a short half-life in the body.

Replacement of the 3-acetoxymethyl group by a wide variety of groups has rendered other cephalosporins much less prone to esterase attack. For example, cephaloridine (9.48) has an internally compensated betaine group at position 3 and

| (9.48) | Cephaloridine | —CH_2CO— | |

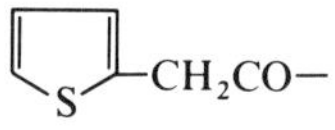

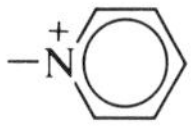

is metabolically stable. It gives higher and more prolonged blood levels than cephalothin.

Cephalosporins such as the 3-acetoxymethyl derivatives (9.45, 9.46 and 9.47), cephaloridine (9.48) and cefazolin (9.49) are inactive when given orally. For good

| (9.49) | Cefazolin | —CH_2CO— | —CH_3 |

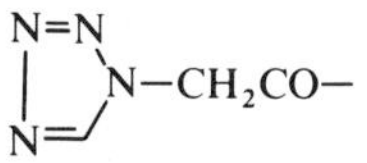

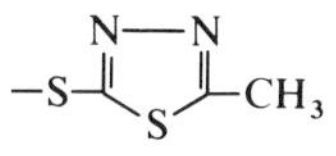

oral absorption, the 7-acyl group must be based on phenylglycine and the amino group must remain unsubstituted. At position 3, the substitutent must be small, non-polar and stable, with a methyl substituent considered desirable (although this can decrease antibacterial activity). Examples of orally absorbable cephalosporins are cephalexin **(9.50)**, cefaclor **(9.51)** and cephradine **(9.52)**. Although cephalexin

(9.50)   Cephalexin   ⬡—CH·CO—   —H
                                   |
                                   NH$_2$

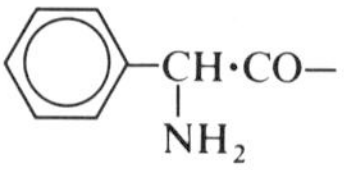

(9.51)   Cefaclor   ⬡—CH·CO—   —Cl
                                   |
                                   NH$_2$

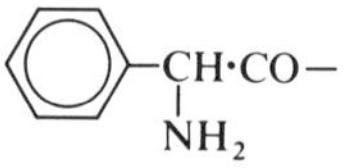

(9.52)   Cephradine   ⬡—CH·CO—   —H
                                   |
                                   NH$_2$

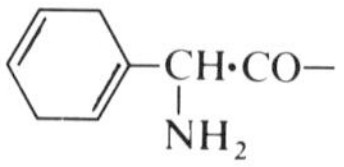

has some degree of resistance to β-lactamases produced by Gram-negative bacteria, there are currently no orally absorbed cephalosporins with a significant degree of resistance to these enzymes.

Parenterally administered cephalosporins which are metabolically stable and which are resistant to many types of β-lactamases include cefuroxime **(9.53)**,

(9.53)   Cefuroxime   [furan]—C·CO—   —OCONH$_2$
                                      ||
                                   N·O·CH$_3$

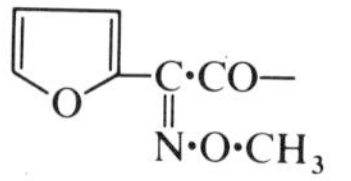

cefamandole **(9.54)**, cefotaxime **(9.55)** and cefoxitin **(9.56)** which has a 7α-methoxy group.

(9.54)   Cefamandole   ⬡—CH·CO—
                                   |
                                   OH

$$-S \overset{5}{\underset{N-N}{\Vert}}\begin{matrix}N{-}N\\ \Vert \\ N\end{matrix}$$
CH$_3$

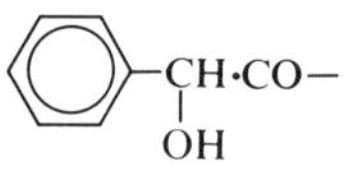

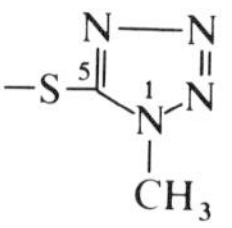

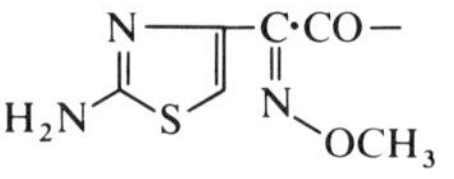

(9.55)   Cefotaxime   [thiazole: N, S, H$_2$N]—C·CO—   —O·COCH$_3$
                                                      N
                                                      OCH$_3$

(9.56)   Cefoxitin   [thiophene: S]—CH$_2$CO—   —OCONH$_2$

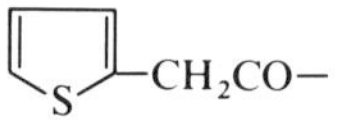

9.5.3 β-Lactamase stability

This short section attempts to summarize the facts presented in Sections 9.5.1 and 9.5.2.

β-lactam antibiotics, both penicillins and cephalosporins, with simple side-chains (Ar—$\overset{\alpha}{C}H_2$—CO—NH—) are usually sensitive to β-lactamases, whereas the incorporation of the α-carbon atom into an aromatic ring (e.g. methicillin) increases resistance.

The presence of an additional substituent, e.g. methoxy, in the 6-(penicillins) or 7α(cephalosporins) position greatly increases β-lactamase resistance, although intrinsic antibacterial activity may be decreased. Cefoxitin **(9.56)**, however, has a broad spectrum of activity and is almost totally resistant to β-lactamases. Newer 7α-methoxycephalosporins have been described that have the same spectrum of activity as cefoxitin but are more active. The new 1-oxacephem antibiotic moxalactam ((**9.57**) *see* Section 9.5.5.1) has oxygen instead of sulphur at position

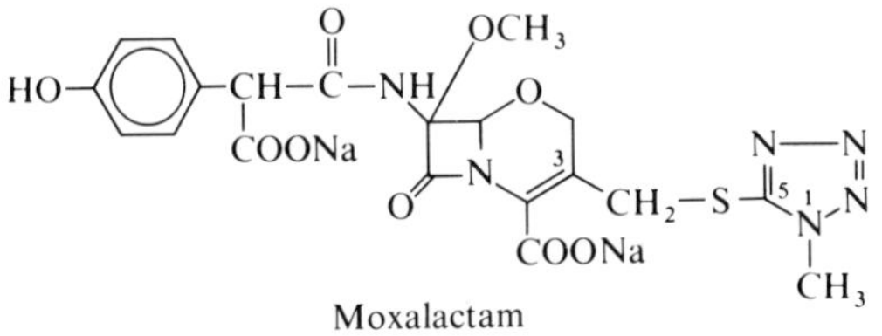

Moxalactam
(**9.57**)

1, which would tend to make it less chemically stable and more enzyme-labile; however, the presence of the 7α-methoxy group, as in cefoxitin (**9.56**) stabilizes the molecule.

Absence of sulphur or oxygen in the fused ring results in increased resistance to β-lactamases (*see* Section 9.5.4). Generally, changes at C2 and C3 in a penicillin or cephalosporin do not affect resistance to a β-lactamase.

9.5.4 β-Lactamase inhibitors

An exciting new concept in antibiotic therapy is the distinct possibility of using β-lactamase inhibitors clinically. This is not, in fact a revolutionary idea, as many of the older penicillins were able to inhibit the enzyme (*see* Section 9.5.4.1). The recent development of clavulanic acid (*see* Section 9.5.4.2) does, however, seem to bridge the gap between theoretical desirability and actual practice, and the recent introduction (1981) of an antibiotic mixture (Augmentin[R], Beecham Research Laboratories) consisting of clavulanic acid with the β-lactamase sensitive penicillin, amoxycillin, provides the clinician with a new weapon in his armoury against microbial infection.

9.5.4.1 *β-Lactams as inhibitors*

Some of the earlier penicillins (e.g. cloxacillin and methicillin) and cephalosporins (such as cephalosporin C) were found to inhibit *Bacillus cereus* β-lactamase and later were shown to be active against some β-lactamases elaborated by Gram-negative bacteria. This inhibition was competitive in nature, and marked potentiation of a β-lactamase sensitive β-lactam antibiotic could be achieved *in vitro*. The problem, nevertheless, was two-fold: (*a*) high concentrations of inhibitor were necessary, (*b*) no single inhibitor was able to inhibit a wide range of β-lactamases.

Thus, it was not possible to design a new antibiotic mixture incorporating a β-lactamase inhibitor for clinical use.

9.5.4.2 *Naturally occurring β-lactamase inhibitors*

The β-lactamase-inhibitory properties of cephalosporin C (described above, Section 9.5.4.1), itself produced by a micro-organism, stimulated a search for other naturally occurring β-lactamase inhibitors. In principle, this technique has involved testing culture fluids in which *Streptomyces* species have been growing for their ability to inhibit the β-lactamase produced by a specific strain of *Klebsiella aerogenes*. Research investigations at Beecham Research Laboratories in the U.K. and studies elsewhere, notably in the United States and in Japan, have shown the production of β-lactamase inhibitors in the culture fluids of *Streptomyces olivaceus* and *Streptomyces clavuligerus*.

Three β-lactamase-inhibiting acidic substances, termed the olivanic acids (general structure (9.58)) have, with some difficulty, been isolated from the culture fluids of *Streptomyces olivaceus*. These possess potent activity against various types

General structure of
olivanic acids
(9.58)

of β-lactamases, when they act as competitive inhibitors, and are also broad-spectrum antibiotics in their own right. The olivanic acids, characterized as closely related members of a new class (1-carbapenems (9.59)) of fused β-lactams, are analogues of penicillins or clavulanic acid (9.60) where sulphur or oxygen, respectively, has been replaced by a methylene group. An antibiotic thienamycin (9.61) with a similar structure to the olivanic acids has been isolated from

1-Carbapenems
(9.59)

Sodium clavulanate
(9.60)

Thienamycin
(9.61)

Streptomyces cattleya. It is of interest to note that thienamycin, a very broad spectrum antibiotic, is often a poor β-lactamase inhibitor, but could well play an important clinical role (*see*, however, Section 9.5.5.2).

It would thus appear logical for a member of the olivanic acid group to be utilized as a β-lactamase inhibitor in the design of a new antibiotic mixture. Unfortunately, the olivanic acids are produced in low yields and, as mentioned above, there have been problems with their isolation.

Attention has thus been focussed on other types of β-lactamase inhibitors. One of these, clavulanic acid, isolated from *Streptomyces clavuligerus*, was sufficiently promising for a comprehensive investigation to be undertaken. Clavulanic acid (9.60) is a fused bicyclic compound containing a β-lactam ring; it is similar in structure to the penicillins except that it contains oxygen in place of sulphur, i.e. an oxazolidine, instead of a thiazolidine, ring. It is produced in higher yields than the olivanic acids, but has a poor antibacterial action; it is, however, a potent inhibitor of staphylococcal β-lactamase and of β-lactamases produced by Gram-negative bacteria, in particular those with a 'penicillinase' rather than a 'cephalosporinase' type of action. Clavulanic acid inhibits β-lactamases of Types II, III, IV and V (Table 9.3) but is a poor inhibitor of Type I. Clavulanic acid effects a progressive inhibition of β-lactamase, the initial effect probably being competitive in nature, and this being followed by a phase of rapid inactivation. Studies with different types of β-lactamases have demonstrated that this inhibitor is a k_{cat} inhibitor (see p. 113) acting in a competitive and irreversible manner.

9.5.4.3   Synthetic β-lactamase inhibitors

Penicillanic acid derivatives are also known to inhibit β-lactamases. Penicillanic acid sulphone **(9.62)** is a β-lactamase inhibitor that protects ampicillin from hydrolysis by staphylococcal β-lactamase and some, but not all, of the Gram-negative types depicted in Table 9.3. It is, however, a less active inhibitor than clavulanic acid. 6-bromopenicillanic acid **(9.63)** inhibits some types of β-lactamases.

Penicillanic acid sulphone,
sodium salt
(9.62)

6-bromopenicillanic acid,
sodium salt
(9.63)

9.5.4.4   Mutual pro-drugs

A pro-drug (see Section 9.5.1 and Chapter 7) is an inactive compound that is converted in vivo to an active form. Pro-drugs of penicillin are usually penicillin esters which are broken down by mammalian esterases. A recent, potentially exciting development has been the synthesis of linked esters of penicillins and β-lactamase inhibitors to produce what are termed mutual pro-drugs. These must be well absorbed and the two active constituents released in equal amounts. One problem is that maximum antibacterial activity is not necessarily achieved at a 1 : 1 ratio. It has been suggested that it might even be possible to develop a mutual pro-drug (an ester of a penicillin with a β-lactamase inhibitor) and combine it with a pro-drug of the non β-lactamase inhibitor moiety. This is an interesting theoretical possibility, but might itself pose many practical problems in formulation.

9.5.5   New β-lactam ring systems

For several years, investigations have been carried out on modifications of β-lactam drugs in order to improve and extend their antibacterial activity or to alter their pharmacokinetic properties. The result has been the development of an impressive array of β-lactam antibiotics with new ring systems which may prove to be of value clinically in their own right, or may serve as starting-points for the design of still more important antibiotics, or, again, may be potent β-lactamase inhibitors (*see* Section 9.5.3).

9.5.5.1   *1-Oxacephems*

A highly active 1-oxacephem (moxalactam **(9.57)**) has been obtained semi-synthetically from penicillin. The sulphur atom in the cephalosporin dihydro-thiazine ring is isosterically replaced by an oxygen atom. Moxalactam shows similarities to other β-lactam antibiotics, e.g. a 7α-methoxy group (as in cefoxitin), a *p*-hydroxybenzyl group (amoxycillin) and an α-carboxylic acid group (car-benicillin) and a 3-(1-methyltetrazol-5-ylthiomethyl) substituent (cefamandole). Moxalactam is an effective k_{cat} inhibitor of some β-lactamases and a competitive inhibitor of others.

9.5.5.2   *Penems*

In the penems, the double bond in the dihydrothiazine ring of the cephalosporins has been placed in the corresponding (thiazolidine) ring of the penicillins. In the carbapenems **(9.59)**, a methylene group has replaced the —S— atom at position 1 in the penicillin molecule. Examples have already been dealt with (olivanic acids, thienamycin) although it must be noted that, despite its high activity and β-lactamase resistance, thienamycin suffers the disadvantage of being chemically unstable. A new *N*-formimidinyl derivative overcomes this problem.

9.5.5.3   *Nocardicins*

A novel group of β-lactam antibiotics, the nocardicins **(9.64)** have been isolated from a strain of *Nocardia*. This group has been characterized into seven closely related compounds (*viz.* nocardicins A–G), with nocardicin A **(9.64)** the most

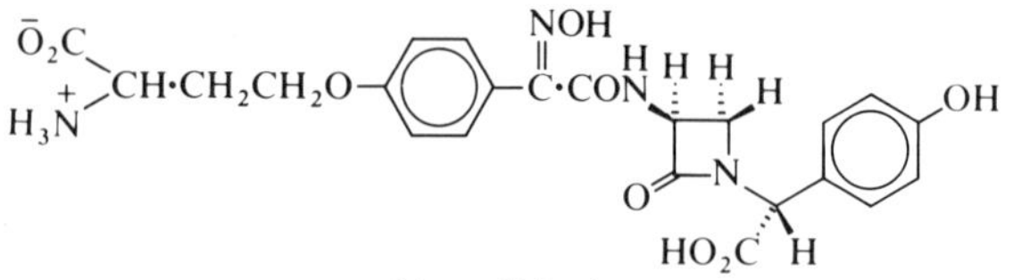

Nocardicin A
(9.64)

active. *In vitro*, nocardicin A is less active than carbenicillin against Gram-negative bacteria and has no effect on Gram-positive organisms. *In vivo*, however, nocardicin A is more active than carbenicillin because the potency of the former is increased in the presence of polymorphonuclear leucocytes.

9.5.5.4   *Monobactams*

The monobactams are monocyclic β-lactam antibiotics produced by bacteria. They have been isolated from bacteria using as test organism a strain of *B. licheniformis* which is specific for, and highly sensitive ($100\,ng\,ml^{-1}$) to, molecules containing a β-lactam ring.

On the basis of the novel nucleus (3-aminomonobactamic acid, 3-AMA, **(9.65)**) possessed by these antibiotics a new, potent monobactam has been synthesized. This is currently known as azthreonam (SQ 26 776 **(9.66)**) and is undergoing

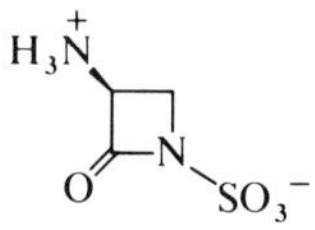

3-AMA
(9.65)

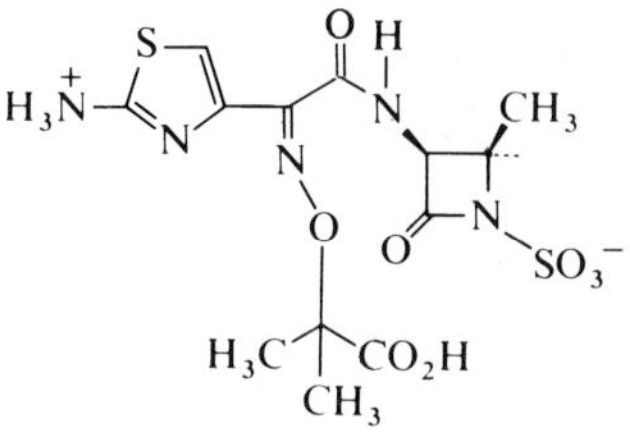

(SQ26776)
(9.66)

clinical evaluation. It is highly active against most Gram-negative bacteria and is very stable to most types of β-lactamases, including staphylococcal, although – interestingly – it is without effect on the growth or viability of *S. aureus* strains. Its lack of effect on staphylococci is believed to result from its predominant effect on PBP 3 in Gram-negative organisms since this PBP is absent from staphylococci.

9.6   DESIGN OF OTHER ANTIBACTERIAL AGENTS

Whilst it is true to state that β-lactam antibiotics are currently occupying the greatest attention in the treatment of bacterial infections, it would be incorrect to imply that other antibiotic agents have an unimportant role to play. Several other groups of antibiotics exist, notably the aminoglycosides, tetracyclines, macrolides, polymyxins, lincomycins, rifamycins together with choramphenicol, vancomycin and bacitracin. In recent years, advances have also been demonstrated in several of these groups, resulting in the production of new antibiotics and these are considered in this section.

9.6.1   Aminoglycoside antibiotics

The general structure of the 2-deoxystreptamine-containing antibiotics (the amino-glycoside antibiotics) is shown in **(9.67)**, together with examples of the different drugs. Streptomycin **(9.68)** does not contain 2-deoxystreptamine. The more important aminoglycoside antibiotics (*see* **(9.21)**, **(9.69)**, **(9.70)**, **(9.22)**, **(9.71)** and **(9.72)**) are kanamycin, gentamicin, tobramycin, amikacin, sisomicin (sissomicin) and netilmicin, respectively. As a group, the aminoglycoside antibiotics are bactericidal to Gram-negative bacteria and to staphylococci. Two of the major problems, however, have been the development of resistance of Gram-negative bacteria, often by virtue of drug-modifying enzymes (acetyltransferases, adenyly-lating enzymes and phosphotransferases: *see* Section 9.4.1.2) and the toxicity associated with a most important member, gentamicin, which has necessitated careful monitoring of blood and body fluid levels. Desirable properties of the

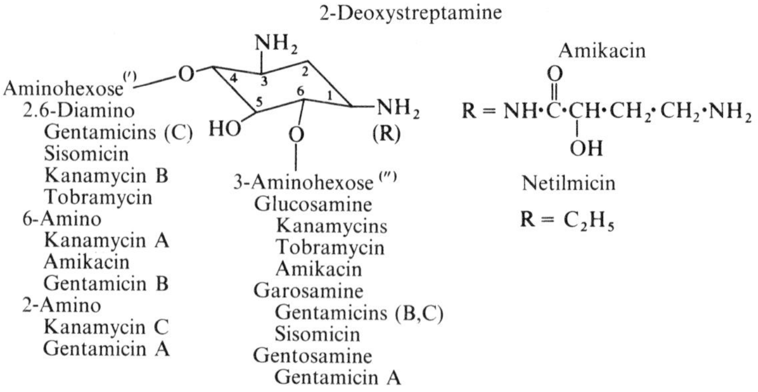

2-Deoxystreptamine

Aminohexose $^{(')}$
2.6-Diamino
  Gentamicins (C)
  Sisomicin
  Kanamycin B
  Tobramycin
6-Amino
  Kanamycin A
  Amikacin
  Gentamicin B
2-Amino
  Kanamycin C
  Gentamicin A

3-Aminohexose $^{(''')}$
Glucosamine
  Kanamycins
  Tobramycin
  Amikacin
Garosamine
  Gentamicins (B,C)
  Sisomicin
Gentosamine
  Gentamicin A

Amikacin

$R = NH \cdot C \cdot CH \cdot CH_2 \cdot CH_2 \cdot NH_2$

Netilmicin

$R = C_2H_5$

Chemical characteristics of aminoglycoside
antibiotics containing streptamine
(Streptomycin contains streptidine, and aminocyclitols,
such as spectinomycin, contain no amino sugar)
(9.67)

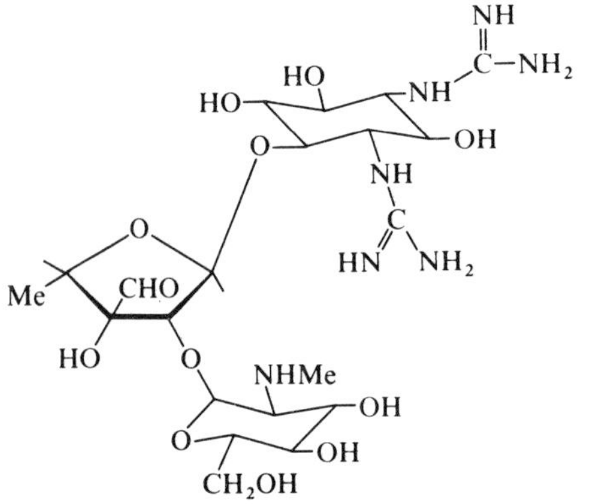

Streptomycin
(9.68)

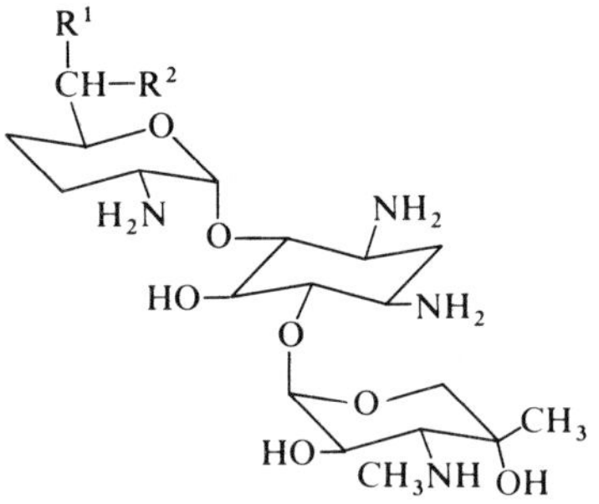

Gentamicins
(9.69)

	R^1	R^2
Gentamicin C_{1a}	H	NH_2
Gentamicin C_1	CH_3	$NHCH_3$
Gentamicin C_2	CH_3	NH_2

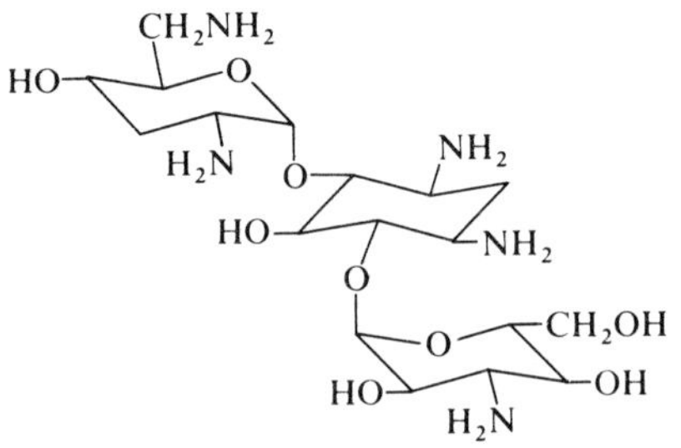

Tobramycin
(9.70)

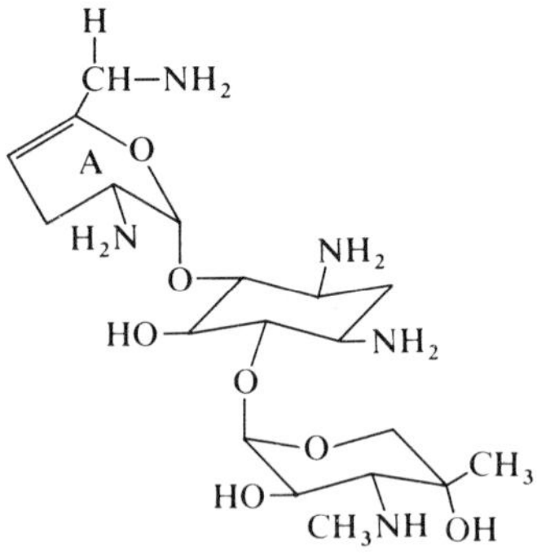

Sisomicin
(Note unsaturation in ring A)
(9.71)

newer (post-gentamicin) types have included increased antimicrobial activity, including improved activity against resistant strains, enhanced pharmacological properties or a reduction in, or freedom from, toxicity.

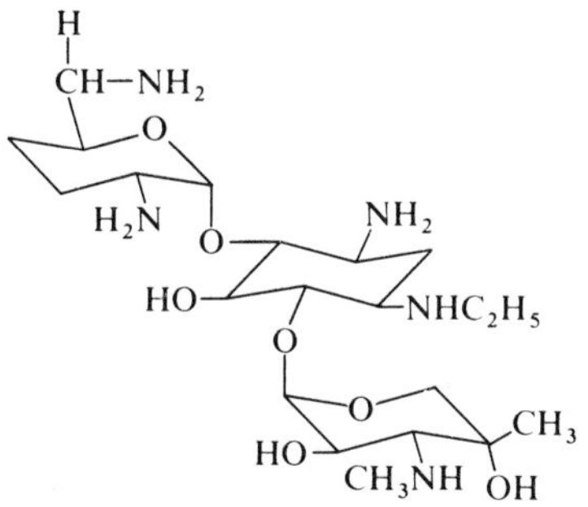

Netilmicin
(9.72)

Aminoglycoside antibiotics have several sites at which chemical substitution can be made. Alteration in the 3′ position of kanamycin B to give 3′-deoxykanamycin B (tobramycin) changes the activity spectrum. Amikacin has a 4-amino-2-hydroxybutanoyl group on the amino group at position 1 in the 2-deoxystreptamine ring, and this enhances the resistance of the molecule to modification by some, but not all, types of aminoglycoside-modifying enzymes. Amikacin is thus effective against several resistant strains because fewer sites on the molecule are modified. Netilmicin (N-ethylsisomicin) is a semisynthetic derivative of sisomicin that is less susceptible to some types of bacterial enzymes.

9.6.2   Tetracyclines

The tetracyclines are no longer used to the same extent as they were some years ago. The most important members of this group are oxytetracycline (9.73), chlortetracycline (9.74), tetracycline (9.75), demethylchlortetracycline (9.76), doxycycline (9.77), methacycline (9.78), clomocycline (9.79) and minocycline (9.80). The microbiological spectrum tends to be similar, with cross-resistance between the individual compounds, except for minocycline. Minocycline is active against some tetracycline-resistant R^+ strains of Gram-negative bacteria and against tetracycline-resistant staphylococci. Against the former, it appears to enter the cells more readily and may be excreted less rapidly.

A recent isosterically related, chemically synthesized thiatetracycline derivative, thiacycline (9.81), is more active than minocycline against tetracycline-resistant R^+ strains. Although some problems have become apparent in the context of its possible clinical use, thiacycline could form a useful fore-runner for a new group of highly active tetracycline antibiotics.

Structure–activity studies in the tetracyclines have shown that inhibitory activity is increased significantly by chlorination at position 7 (e.g. 9.74). Conversely,

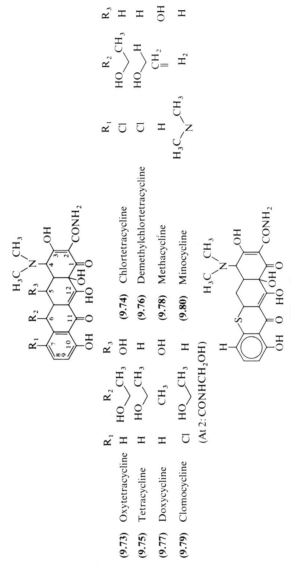

	R_1	R_2	R_3
(9.73) Oxytetracycline	H	HO–CH$_3$	OH
(9.75) Tetracycline	H	HO–CH$_3$	H
(9.77) Doxycycline	H	CH$_3$	OH
(9.79) Clomocycline	Cl	HO–CH$_3$	H

(At 2: CONHCH$_2$OH)

	R_1	R_2	R_3
(9.74) Chlortetracycline	Cl	HO–CH$_3$	H
(9.76) Demethylchlortetracycline	Cl	HO–H	H
(9.78) Methacycline	H	=CH$_2$	OH
(9.80) Minocycline	H$_3$C–N–CH$_3$	H$_2$	H

Thiacycline
(9.81)

decreased potency occurs with epimerization of the 4-dimethylamino group (as in 4-epitetracycline) or with ring opening, e.g. in isotetracycline or *apo*-oxytetracycline. In acid conditions, tetracycline hydrochloride is converted to the inactive 5a,6-anhydro and epi-anhydro compounds. Chlortetracycline (with a 7-chloro substituent) is more resistant to acid-catalysed decomposition.

9.6.3   Macrolides

The most important of the antibacterial macrolide antibiotics is erythromycin **(9.82)**. This is active generally against Gram-positive bacteria and some Gram-negative ones, including *Legionella pneumophila*. The design of an antibacterial

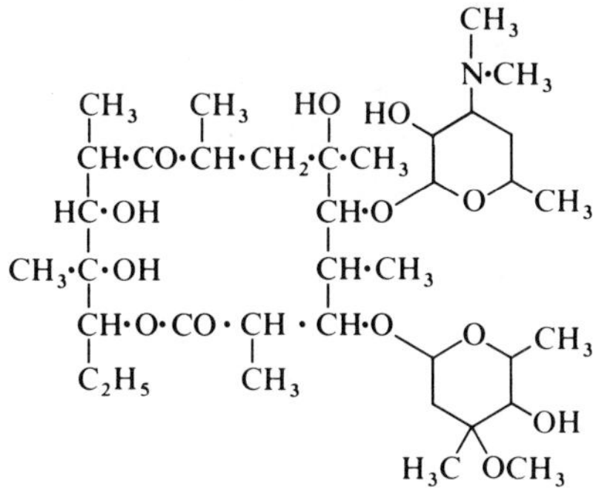

Erythromycin
(9.82)

formulation is more a pharmaceutical than a microbiological challenge, since erythromycin is unstable and inactive in acidic media. It is thus administered in enteric-coated tablets or as the more acid stable esters and ester salts, e.g. ethyl estolate and succinate. These form a stable suspension in water and do not possess the bitter taste of the base.

   The estolate produces higher and more prolonged blood levels and distributes into some tissues more efficiently than other dosage forms. It is hydrolysed *in vivo* to give the free base but at a slower rate than the ethyl succinate.

9.6.4   Chloramphenicol

Chloramphenicol **(9.23)** possesses a broad spectrum of activity against Gram-positive and Gram-negative bacteria, and acts by inhibiting the peptidyl trans-ferase reaction in protein synthesis. The active form is the D-threo isomer; the L-erythro, D-erythro and L-threo isomers do not inhibit protein synthesis and are all inactive as antibacterial agents. Some bacteria possess an enzyme, chloramphe-nicol acetyltransferase, that can inactivate the antibiotic (Section 9.4.1.3). This can pose a problem, and the practical use of chloramphenicol for systemic infections is reduced because of its tendency to cause blood dyscrasias, notably aplastic anaemia.

Chloramphenicol is administered orally as the tasteless palmitate, which is hydrolysed to chloramphenicol in the gastrointestinal tract. The highly water-soluble chloramphenicol sodium succinate comprises the injectable form; this acts as a pro-drug, and chloramphenicol is rapidly liberated, although it has been stated that only $c.$ one-half of the antibiotic in blood is in an active form and that plasma concentrations are lower than those achieved with a comparable oral dose of chloramphenicol.

9.6.5 Folate inhibitors

It was found in 1948 that alkyl or phenyl substituted diaminopyrimidines were antifolate in action. 'Small molecule' inhibitors (collectively, diaminopyrimidine derivatives) were thus studied extensively, leading to the development of compounds that were highly active against bacteria or protozoa and also to agents that were selectively toxic for the parasite rather than the host (mammalian) cells (*see* Section 4.3.2.2). In 1965 it was demonstrated that trimethoprim **(9.15)** inhibits dihydrofolate reductase (DHFR) and that its specificity of action is at the molecular level (Table 9.5). Unsubstituted diaminobenzylpyrimidines ((**9.83**)

Table 9.5   Inhibitors of dihydrofolate reductase (DHFR) in clinical use

| Type of compound | Compound | Concentrations[a] binding to DHFR in | | Specific use |
		E. coli	Rat	
Benzylpyrimidine	Trimethoprim	0·5	40 000	Antibacterial
	Tetroxoprim	8	40 000	Antibacterial
	Ormetroprim	5	34 000	Antiprotozoal
	Diaveridine	10	7000	Antiprotozoal
Diaminopteridine	Triamterene	170	150	Diuretic
Phenylpyrimidine	Pyrimethamine	250	70	Antimalarial
Conjugated pteridine	Methotrexate			Anticancer

[a] As 50% inhibitory concentration ($I_{50} \times 10^{-8}$ M), the concentration that effects 50% binding to DHFR.

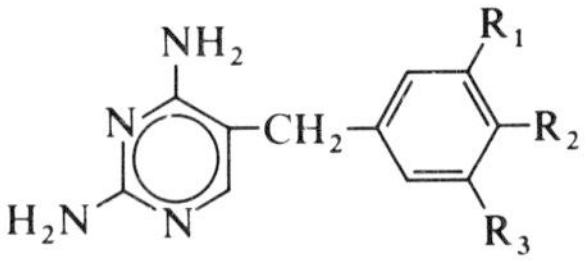

Diaminobenzylpyrimidines
(9.83)

$R_1 = R_2 = R_3 = H$) bind poorly to *E. coli* DHFR; the introduction of a single methoxy group (R_1 (**9.83**)) improves binding to some extent, whereas two methoxy groups (R_1 and R_2 (**9.83**)) improves it still further, and three methoxy groups (R_1,

R_2 and R_3, as in trimethoprim) produces a highly selective antibacterial agent. Diaminobenzylpyrimidines with good antibacterial activity can be obtained if a methoxy group is retained at R_1 and R_3 and a methoxyethoxy or methoxymethoxy group at R_2. One of the most active compounds is 2,4-diamino-5-(3',5'-dimethoxy-4'-methoxyethoxybenzyl) pyrimidine known as tetroxoprim **(9.17)**.

The rationale for combining trimethoprim with a sulphonamide (as in co-trimoxazole) is based upon the *in vitro* assertion that the mixture has a markedly increased activity in comparison to that of either drug alone, i.e. a 'sequential blockade' in which a sulphonamide acts as a competitive inhibitor of dihydropteroate synthetase and trimethoprim inhibits DHFR (*see* also Section 4.3.2.2). It has, moreover, often been stated that the use of such a combination reduces the risk of the emergence of resistance. Arguments about the clinical use of co-trimoxazole, however, continue and it has also been shown that the two components simultaneously bind to DHFR rather than causing the sequential blockade referred to above. Sulphamethoxazole has been found to bind to the purified *E. coli* DHFR, thereby preventing the conversion of dihydrofolate to tetrahydrofolate. Furthermore, synergism between trimethoprim and sulphamethoxazole is not demonstrated against sulphonamide-resistant bacteria and it is uncommon for an organism with acquired trimethoprim resistance to show sulphonamide sensitivity.

Resistance to trimethoprim, by R-factor or chromosomal mediation, results from an insusceptible target site, *viz.* an altered DHFR. Future design of diaminopyrimidines as drugs may well have to concentrate on this aspect.

9.7 DESIGN OF ANTIFUNGAL AGENTS

The design of antifungal agents poses problems different from those associated with the design of antibacterial drugs. Whereas lack of human toxicity with both types of drug is a factor of paramount importance, the differences in structure of, and some biosynthetic processes in, the fungal cell mean that antibacterial antibiotics are usually without action against fungi. Fungal infections are normally less virulent in nature than are bacterial or viral. Furthermore, the fungal cells are eucaryotic, as are human cells, and consequently difficulties arise in designing appropriate chemotherapeutic drugs. One possible target is the fungal cell wall, and considerable advances have been made in understanding its structure and biosynthesis. Another is the cytoplasmic membrane.

The most important chemotherapeutic antifungal agents are the macrolide polyenic antibiotics, imidazole derivatives, flucytosine and griseofulvin, a very small number of useful agents in comparison to the very large number of antibacterial antibiotics.

9.7.1 Polyene antibiotics

The great majority of polyene antibiotics are produced by *Streptomyces* species, with nystatin **(9.84)** the first to be isolated. The macrolide ring of the polyenes is larger than that of the other macrolide group (exemplified by erythromycin **(9.82)**) and contains a series of conjugated double bonds. An ultraviolet absorption spectrum enables a polyenic antibiotic to be classified, on the basis of the number

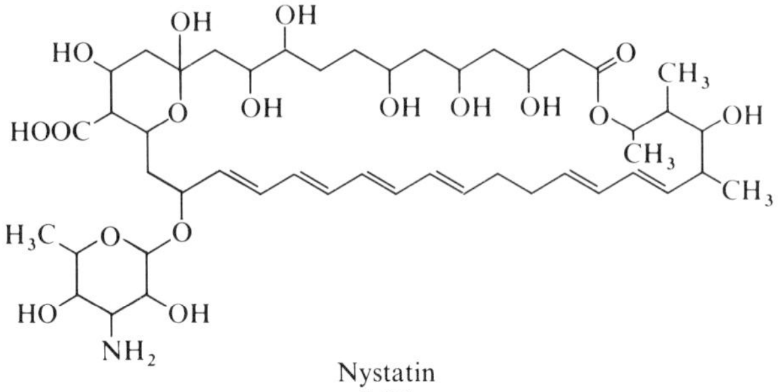

Nystatin
(9.84)

of olefinic (alkenylic) bonds present, into trienes, tetraenes, pentaenes, hexaenes and heptaenes. Generally, antifungal activity increases with the number of conjugated olefinic bonds, although solubility decreases from the tetraenes to the heptaenes.

The polyenes act by combining with the cytoplasmic membrane; this is achieved by an interaction between the antibiotic and membrane sterol. Consequently, only those organisms containing sterol in the membrane are sensitive. The antifungal activity of the polyenes can be reduced by the addition of sterols or in the presence of sterol-complexing agents.

Very few polyenes are used clinically, and two of the most important are nystatin and amphotericin B ((**9.85**) R = H). They show activity against yeasts and fungi but not against bacteria. The therapeutic usefulness of the polyenes as a group is limited by their solubility and stability and especially by their toxicity. Polyene methyl esters have been synthesized and this is a definite advance. For example, amphotericin B methyl ester ((**9.86**) R = CH$_3$) is water-soluble and can be

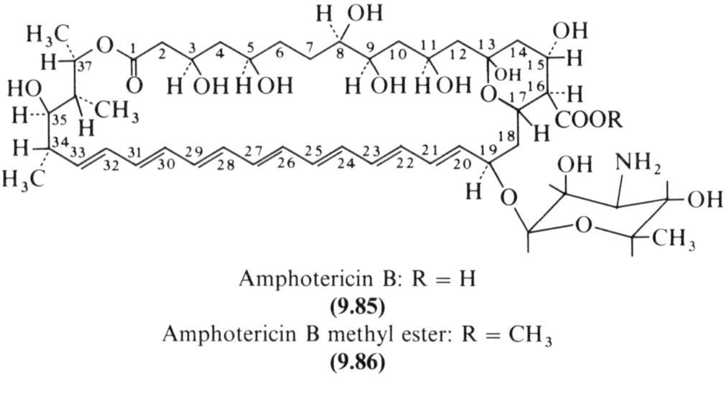

Amphotericin B: R = H
(9.85)
Amphotericin B methyl ester: R = CH$_3$
(9.86)

administered intravenously as a solution, whereas amphotericin B is insoluble in water and is formulated as a colloidal form with sodium deoxycholate. The two forms have equal antifungal activity, but much higher serum peak levels are obtained with the ester which is also considerably less toxic. Amphotericin is eliminated via the bile, whereas the methyl ester is also excreted in the urine. Other esters are less active than the methyl ester. *N*-acyl derivatives are water-soluble and less toxic, but are less active.

Future design of polyenic antibiotics might be related to an improved understanding of the nature of their interaction with sterols. In this context, it is pertinent to record the principle of increased interaction between polyene and fungal membrane ergosterol and decreased interaction between polyene and mammalian membrane cholesterol. Filipen, for example, has a greater affinity for cholesterol than for ergosterol and thus has cytotoxic and haemolytic properties.

9.7.2 Imidazole derivatives

The antifungal imidazoles comprise a large and diverse group of compounds. Some have antibacterial properties (e.g. metronidazole **(9.87)** is of importance in treating anaerobic bacterial infections), others are antihelminthic agents (such as mebendazole) and some, notably clotrimazole **(9.88)**, miconazole **(9.89)** and econazole **(9.90)** are potent antifungal agents. These agents have resulted from the

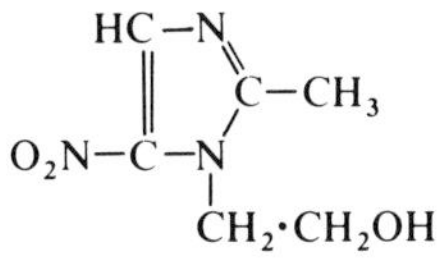

Metronidazole
(9.87)

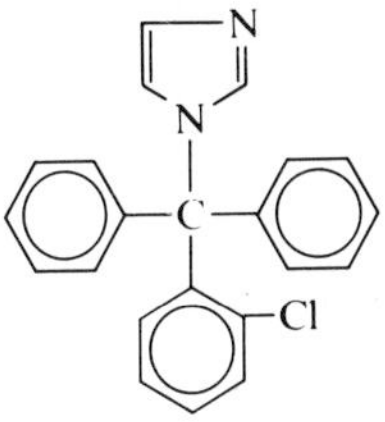

Clotrimazole
(9.88)

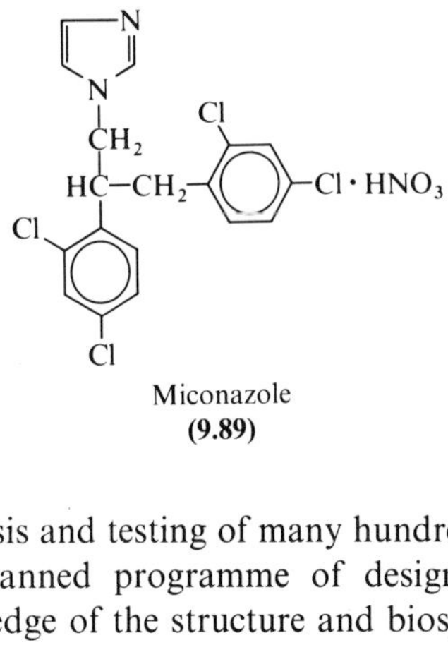

Miconazole
(9.89)

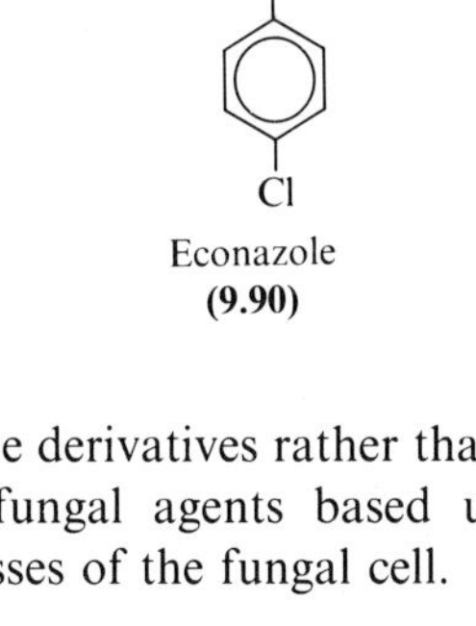

Econazole
(9.90)

synthesis and testing of many hundreds of imidazole derivatives rather than from any planned programme of designing new antifungal agents based upon a knowledge of the structure and biosynthetic processes of the fungal cell.

9.7.3   Griseofulvin

Griseofulvin **(9.91)** was isolated from the mould *Penicillium griseofulvum* in 1939, but because of its lack of antibacterial activity was not then investigated further.

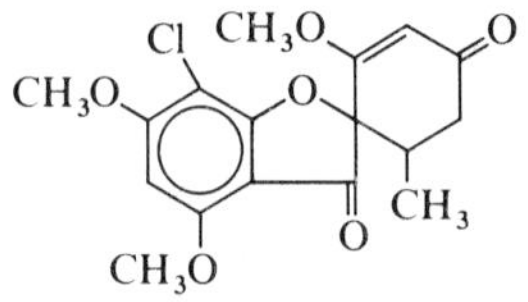

Griseofulvin
(9.91)

Several years later, it was found to be a potent antifungal antibiotic, albeit with a fungistatic rather than fungicidal action, with significant activity against derm-atophytic fungi (e.g. *Trichophyton*, *Epidermophyton* and *Microsporum* species) but not against *Cryptococcus*, *Aspergillus* or *Candida* species or against bacteria.

Successful antifungal therapy of certain conditions requires adequate penetra-tion of nail keratin. Orally administered griseofulvin is deposited in the deeper layers of the skin, in hair and in keratin of the nails, and is used in the treatment of fungal infections of the skin, hair and nails caused by susceptible organisms.

Griseofulvin is not totally absorbed when given orally, and one method of increasing absorption is to reduce the particle size of the drug.

9.7.4   Flucytosine

Flucytosine (5-fluorocytosine **(9.92)**) has a relatively narrow spectrum of activity, with yeasts (including *Candida*, *Cryptococcus* and *Torulopsis*) being most sensitive. Its precise mechanism of action is unknown, but it seems likely that it inhibits both RNA and DNA syntheses. It is believed that, once inside the fungal cell, flucytosine is deaminated to 5-fluorouracil **(9.93)** which cannot itself be used because of (*a*) its poor penetration into fungi, and (*b*) its toxicity to human cells.

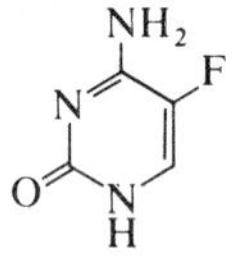

Flucytosine
(9.92)

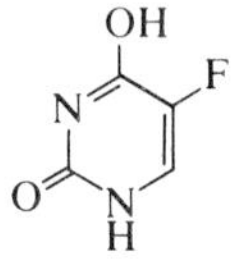

5-fluorouracil
(9.93)

This intracellular deamination is important because 5-fluorouracil replaces uracil in fungal RNA. Furthermore, *Candida albicans* has been shown to convert flucytosine to 5-fluorodeoxyuridine monophosphate (FUdRMP, *see* **(4.44)**) which inhibits thymidylate synthetase and thence DNA synthesis.

It seems logical, at least on paper, to propose that such information coupled with the known mechanisms whereby resistance (which may be a problem) to flucytosine arises, might lead to the development and design of more potent antifungal inhibitors.

Sub-inhibitory concentrations of amphotericin enhance the fungicidal properties of flucytosine against *Candida albicans*, with a markedly increased incorporation of 5-fluorouracil into RNA. It is interesting to speculate that polyenic-induced damage to the fungal cell membrane is responsible for an increased intracellular uptake of flucytosine with a consequent increased deamination to 5-fluorouracil. The effect is most pronounced in flucytosine-resistant *Candida albicans*. Certainly the mixture has proved to be of value in experimental chemotherapy in animals. One problem always associated with flucytosine, however, is the risk of bone-marrow depression.

9.7.5   Conclusions and comments

Studies on antifungal chemotherapy have lagged behind those on antibacterial agents. As further information is gleaned as to the structural complexity of and biosynthetic processes in fungal cells, it is to be hoped that a more logical design of powerful new antifungal compounds can be achieved.

9.8   DESIGN OF ANTIVIRAL AGENTS

The design of antiviral agents presents yet another problem. Since viruses literally 'take over' the machinery of the infected human cell, an antiviral agent must show a remarkable degree of selective toxicity to inhibit the viral cell without having a concomitant action on the human cell. In contrast, the metabolism of pathogenic bacteria is sufficiently different from that of human host cells to render these micro-organisms sensitive to inhibitors (e.g. penicillins) which have little or no effect on the metabolism of the host.

9.8.1   Mechanisms of inhibition

The genetic information for viral reproduction resides in its nucleic acid (RNA or DNA) portion. The viral particle (virion) does not contain the enzymes required for its own reproduction and after penetration into the host cell the virion either uses the enzymes already present or induces the formation of new ones. Unlike bacteria, viruses multiply by synthesis of their separate components, followed by assembly.

A typical sequence of events is depicted in Fig. 9.5. The first stage is adsorption of the virus particle to the cell, followed by penetration into the cell and uncoating. After the viral protein coat (capsid) has been shed, the naked viral genome is released and comes into contact with the appropriate cell machinery. Viral nucleic acid replication is followed by capsid protein specifying mRNA formation, the mRNA molecules being transported on cytoplasmic ribosomes. The proteins produced are then rapidly returned to the nucleus where capsid assembly takes

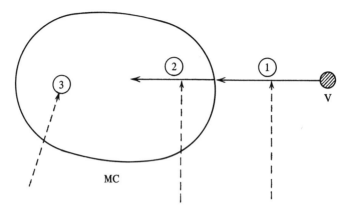

Fig. 9.5   Possible sites of viral inhibition (denoted by dotted lines): (1) Adsorption, (2) Penetration, (3) Synthesis. MC, mammalian cell; V, virus particle (not to scale).

place. This is a typical pattern of events of DNA virus replication (an exception occurs with vaccinia virus). With some (but not all) RNA viruses, the viral RNA acts directly as mRNA.

From the fore-going, it is apparent that possible sites of inhibition by an antiviral agent are adsorption (*see* Fig. 9.5 (1)), prevention of penetration of the adsorbed virus particle (*see* Fig. 9.5 (2)) and inhibition of synthesis (*see* Fig. 9.5 (3)). The amantadines **(9.94)** do not prevent adsorption, but inhibit viral penetration. Amantadine hydrochloride **(9.94)** has a very narrow antiviral spectrum and its use is usually restricted to prevention of influenza A. Methisazone, idoxuridine and cytarabine inhibit DNA, but not RNA, viruses. Idoxuridine (IUdR; 2'-deoxy-5-iodouridine **(9.95)**) is a thymidine analogue which inhibits the utilization of

Amantadine
(9.94)

Idoxuridine
(9.95)

thymidine in the rapid synthesis of DNA that normally occurs in herpes-infected cells. Cytarabine (cytosine arabinoside; Ara-C **(9.96)**) also acts by inhibiting DNA synthesis (*see* also Section 4.3.4). Methisazone (1-methylindoline-2,3-dione-3-thiosemicarbazone, **(9.97)**) is active against variola; it does not prevent adsorption of the virus, or its penetration or synthesis of viral DNA, and appears to inhibit synthesis of viral proteins (*see* also p. 157).

Because of its toxicity, idoxuridine is unsuitable for systemic use, and it is restricted to topical treatment of herpes-infected eyes. Cytarabine is significantly more toxic than idoxuridine.

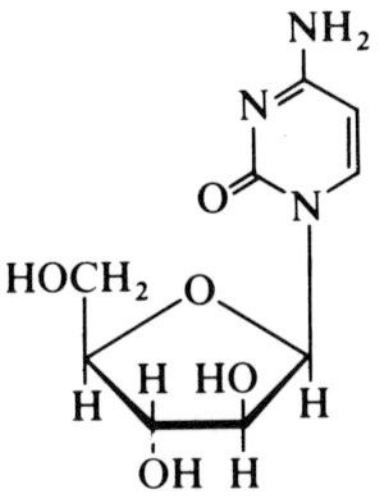

Cytarabine
(9.96)

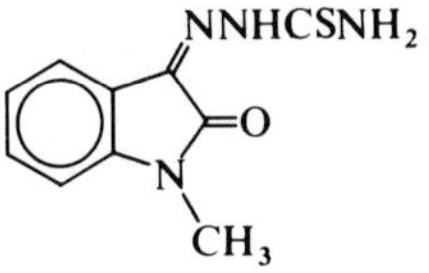

Methisazone
(9.97)

Other nucleoside analogues have been developed that are at least as active as idoxuridine, e.g. adenosine arabinoside (Ara-A). A water-soluble nucleotide based on hypoxanthine monophosphate (Ara-HXMP) has given promising results in the treatment of herpes encephalitis in mice. Ribavirin (1-β-D-ribofuranosyl-1,2,4-triazole-3-carboxamide (9.98)) is a synthetic nucleoside with a broad spectrum of activity, inhibiting both RNA and DNA viruses (see also p. 107).

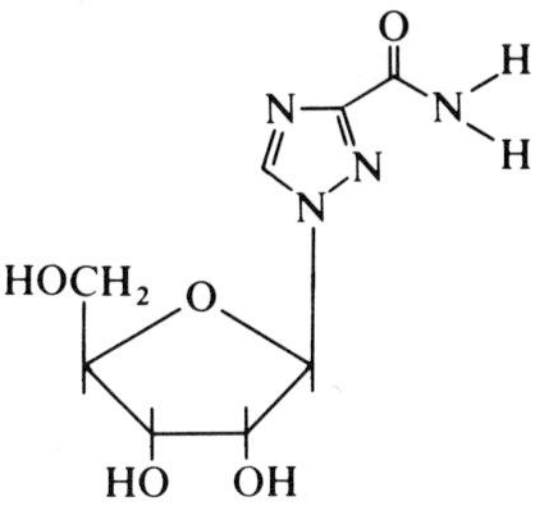

Ribavirin
(9.98)

9.8.2 Selective toxicity

Selectively toxic agents in the chemotherapy of viral diseases are notoriously difficult to design. This section will consider briefly what progress has been made to date.

9.8.2.1 Interferons (see also Section 6.9)

The phenomenon of 'viral interference' means that one virus greatly modifies the response of the host to infection with a second, immunologically distinct virus. The term Interferon is applied to a class of basic polypeptides of molecular weights c. 20 000–30 000 induced by viruses; but it (interferon) is also applied to materials (molecular weights c. 87 000) not induced by viruses. Interferons are thus produced by the host cell in response to the virus particle, the viral nucleic acid and non-viral agents (including synthetic polynucleotides such as polyinosine: polycytidylic acid (poly I : C)). The interferon system involves the induction of an antiviral protein (interferon) by a well-defined inducer and its subsequent interaction with the cell leading to the development of an antiviral state.

Type I interferons are acid-stable, and comprise two major classes, *viz.* leucocyte interferon (Le-IF) released by stimulated leucocytes, and fibroblast interferon (F-IF) produced by stimulated fibroblasts. Le-IF and F-IF differ immunologically and also in their target cell specificity, although both induce a virus-resistant state in human cells. Type II interferons are acid-labile and are also known as 'immune' interferons since they are produced by T-lymphocytes in the cellular immune system to specific antigens. Type II are more active than Type I in inhibiting growth of tumour cells.

Yields of Le-IF and F-IF from eukaryotic cells have usually been disappointingly low. Recently, however, recombinant DNA technology has been employed as an alternative method of producing large quantities of interferon in prokaryotic cells (bacteria). Human F-IF copy DNA (cDNA) has been cloned and biologically active mature F-IF expressed in *E. coli*. Similarly, a species of human Le-IF cDNA has been cloned in this organism. Techniques have been published describing the construction of a plasmid directing the high level expression in *E. coli* of a human Le-IF which exhibits *in vivo* antiviral activity.

This work is potentially one of the most exciting applications of molecular biology to the design of a potent new antiviral (and anticancer: *see* Section 6.9) agent.

9.8.2.2 *Acycloguanosine*

Acycloguanosine (Acyclovir) is a nucleoside analogue **(9.99)** which becomes activated only in infected host cells. It is claimed to be highly active against *Herpes*

Acyclovir
(9.99)

simplex virus Types I and II and rather less active against *Varicella zoster* (shingles). Initially, acycloguanosine is being marketed as an ophthalmic product, but later an intravenous formulation is being planned for treatment in life-threatening herpes infections in immunocompromised patients.

In brief, acyclovir is active only against replicating viruses. It is activated in infected cells by a herpes-specific enzyme, thymidine kinase. This enzyme initiates conversion of acyclovir initially to a monophosphate and then to the antiviral triphosphate which inhibits viral (but not, to the same extent, host cell) DNA polymerase. The triphosphate is not produced in uninfected cells.

Another nucleoside analogue currently under investigation is bromovinyl-deoxyuridine which also becomes active only in infected host cells.

9.8.2.3   *Phosphonoformate*

Sodium phosphonoformate is a simple molecule **(9.100)** which has potent activity against *Herpes simplex labialis* (cold sores) and is non-toxic when applied to the

$$\text{HO}-\overset{\overset{\displaystyle O}{\|}}{\underset{\underset{\displaystyle OH}{|}}{P}}-\text{COOH}$$

Phosphonoformate
(9.100)

skin. It inhibits herpes DNA polymerase and promises to be a useful product once clinical trials have been completed.

9.9   OVERALL CONCLUSIONS AND COMMENTS

In many instances (e.g. penicillins, cephalosporins), the development of chemotherapeutic agents for use in the treatment of bacterial, fungal or viral infections has generally followed an enlightened empirical pattern, based upon experimental testing and observations of series of compounds, rather than upon theoretical design.

With antibacterial drugs, for example, screening of moulds or *Streptomyces* for the production of antibiotics or enzyme inhibitors has often been followed by the isolation, by further chemical means, of material that is suitable for the design of additional drugs. As more information becomes available about their action at the molecular level, it should be possible at some time in the future to design more sophisticated drugs, with, for example, improved intracellular penetration, increased enzyme resistance or increased binding at the sensitive site in the cell. Other possibilities include the improved design of pro-drugs and the design of more logical combinations of antibiotics to delay or prevent the onset of bacterial resistance.

Antifungal compounds have often been developed following chance observations, the screening of antibacterial agents or of substances that have been discarded because of a lack of effect on bacteria. Modifications of chemical structure and an empirically based testing procedure have usually followed. Information on the mechanism of action of antifungal compounds has increased considerably, as has that on the underlying reasons for tissue toxicity. Taken with an improved knowledge of the fungal cell wall structure and of its biosynthesis, these facts lead to the hope that more effective, less toxic antifungal agents can be designed.

Antiviral drugs have often proved to be disappointing, with the major problem being the achievement of a selectively toxic effect on the infecting virus without a concomitant harmful effect on the host. Important developments include the recent design of a selectively toxic agent (acycloguanosine) and the possibility of using interferon as an antiviral drug. What is still needed, however, is an improved knowledge of the mechanism of action of existing drugs.

Finally, two other points should be mentioned. First, *in vivo* the adherence of pathogenic bacteria such as *Ps. aeruginosa* to human tissue is mediated by an outer covering (glycocalyx) on the bacterial cell. Thus, any future antibiotic design might well be considered from the point of view of preventing this adherence. Second, a fresh approach to new antibiotic production has been advocated; in brief, this involves recombination between strains (e.g. polyethylene glycol-induced fusion of protoplasts) that produce different secondary metabolites.

FURTHER READING

1. Brown A. G. (1981) New naturally occurring β-lactam antibiotics and related compounds. *J. Antimicrob. Chemother.* **7**, 15–48.
2. Cole M. (1980) 'β-lactams' as β-lactamase inhibitors. *Phil. Trans. Roy. Soc. Lond.* **B289**, 207–23.
3. Collier L. and Oxford J. S. (1980) *Developments in Antiviral Chemotherapy.* London and New York, Academic Press.
4. D'Arcy P. F. and Scott E. M. (1978) Antifungal agents. In Jucker E. (ed.), *Progress in Drug Research*, Vol. 22. Basel and Stuttgart, Birkhäuser Verlag, pp. 93–147.
5. Davies J., Courvalin P. and Berg D. (1977) Thoughts on the origins of resistance plasmids. *J. Antimicrob. Chemother.* **3** (Suppl. C) 7–17.
6. Davies J. and Smith D. I. (1978) Plasmid-determined resistance to antimicrobial agents. *Ann. Rev. Microbiol.* **32**, 469–518.
7. Fisher J., Belasco J. G., Charnas R. L., Khosla S. and Knowles J. R. (1980) β-lactamase inactivation by mechanism-based reagents. *Phil. Trans. Roy. Soc. Lond.*, **B289**, 309–19.
8. Franklin T. J. and Snow G. A. (1981) *Biochemistry of Antimicrobial Action*, 3rd ed. London and New York, Chapman & Hall.
9. Nikaido H. and Nakae N. (1979) The outer membrane of Gram-negative bacteria. *Adv. Microb. Physiol.* **20**, 163–250.
10. O'Callaghan C. H. (1980) Structure–activity relations and β-lactamase resistance. *Phil. Trans. Roy. Soc. Lond.*, **B289**, 197–205.
11. Oxford J. S. (1979) Inhibition of herpes virus by a new compound – acyclic guanosine. *J. Antimicrob. Chemother.* **5**, 333–4.
12. Richmond M. H. (1978) Factors influencing the antibacterial action of β-lactam antibiotics. *J. Antimicrob. Chemother.* **4** (Suppl. B) 1–14.
13. Russell A. D. (1982) Modification of the bacterial cell envelope and enhancement of antibiotic susceptibility. In Stuart-Harris C. H. and Harris D. M. (eds), *The Control of Antibiotic-resistant Bacteria*. Beecham Research Colloquium No. 4. London and New York, Academic Press.
14. Sammes P. G. (ed.) *Topics in Antibiotic Chemistry*. Volumes 1–5. (This excellent series contains many very useful review articles.) Chichester, Ellis Horwood.
15. Spratt B. G. (1980) Biochemical and genetical approaches to the mechanism of action of penicillin. *Phil. Trans. Roy. Soc. Lond.* **B289**, 273–83.
16. Sykes R. B. and Matthew M. (1976) The β-lactamases of Gram-negative bacteria and their role in resistance to β-lactam antibiotics. *J. Antimicrob. Chemother.* **2**, 115–57.
17. Wise R. and Reeves D. S. (1979) (ed.) Proceedings of a Symposium: Advances in Therapy with Antibacterial Folate Inhibitors. *J. Antimicrob. Chemother.* **5**, Suppl. B.

Index

Geometrical isomerism (alkenylic), 78, 79–80
GFR, 30
Glomerular filtration rate, 30
Glucuronide, formation, 25
Glutamyl transpeptidase inhibitor, 122
Glutathione, conjugation, 26
Glutethimide, 29, 45
Glyceryl trinitrate, 10, 12, 13, 16
Gramine, 156
Griseofulvin, 11, 29, 43, 278
Guanethidine, 19, 24
Guanylic acid, 85

Half-life, 32
Halothane, 24, 37
Hammett constants, 216
Hansch C., 214
Hansch, substituent constants, 225– analysis, 228
Hecogenin (steroid production), 190
Henderson equation, 54
Heparin, 17
Heroin (diamorphine, diacetylmorphine), 59
Hetacillin, 205
Hexamethonium, 10
Hexobarbitone, 27, 28
Histamine,
  conformations, 68
  ionization, 69
  2-methyl, 69
  5-methyl, 69
Histamine, H_1-receptor antagonists, 152–4, 158–9
Histamine, H_2-receptor antagonists, 68–71, 155
  conformation, 70
  ionization of, 69
Hydrallazine, 28
Hydrallazine (iron complex), 143
Hydrogen bonding, 55
Hydrogentartrate, adrenaline, 161
Hydrophobic binding, 55–6
11β-Hydroxylase inhibitors, 89
Hydroxylation,
  aromatic, 21
  aliphatic, 21
17α-Hydroxyprogesterone, 187
8-Hydroxyquinoline (iron complex), 143–4
  halogenated derivatives, 144
Hydroxyurea (anti-cancer), 143

Idoxuridine, 89, 106
Imidazole derivatives, antifungal, 277
Imipramine, 11, 27, 28, 76, 153
Indapamide, 19

Indomethacin, 13, 36, 154–5
Inductive substituent constants, 219
Inhibitors (see enzyme inhibitors, reversible inhibitors, irreversible inhibitors and specific enzymes)
Inosine, 123
Insulin, 12
Intercalation, activity related to, 71–5
Interferons, chemotherapy,
  cancer, 192–4
  nomenclature, 193
  virus, 281–2
Intestine, motility of, 11
Intravenous injection, 14
Inulin, 33
7-Iodo-5'-amino-2',5'-dideoxyuridine, 106
Ionization,
  aminoacridines, 71–2
  constants, 54
  in drug action, 54
  of histamine and H_2-receptor antagonists, 69–70
  sulphonamides, 97–9
  tetrazole, 160
Iprindole, 79
Iron, medicinal preparations,
  absorption, 146
  choline dihydrogen citrate complex, 146
  dextran complex, 146
  sorbitol complex, 147
Irreversible inhibitors, 90
  (see specific enzymes)
  active site-directed, 90, 91
  as drugs, 93
  k_{cat} inhibitors, 90
  kinetics, 90
Isoniazid, 26, 28, 143, 144
Isoprenaline, 12, 13, 15, 27
Isosteres, 150
Isosteric modifications in drug design, 149–61
  classical, 151–5
  non-classical, 155–61
  similar polar effects, 159
Isothipendyl, 154

pK_a, 7, 54
Kallikrein, 117
k_{cat} inhibitors, 124–31
  flavin-linked monoamine oxidase, 125
  pyridoxal phosphate-dependent enzymes, 127
K_i, 87

β-Lactam antibiotics,
  cephalosporins, 261–4